T0276590

Celiac Disease: F

Celiac Disease: Recent Advances

Edited by **Brianna Gray**

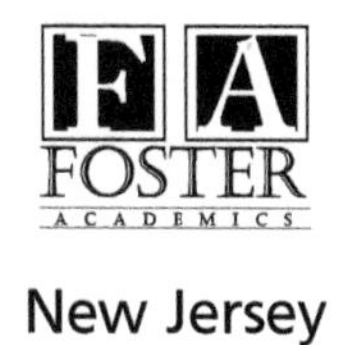

New Jersey

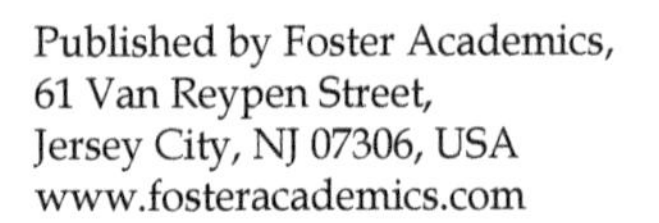

Published by Foster Academics,
61 Van Reypen Street,
Jersey City, NJ 07306, USA
www.fosteracademics.com

Celiac Disease: Recent Advances
Edited by Brianna Gray

International Standard Book Number: 978-1-63242-073-2 (Hardback)

Printed in the United States of America.

Contents

Preface

This book, written by renowned experts, comprises advanced studies and researches concerning Celiac Disease (CD). CD is an immune-mediated enteropathy triggered by the ingestion of gluten-containing grains in genetically vulnerable people. CD can manifest itself with a formerly unacknowledged variety of clinical symptoms, inclusive of the usual malabsorption syndrome and a range of symptoms potentially disturbing any organ structure. As CD often manifests itself in an uncommon manner, many cases remain undiagnosed and carry the risk of long-term difficulties, including anemia and other hematological disorders, neurological disorders or cancer. The pervasiveness of the disorder and its range of clinical outcomes pose a number of questions. This book presents answers to these questions by compiling researches conducted by prominent experts in this field.

After months of intensive research and writing, this book is the end result of all who devoted their time and efforts in the initiation and progress of this book. It will surely be a source of reference in enhancing the required knowledge of the new developments in the area. During the course of developing this book, certain measures such as accuracy, authenticity and research focused analytical studies were given preference in order to produce a comprehensive book in the area of study.

This book would not have been possible without the efforts of the authors and the publisher. I extend my sincere thanks to them. Secondly, I express my gratitude to my family and well-wishers. And most importantly, I thank my students for constantly expressing their willingness and curiosity in enhancing their knowledge in the field, which encourages me to take up further research projects for the advancement of the area.

Editor

Section 1

New Insights on Pathophysiology of Celiac Disease

1

Mucosal Expression of Claudins in Celiac Disease

Dorottya Nagy-Szakál[1], Hajnalka Győrffy[2], Katalin Eszter Müller[1], Kriszta Molnár[1], Ádám Vannay[1,3], Erna Sziksz[1,3], Beáta Szebeni[1,3], Mária Papp[4], András Arató[1] and Gábor Veres[1]
[1]First Department of Pediatrics, Semmelweis University, Budapest,
[2]Second Department of Pathology, Semmelweis University, Budapest,
[3]Research Group for Pediatrics and Nephrology, Semmelweis University and Hungarian Academy of Sciences, Budapest,
[4]Department of Medicine, University of Debrecen, Hungary

1. Introduction

Celiac disease is an autoimmune gluten-sensitive enteropathy or nontropical sprue occurring in genetically susceptible individuals, triggered by dietary gluten and related prolamins, which damage small intestine and interfere with absorption of nutrients. Tight junctions play an important role in the pathomechanism of different gastrointestinal diseases. Claudins, the main tight junction proteins are found in the monolayer of the gastrointestinal epithelium (Bornholdt et al., 2011). The presence and distribution of claudin depend on the organs and the function of the tissues (Gonzales-Mariscal et al., 2003). The expression levels of various claudins correlate to the distinct physiological and pathological conditions. Claudins modulate the permeability of the epithelial barrier (Bornholdt et al., 2011). Surprisingly, there is only one study analyzing different claudins at protein level of intestinal biopsies in patients with celiac disease. At first, general information of tight junctions and the characteristics of claudins in different gastrointestinal disorders will be highlighted for a better understanding of the role of claudins in celiac disease.

2. Characteristics of tight junctions

Intercellular junctions are presented in multicellular organism as linking cells and maintaining barrier function between the two sides of cell layer (Staehelin et al., 1974). It plays a structural role in maintaining biological compartments, cell polarity, and a barrier function separating the internal and external environments (Krause et al., 2008). It also controls the paracellular transport (Balda et al., 1996). The barrier and fence function are dynamically changing and guide cell behavior. Three major types of intercellular junctions are the zonula occludens (tight junction), the zonula adherens (adherens junction) and the macula adherens (desmosome). The tight junction is an intercellular junction by interlinked rows of integral membrane proteins limiting the intercellular transport. One of the most important components of tight junction is claudin (Figure 1).

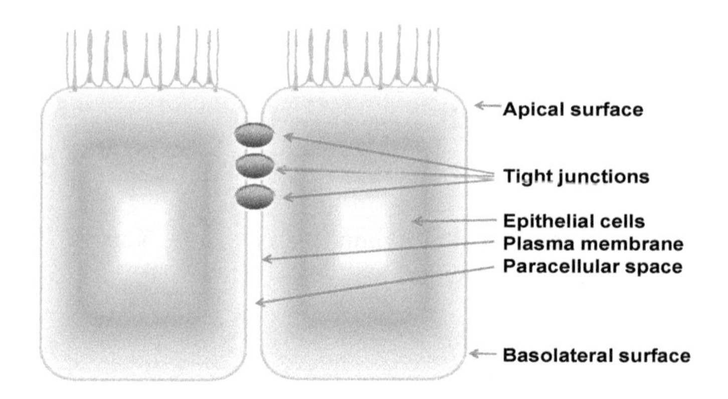

Fig. 1. Schematic structure of tight junctions.

The adherent junction links cell membranes and cytoskeletal elements connecting cells mechanically. The gap junction containing channels regulates trespassing of ions and microelements through the cell layer. Tight junction, as the most apical component of intercellular junctional complexes in basolateral spaces, constitutes the barrier between cells and has a fundamental function to separate different compartments within the organism (Farquhar et al., 1963). Tight junctions were first described in epithelia and endothelia (Stevenson et al., 1988). However, recent studies suggest that they are also found in myelinated cells. There are more than 40 different tight junction proteins in epithelia or endothelia (Gonzalez-Mariscal et al., 2003). Tight junctions have a complex structure - cortical or transmembrane protein -, and form a continuous, circumferential belt separating apical and basolateral plasma membrane domains. Tight junctions play a role not only in the maintenance of paracellular transport, but also in the cell growth and differentiation via signaling cascades. Altered tight junction structures and ratios present distinct permeability in different tissues and have a dynamic capacity responding to the altered environmental conditions. Furthermore, extracellular stimuli, such as cytokines and growth factors, also affect the distribution of tight junctions (Steed et al., 2010). Interferon-gamma, tumor necrosis factor-alpha, insulinlike growth factor-I and insulinlike growth factor -II, vascular endothelial growth factor, interleukin-1, interleukin -4, interleukin -13, and hepatocyte growth factor decrease the barrier function. Adverse effect (increased or protected barrier function) is known by transforming growth factor-beta, epidermal growth factor, interleukin-10 and interleukin-17 (Dignass et al., 1993).

Tight junctions are integral components of cells and the disturbance of the barrier function can lead to diseases (Sawada et al., 2003). The loss of fence function (decreased cell polarity) is known in cancer cells and oncogenic papillomavirus infection (Tobioka et al., 2002; Glaunsinger et al., 2000). The defect of barrier function and consequential deficiency of paracellular transport can affect the vascular system (edema, endotoxinemia, cytokinemia, blood-borne metastasis), liver (jaundice, primary biliary cirrhosis, primary sclerosing cholangitis), respiratory tract (asthma), and hereditary diseases (hypomagnesaemia, deafness, cystic fibrosis) (Sawada et al., 2003; Forster et al., 2008; Furuse et al., 2009). The gastrointestinal tract can be affected and the deterioration of tight junctions is responsible, at least in part, for the increased permeability in patients with bacterial gastritis, pseudomembranous or collagenous colitis, Crohn's disease, ulcerative colitis, and celiac disease (Schulzke et al., 2000, 2009).

Integral proteins, such as occludins, claudins and junctional adhesion molecules, constitute the tight junctions, and responsible together for the maintenance of barrier function. Occludin was identified as the first integral membrane protein (Furuse et al., 1993). It appears to interact with claudins and form long tight junction strands. Its overexpression increases transepithelial resistance and affects the polarization and diffusion through the membrane. Claudins are the most important components of the backbone tight junction strain (Furue et al., 1998). In this chapter, claudins and their role in different gastrointestinal diseases will be highlighted.

3. Characteristics of claudins

As an integral component of tight junctions, claudins play a central role in the regulation of cell-cell adhesion, cell polarity and transportation of paracellular ion, water, and molecules (Gonzalez-Mariscal et al., 2003). Twenty-four subgroups are known (Table 1). In general, claudin genes contain only some introns and several lack introns altogether. All claudin genes are typically small and their sequences are similar to each other. Some claudins are located close to each other in the human genome (Lal-Nag et al., 2009). For instance, claudin22 and -24 is located on chromosome 4, claudin3 and -4 on chromosome 7, claudin6 and -9 on chromosome 16, and claudin8 and -17 on chromosome 21 (Gupta IR et al., 2010). Their close proximity results simultaneous regulation and expression following different responses. The others are located on different chromosomes giving them a slightly different regulation and properties. All claudins encode 20-27 kDa proteins with four transmembrane domains and two extracellular loops where the first one is significantly longer (around 60 residues) than the second one (24 residues) (Krause et al., 2008). The first loop contains charged amino acids influencing paracellular charge selectivity. The highly conserved cysteine residues are present increased protein stability as formation of intermolecular disulfide bond. The second loop is responsible for confirmation through hydrophobic interactions. The short intracellular cytoplasmatic amino-terminal sequence (4 to 5 residues) is more conserved than the short intracellular carboxyl tail (Figure 2). The latter comprises a PZD-domain-binding motif (Guillemot et al, 2008). This part of claudins interacts directly with the tight junction-associated proteins, and determines the stability and function of proteins. Although claudins are known as the main component of the apical tight junctions, claudin can be localized in the cytoplasm as well (Acharya et al., 2004). The role of cytoplasm claudin is concluded in cell-matrix interactions and vesicle trafficking. Claudins appear to be expressed in a tissue-specific behavior. Variations in the tightness of the tight junction appear to be determined by the combination and mixing ratios of different claudins. Different tissues have altered claudin profile, and it can be also changed by abnormal conditions. Claudins have a crucial role in the regulation of the selectivity of paracellular permeability; and their lack or overexpression can influence these changes (permeability and resistance). The nephron is a representative model of illustration the different functions of claudin (Li et al., 2004). The renal epithelia contain mostly all of the subgroups of claudins according to the function of different areas of the nephron. Although claudins are expressed in all epithelial and endothelial tissues, mutations are frequently associated with diseases of the kidney, the skin and the ear.

CLAUDINS	CHARACTERISTICS, EXPRESSION IN DIFFERENT TISSUES (INCREASED ↑ OR DECREASED ↓)
CLDN1 'tight' epithelia	Renal epithelia (collecting segment and proximal tubule), Epidermal barrier, Gallbladder, Ovarium, Inner ear, Brain capillary endothelium Breast cancer cell lines↓, Squamous cell cancer↓, Glioblastoma↓, Prostate AC↓
CLDN2 'leaky' epithelia	Renal epithelia (collecting segment and proximal tubule), Choroids plexus epithelium, Ovarium surface epithelium, Inner ear. Crohn's disease↑
CLDN3 RVP1	Capable of CPE binding Tighter segment of nephron, Gallbladder, Inner ear, Brain capillary endothelium, Liver and intestinal epithelial cells. Prostate AC↑, Ovarian CC↑, Colorectal CC↑, Breast CC↑, Glioblastoma↓, Encephalomyelitis↓
CLDN4 CPE-R	Selective CPE binding Tighter segment of nephron, Gallbladder. Pancreatic CC↑, Prostate AC↑, Ovarian CC↑, Colorectal CC↑, Breast CC↑
CLDN5	Endothelial cells (e.g. brain), Ovarium surface epithelium, Colon epithelium, Retinal pigment epithelium during development. Glioblastoma↓, Cardiofacial syndrome↓, Crohn's disease↓, Pancreatic CC↑
CLDN6	Embryonic epithelia
CLDN7	Gastrointestinal tract, Tonsillar epithelium Head and neck squamous cell carcinoma↓, Stomach CC↑
CLDN8	Tighter segment of nephron, Gastrointestinal tract Crohn's disease↓
CLDN9	Inner ear, Neonatal kidney
CLDN10	Inner ear, Most segments of nephron
CLDN11 OSP	Oligodendrocytes, Sertolli cells
CLDN12	Inner ear, Brain endothelial cells, Gastrointestinal tract
CLDN13	Gastrointestinal tract, Neonatal kidney
CLDN14	Sensory epithelium (organ of Corti), Inner ear Nonsyndromic deafness↓
CLDN15	Kidney and Gastrointestinal tract endothelial cells
CLDN16 Paracellin-1	Thick ascending limb of Henle (Mg^{2+} and Ca^{2+} resorption) Hypomagnesaemia, Hypercalciuria, nephrocalcinosis
CLDN17	Kidney, Taste receptor cells
CLDN18	Lung and stomach, Inner ear Gastric CC↓
CLDN19	Kidney, Retina, Myelinated peripheral neurons, Schwann cells
CLDN20	mRNA in skin
CLDN21	Human DNA sequence
CLDN22	mRNA in trachea
CLDN23	mRNA in colon, stomach, placenta, skin
CLDN24	Human DNA sequence

Table 1. The characteristics and altered expression of claudins in different human tissues and cancers. Claudins were mostly investigated in the renal epithelium where the claudin pattern and the subsequent changes of permeability are easily followed by. (Abbreviations: CLDN: Claudin, AC: Adenocarcinoma, CC: Carcinoma, RVP: Rat Ventral Prostate, CPE: Clostridium Perfringens Enterotoxin, CPE-R: Clostridium Perfringens Enterotoxin Receptor, OSP: Oligodendrocyte Specific Protein)

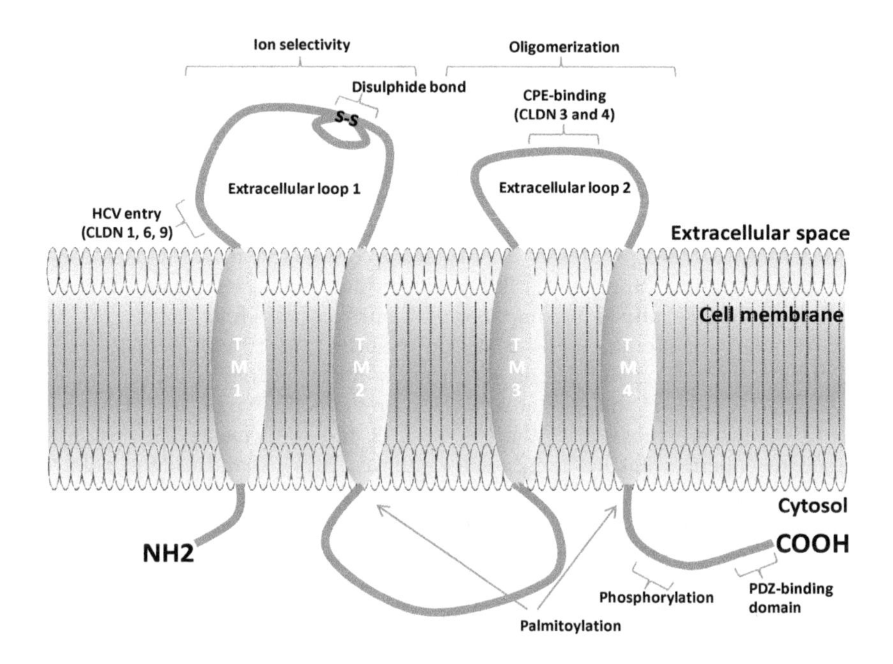

Fig. 2. Schematic structure of claudin.

3.1 Claudins and tumour of the gastrointestinal tract

Altered claudin expression is associated with different disorders of the intestine (Table 2).

Gastrointestinal tract	Disorders and altered CLDN pattern (increased↑ or decreased↓ expression)
Esophagus	Barrett's epithelia: CLDN2 and -3 ↑ Adenocarcinoma: CLDN2 and -3 ↑
Stomach	Gastric metaplasia CLDN2,-3 and -4 ↑
Duodenum, Ileum, Jejunum	Adenocarcinoma: CLDN2 ↑ GIST: CLDN2,-3, -4, -5 and -7 ↑ Angiosarcoma: CLDN2 and -5 ↑ Hemangioma: CLDN2 ↑ Leiomyoma: CLDN2 ↑ Leiomyosarcoma: CLDN1, -2, -3, -4, -5 and 7 ↑ Celiac disease: CLDN2 and -3 ↑ Gluten-intolerance: CLDN4 ↑
Colon	Adenocarcinoma: CLDN2 ↑ IBD: CLDN2 ↑ and CLDN3, -4, -5 and -8 ↓

Table 2. Claudin expression in the gastrointestinal tract in different disorders. (Abbreviations: CLDN: Claudin, GIST: gastrointestinal stromal tumour, IBD: inflammatory bowel disease)

Since the damage of the cell-cell adhesion is an important role in the carcinogenesis, several papers have studied changes of claudins during tumor development and progression. All claudins were found in gastrointestinal carcinomas, and their expression was tumour-specific. The Barrett's metaplasia of the esophagus requests attention for its precancerous behaviour (Thomson et al., 1983). Claudin2 and -3 expressions in Barrett's esophagus were higher compared to the normal foveolar epithelium. The esophageal adenocarcinoma showed higher claudin2 and -3 expression compared with normal and Barrett's epithelia. The similar claudin expression profile of Barrett's esophagus and adenocarcinoma supports their sequential development (Győrffy et al., 2005). The low expression of the claudin4 is associated with the poor prognosis in the most common tumour of the esophagus, squamous cell carcinoma (Sung et al., 2011). Gastric intestinal metaplasia showed higher expression of claudin2, -3 and -4 as compared with normal antral foveolar mucosa (Győrffy, 2009). Gastric adenocarcinoma expresses various claudin. Lower expression of claudin1 is common in the intestinal type of gastric adenocarcinoma according to Lauren classification (Jung et al., 2011). Claudin3 and -4 overexpression prevents the lymphatic invasion (Jung et al., 2011), but the overexpression of the claudin6, -7 and -9 increases the invasiveness of tumour cells in experimental model (Zavala-Zendejas, 2011). Claudin4 is a good general prognostic marker in the gastric adenocarcinoma (Jung et al., 2011). Autoantibodies against claudin18 prevent the development of the lung metastasis (Klamp et al., 2011). Tumours of small and large bowels exhibited higher claudin2 expression compared to normal epithelia (Győrffy, 2009). Decreased claudin4 expression correlates with the invasiveness and metastasis (Ueda et al., 2007). In addition, claudin18 overexpression is associated with poor prognosis of the colorectal cancer (Matsuda et al., 2010). However, colorectal adenoma and adenocarcinoma could not be differentiated according to their claudin profile (Győrffy, 2009).

3.2 Claudins and inflammatory bowel disease

Beside the neoplastic or precancerous lesions, some of the inflammatory processes show alteration of the tight junctions. In inflammatory bowel diseases, including Crohn's disease and ulcerative colitis, the intestinal barrier function is impaired due to deterioration in the structure of the epithelial tight junction. Claudin, as a key component of tight junction, might play an important role in the pathogenesis of inflammatory bowel diseases. In addition, tumour necrosis factor in inflammatory bowel diseases is upregulated, which induces barrier defects and is associated with the induction of claudin2 expression. Increased expression of claudin2 is detected along the inflamed crypt epithelium, whilst absent or barely detectable in normal colon (Weber et al., 2010). This higher expression of channel-forming claudin2 can cause reduced epithelial barrier in inflammatory bowel diseases (Suzuki et al., 2011). In the inflamed colonic mucosa of patients with ulcerative colitis, the protein expression of claudin1 was increased compared to non-inflamed ulcerative colitis colon and normal colon (Poritz et al., 2011). In addition, the higher expressions of claudin1 and -2 correlated positively with inflammatory activity of inflammatory bowel diseases and this increased expression may be involved at early stages of transformation in inflammatory bowel diseases -associated neoplasia (Weber et al., 2008). In experimental model of colitis in rats, significant decrease of claudin2, -12, -15 levels were detected in the colonic mucosa after dextrane-sodium sulphate induces colitis (Arimura et al., 2011). In contrast, some members of the claudin family such as claudin3 and -4 were present throughout normal colonic epithelium and were reduced or redistributed in the inflamed surface epithelium (Prasad et al., 2005). Food components can strengthen the epithelial barrier as for example the flavonoid quercetin. Quercetin has been shown to upregulate claudin4 within the epithelial tight junction. This might be a therapeutic option in inflammatory bowel diseases patients to rebuild the tight junction complex (Hering et al., 2009).

3.3 Claudins and intestinal infections

Claudins may serve as cell surface receptors for epithelial pathogens. Intestinal pathogens such as Vibrio cholerae, Salmonella, E. coli, Shigella, Giardia lamblia, and Rotavirus were found to directly alter tight junction permeability. Claudin3 and -4 have been shown to act as a receptor for C. perfringens enterotoxin (Katahira et al., 1997). Rotavirus infection of Caco-2 intestinal cells altered distribution of claudin1 and other tight junction proteins (Dickmann et al., 2000). In the pathogenesis of Helicobacter pylori infection, disruption of the tight junction implicated host cell signaling pathways including the dysregulation of claudin4 and -5 was observed (Fedwick et al., 2005). Moreover, claudin1, -6, and -9 are coreceptors for cellular entry of hepatitis C virus (Angelow et al., 2008). The importance of intestinal barrier function in the pathogenesis of necrotizing enterocolitis has been suggested in a rat model, where necrotizing enterocolitis was associated with increased claudin3 mRNA levels in both jejunum and ileum (Clark et al., 2006).

3.4 Claudins in food allergy, obstructive jaundice and obesity

In food allergy, mast cells are classically associated with allergen-induced immunoglobulin E mediated responses. Concerning our topic, mast cell deficient mice-model demonstrated dysregulation of claudin3 expression (Gorschwitz et al., 2009). Furthermore, claudin1 expression was elevated in the small intestine in patients with food allergy (Pizzuti et al., 2011). Experimental and clinical studies have shown that there is an increased intestinal permeability permitting the escape of endotoxin from gut lumen in patients with obstructive jaundice. In these subjects, claudin1 and -7 were significantly decreased whereas claudin4 expression was increased. This pattern may be a key factor contributing to the disintegration of mucosal barrier (Assimakopoulos et al., 2011). Recently, obesity and diabetes have been characterized by low-grade chronic systemic inflammation. According to a novel hypothesis, this systemic inflammation is closely linked to the plasma endotoxemia due to increased intestinal permeability in obese animals (Cani et al., 2008). It is of interest, that excessive dietary fat increased small intestinal permeability resulting from the suppression of tight junction protein expression. Claudin1 and -3 were influenced by diet.

4. Tight junctions and its effect on intestine in celiac disease

4.1 Celiac disease and intestinal barrier function

Deterioration of intestinal barrier function is one of the most important steps in the pathomechanism of celiac disease (Sapone et al, 2011). According to functional, structural and molecular analyses, intercellular junctions between epithelial cells are abnormal in the gut of patients with celiac disease (Madara et al, 1987; Poritz et al, 2011). Decreased intestinal barrier function leads to a continuous abnormal passage of antigens through the epithelial layer. The main antigen of gluten in wheat, the gliadin can regulate cell activation, especially inhibits cell development and induces apoptosis. Gliadin almost immediately can change the barrier function of the intestinal mucosa inducing a reorganization of actin filaments and altered expression of different tight junction proteins (Drago et al, 2006; Fasano et al., 2000). In a human Caco-2 intestinal epithelial cell-model, gliadin altered barrier function almost immediately by decreasing transepithelial resistance and increasing permeability to small molecules (4 kDa). In addition, gliadin induced a reorganisation of actin filaments and altered expression of the tight junction proteins occludin, claudin3 and -4, the tight junction-associated protein zonula occludens-1 and the adherens junction protein E-cadherin (Sander et al., 2005). The activation of T helper 1 and T helper 17 cells results tissue damage and disrupts barrier function. Namely, expression of interleukin-17A, interferon-gamma and interleukin-6 is enhanced and leads to increased immune reaction and promotes differentiation. On the other hand, reduced function of adaptive immunity is also detected. Decreased regulatory T cells in the epithelial mucosa are related to disturbed adaptive capacity. In addition, upregulation of regulatory T cell markers (like FoxP3 and tranforming growth factor-beta) was reported which phenomenon may be explained as a secondary compensatory response to injury.

4.2. Claudins and the gut microbiota

The intestinal epithelium is one of the most immunologically active surfaces in the body. Beside the barrier function, immunological reactions against food antigens and toxins are involved in the maintenance of healthy gut status. However, inappropriate increase of the immune response can lead to decreasing tolerance and intestinal immune disorders (e.g. celiac disease). The commensal bacteria and their dynamic interaction of the host gut play an essential role in the preservation of gut homeostasis. Intestinal flora is involved in the regulation of gut intestinal epithelial cells, maintenance of barrier function, and also in the restitution and reformation (stabilization) of tight junctions (Yu et al., 2012).

Highlighting the importance of claudins, recent studies suggested that invasive bacterial pathogens (e.g. *Streptococcus pneumonia* and *Haemophilus influenza*) decrease the CLDN7 and -10 expression via TLR-dependent pathway leading decreased integrity of the epithelial cells (Clarke et al., 2011). This mechanism due to epithelial opening and bacterial translocation through the epithelial layer leads increased permeability and bacterial invasion.

Recent studies suggested that the altered intestinal microbiota plays a role in the development of different disorders such as celiac disease, inflammatory bowel diseases and irritable bowel syndrome. In celiac disease, rodent studies suggest that gut microbiota influences mucosal integrity and plays a role in the early pathogenesis of CD (Cinova et al., 2011). In human celiac disease, intestinal flora may be a key component switching oral tolerance to immune response against gliadin (Ray et al., 2012). In celiac disease, intestinal dysbiosis, along with increased Gram-negative bacteria and decreased Bifidobacteria was determined (Sanz et al., 2011). Infants who developed CD later in life had an unstable and immature microbiome with decreased abundance of the phylum Bacteriodetes along with high amount of Firmicutes compared to healthy individuals (Sellitto et al., 2012). The metabolomic analysis reveals increased lactate in CD which may be a predicting factor of CD.

5. Claudins and celiac disease

5.1. Claudin-protein level in patients with celiac disease

To the best of our knowledge, there is only one study to address the question to determine the expression of different claudin proteins in patients with celiac disease. The aim of this prospective study was to compare claudin2, -3 and -4 expressions in proximal and distal part of duodenum in children with celiac disease and in controls (Szakal et al., 2010). Biopsy samples from the proximal and distal part of duodenum were taken from newly diagnosed children with celiac disease. The villous/crypt ratio and the percentage of lymphocytes in the intraepithelial region using monoclonal CD3 antibodies were determined (Marsh scoring). The expression pattern of claudins in the duodenal mucosa was investigated by immunohistochemistry. The monoclonal anti-claudin2 and -4 and the polyclonal anti-claudin3 antibodies were purified from rabbit antiserum. For visualization, biotinilated goat anti-rabbit secondary antibody and standard avidin-biotin peroxidase technique with diaminobenzidine were used as chromogen. The number of positive cells was calculated in the surface epithelium (with 100 enterocytes) on the top of the villi. Increased expression of claudin2 and -3 was detected in distal part of duodenal mucosa in pediatric patients with celiac disease compared to the proximal region and controls. It should be emphasized that claudin4 expression was comparable between the different groups studied (see later).

Moreover, there was an association between expression of claudin and the grade of atrophy. Changes in the composition and the overturn of the different types of claudin may lead to structural alteration of tight junctions. This phenomenon may be responsible for the increased permeability and the modified cell-to-cell adhesion in the pathomechanism of celiac disease. In addition, comparative substudy showed that both proximal and distal parts of duodenum are also reliable for taking biopsy sample to prove villous atrophy. However, using sensitive methods, the distal part of duodenum depicted earlier signs of mucosal deterioration. Histological scoring grade (Marsh classification), the percentage of CD3 positive T cells and the expression of different claudin showed slightly more severity in the distal part of duodenum compared to the bulbus duodeni.

5.2 Claudin-mRNA expression in celiac disease and gluten-sensitive disease

As described previously, celiac disease is an autoimmune enteropathy triggered by the ingestion of gluten. Gluten sensitive individuals cannot tolerate gluten and may develop gastrointestinal symptoms similar to those in celiac disease. However, in contrast to celiac disease, the overall clinical picture is generally less severe and is not accompanied by the elevation of tissue transglutaminase autoantibodies or autoimmune comorbidities (Sapone, 2011). In this study, innate and adaptive immunity in celiac disease were compared with gluten sensitivity. Intestinal permeability was evaluated using a lactulose and mannitol probe, and mucosal biopsy specimens were collected to study the expression of genes involved in barrier function and immunity. In contrast to celiac disease, gluten sensitivity was not associated with increased intestinal permeability. In fact, this was significantly reduced in gluten sensitive individuals compared to controls paralleled by significantly increased mRNA expression of claudin4. In comparison to controls, adaptive immunity markers interleukin-6 and interleukin-21 were significantly increased in celiac disease but not in gluten sensitivity, while expression of the innate immunity marker Toll-like receptor 2 was increased in gluten sensitive individuals but not in celiac disease. In addition, expression of the T-regulatory cell marker FOXP3 was significantly reduced in gluten sensitive individuals relative to controls and celiac disease patients. Authors concluded, that the two gluten-associated disorders, celiac disease and gluten sensitivity, are different clinical entities, and it contributes to the characterization of gluten sensitivity as a condition associated with prevalent gluten-induced activation of innate, rather than adaptive immune responses. In addition, previous study conducted by Szakal et al showed no elevation of claudin4 in the intestinal mucosa of patients with celiac disease (Szakal, 2010). This finding strengthen the hypothesis of Sapone et al that claudin4 could be an important marker to differentiate between celiac disease and gluten sensitivity (Sapone, 2011). Further studies are necessary to characterize gluten sensitivity as a well-defined entity in the family of celiac-related disorders.

6. Conclusion and future remarks

Gluten-induced changes in the tight junction and the ratio of claudins influence immune processes and barrier mechanism underlying celiac disease pathogenesis. As sensitive methods, detection of claudins in the upper gastrointestinal tract may help to detect abnormalities in an early stage and provide information to determine the prognosis of celiac disease (Szakal et al., 2010; Prasad et al, 2005; Visser et al, 2009). Nevertheless, modification of claudins and tight junction might be therapeutic approach in the future. Furthermore, influence of tight junctions' regulation may be a novel approach of treatment in several diseases due to the fact that celiac disease may serve as a model for other autoimmune disorders. The advantage in celiac disease is that the causative agent (gluten) is well known compared to other autoimmune disorders such as in inflammatory bowel diseases. Development of agents making tight junctions close might be used as anti-inflammatory, anti-metastatic and anti-diarrhea drugs. In contrast, drugs opening tight junctions are new applications of treating tumors and help reaching closed compartment of the body (e.g. brain-blood barrier).

7. Acknowledgments

This work was financially supported by OTKA-K81117 and Janos Bolyai grant (2011-2014) of Gabor Veres and Adam Vannay.

8. References

Acharya, P., Beckel, J., Ruiz, WG., Wang, E., Rojas, R., Birder, L., Apodaca, G. (2004). Distribution of the tight junction proteins ZO-1, occludin, and claudin-4, -8, and -12 in bladder epithelium. Am J Physiol Renal Physiol. 287(2):F305-18.

Angelow, S., Ahlstrom, R., & Yu, AS. (2008). Biology of claudins. *Am J Physiol Renal Physio,* 295 : F867-F876.

Arimura Y, Nagaishi K, & Hosokawa M. (2011). Dynamics of claudins expression in colitis and colitis-associated cancer in rat. *Methods Mol Biol.* 762:409-25.

Assimakopoulos, SF., Tsamandas, AC., Louvris, E., Vagianos, CE., Nikolopoulou, VN., Thomopoulos, KC., Charonis, A., & Scopa, CD. (2011). Intestinal epithelial cell proliferation, apoptosis and expression of tight junction proteins in patients with obstructive jaundice. *Eur J Clin Invest.* 41:117-125.

Balda, MS., Whitney, JA., Flores, C., Gonzalez, S., Cereijido, M., & Matter, K. (1996). Functional dissociation of paracellular permeability and transepithelial electrical resistance and disruption of the apical-basolateral intramembrane diffusion barrier by expression of a mutant tight junction membrane protein. *J Cell Biol.* 134(4):1031-49.

Bornholdt, J., Friis, S., Godiksen, S., Poulsen, SS., Santoni-Rugiu, E., Bisgaard, HC., Lothe, IM., Ikdahl, T., Tveit, KM., Johnson, E., Kure, EH., & Vogel LK. (2011). The level of claudin-7 is reduced as an early event in colorectal carcinogenesis. *BMC Cancer.* 11:65.

Cani, PD., Bibiloni, R., Knauf, C., Waget, A., Neyrinck, AM., Delzenne, NM., & Burcelin R. (2008). Changes in gut microbiota control metabolic endotoxemia-induced inflammation in high fat diet induced obesity and diabetes in mice. *Diabetes.* 57:170-181.

Cinova, J., De Palma, G., Stepankova, R., Kofronova, O., Kverka, M., Sanz, Y., Tuckova, L. (2011). Role of intestinal bacteria in gliadin-induced changes in intestinal mucosa: study in germ-free rats. *PLoS One.* 6(1):e16169.

Clark, JA., Doelle, SM., Halpern, MD., Suanders, TA., Holubec, H., Dvorak, K., Boitano, SA., & Dvorak B. (2006). Intestinal barrier failure during experimental necrotizing enterocolitis: protective effect of EGF treatment. *Am J Physiol Gastrointest Liver Physiol.* 291;G938-G949.

Clarke ,TB., Francella, N., Huegel, A., Weiser, JN. (2011). Invasive bacterial pathogens exploit TLR-mediated downregulation of tight junction components to facilitate translocation across the epithelium. *Cell Host Microbe.* 9(5):404-14.

Dickmann, KG., Hempson, SJ., Anderson, J., Lippe, S., Zhao, L., Burakoff, R., & Shaw, RD. (2000). Rotavirus alters paracellular permeability and energy metabolism in Caco-2 cells. *Am J Physiol Gastrointest Liver Physiol.* 279:G757-G766.

Dignass, AU., & Podolsky DK. (1993). Cytokine modulation of intestinal epithelial cell restitution: central role of transforming growth factor beta. *Gastroenterology.* 105(5):1323-32.

Drago, S., El Asmar, R., Di Pierro, M., Grazia Clemente, M., Tripathi, A., Sapone, A., Thakar, M., Iacono, G., Carroccio, A., D'Agate, C., Not, T., Zampini, L., Catassi C., Fasano, A. (2006). Gliadin, zonulin and gut permeability: Effects on celiac and non-celiac intestinal mucosa and intestinal cell lines. *Scand J Gastroenterol.* 41(4):408-19.

Farquhar, MG., & Palade, GE. (1963). Junctional complexes in various epithelia. *J Cell Biol.* 17:375-412.

Fasano, A., Not, T., Wang, W., Uzzau, S., Berti, I., Tommasini, A., Goldblum, SE. (2000). Zonulin, a newly discovered modulator of intestinal permeability, and its expression in celiac disease. *Lancet.* 355(9214):1518-9.

Fedwick, JP., Lapointe, TK., Meddings, JB., Sherman, PM., & Buret, AG. (2005). Helicobacter pylori activates myosin light chain kinase to disrupt claudin-4 and claudin-5 and increase epithelial permeability. *Infection and immunity.* 7844-7852.

Forster, C. (2008). Tight junctions and the modulation of barrier function in disease. *Histochem Cell Biol.* 130(1):55-70.

Furuse, M., Fujita, K., Hiiragi, T., Fujimoto, K., & Tsukita S. (1998). Claudin-1 and -2: novel integral membrane proteins localizing at tight junctions with no sequence similarity to occludin. *J Cell Biol.* 141(7):1539-50.

Furuse, M., Hirase, T., Itoh, M., Nagafuchi, A., Yonemura, S., & Tsukita, S. (1993). Occludin: a novel integral membrane protein localizing at tight junctions. *J Cell Biol.* 123(6 Pt 2):1777-88.

Furuse, M. (2009). Knockout animals and natural mutations as experimental and diagnostic tool for studying tight junction functions in vivo. *Biochim Biophys Acta.* 1788(4):813-9.

Glaunsinger, BA., Lee, SS., Thomas, M., Banks, L., & Javier, R. (2000). Interactions of the PDZ-protein MAGI-1 with adenovirus E4-ORF1 and high-risk papillomavirus E6 oncoproteins. *Oncogene.* 19(46):5270-80.

Gonzalez-Mariscal, L., Betanzos, A., Nava, P., & Jaramillo, BE. (2003). Tight junction proteins. *Prog Biophys Mol Biol.* 81(1):1-44.

Gonzalez-Mariscal, L., Lechuga, S., & Garay, E. (2007). Role of tight junctions in cell proliferation and cancer. *Prog Histochem Cytochem.* 42:1-57

Gorschwitz, KR., Ahrens, R., Osterfeld, H., Gurish, MF., Han, X., Abrink, M., Finkelman, FD., Pejler, G., & Hogan, SP. (2009). Mast cells regulate homeostatic intestinal epithelial migration and barrier function by a chymase/Mcpt4-dependent mechanism. *PNAS.* 106:22381-22386.

Guillemot, L., Paschoud, S., Pulimeno, P., Foglia, A., & Citi, S. (2008). The cytoplasmic plaque of tight junctions: a scaffolding and signalling center. *Biochim Biophys Acta.* 1778(3):601-13.

Gupta, IR., & Ryan, AK. (2010). Claudins: unlocking the code to tight junction function during embryogenesis and in disease. *Clin Genet.* 77(4):314-25.

Győrffy, H., Holczbauer, Á., Nagy, P., Szabó, Zs., Kupcsulik, P., Páska, Cs., Papp, J., Schaff, Zs., & Kiss, A. (2005). Claudin expression in Barrett's esophagus and adenocarcinoma. *Virchows Arch.* 447: 961–8

Győrffy H. (2009). Study of claudins and prognostic factors in some gastrointestinal diseases. *Magy Onkol.* 53:377-83.

Hering, NA., & Schulzke, JD. (2009). Therapeutic options to modulate barrier defects in inflammatory bowel disease. *Dig Dis.* 27:450-4.

Jung, H., Jun, KH., Jung, JH., Chin, HM., & Park, WB. (2011). The expression of claudin-1, claudin-2, claudin-3, and claudin-4 in gastric cancer tissue. *J Surg Res.* 167:e185-91.

Katahira, J., Sugiyama, H., Inoue, N., Horiguchi, Y., Matsuda, M., & Sugimoto, N. (1997). Clostridium perfringens enterotoxin utilizes two structurally related membrane proteins as functional receptors in vivo. *J Biol Chem.* 272:26652-26658.

Klamp, T., Schumacher, J., Huber, G., Kühne, C., Meissner, U., Selmi, A., Hiller, T., Kreiter, S., Markl, J., Türeci, Ö., & Sahin, U. (2011). Highly specific auto-antibodies against claudin-18 isoform 2 induced by a chimeric HBcAg virus-like particle vaccine kill tumor cells and inhibit the growth of lung metastases. *Cancer Res.* 71:516-27.

Krause, G., Winkler, L., Mueller, SL., Haseloff, RF., Piontek, J., & Blasig, IE. (2008). Structure and function of claudins. *Biochim Biophys Acta.* 1778(3):631-45.

Lal-Nag, M., & Morin, PJ. (2009). The claudins. *Genome Biol.* 10(8):235.

Li, WY., Huey, CL., & Yu, AS. (2004). Expression of claudin-7 and -8 along the mouse nephron. *Am J Physiol Renal Physiol.* 286(6):F1063-71.

Madara, JL., & Pappenheimer, JR. (1987). Structural basis for physiological regulation of paracellular pathways in intestinal epithelia. *J Membr Biol.* 100(2):149-64.

Matsuda, M., Sentani, K., Noguchi, T., Hinoi, T., Okajima, M., Matsusaki, K., Sakamoto, N., Anami, K., Naito, Y., Oue, N., & Yasui W. (2010). Immunohistochemical analysis of colorectal cancer with gastric phenotype: claudin-18 is associated with poor prognosis. *Pathol Int.* 60:673-80.

Pizzuti, D., Senzolo, M., Buda, A., Chiarelli, S., Giacomelli, L., Mazzon, E., Curioni, A., Faggian, D., & De Lazzari, F. (2011). In vitro model for IgE mediated food allergy. *Scand J Gastroenterol.* 46:177-87.

Poritz, LS., Harris, LR., Kelly, AA., & Koltun WA. (2011). Increase in the Tight Junction Protein Claudin-1 in Intestinal Inflammation. *Dig Dis Sci.* 2011 Jul 12. (Epub ahead of print)

Prasad, S., Mingrino, R., Kaukinen, K., Hayes, KL., Powell, RM., MacDonald, TT, & Collins, JE. (2005). Inflammatory processes have differential effects on claudins 2, 3 and 4 in colonic epithelial cells. *Lab Invest.* 85:1139-62.

Ray, K. (2012) Microbiota: Tolerating gluten-a role for gut microbiota in celiac disease? *Nat Rev Gastroenterol Hepatol.* 9(5):242.

Sander, GR., Cummins, AG., Henshall, T., & Powell, BC. (2005). Rapid disruption of intestinal barrier function by gliadin involves altered expression of apical junctional proteins. *FEBS Lett.* 579(21):4851-5.

Sanz, Y., De Pama,, G., Laparra, M. (2011). Unraveling the ties between celiac disease and intestinal microbiota. *Int Rev Immunol.* 30(4):207-18.

Sapone, A., Lammers, KM., Casolaro, V., Cammarota, M., Giuliano, MT., De Rosa, M., Stefanile, R., Mazzarella, G., Tolone, C., Russo, MI., Esposito, P., Ferraraccio, F., Cartenì, M., Riegler, G., de Magistris, L., & Fasano A. (2011). Divergence of gut permeability and mucosal immune gene expression in two gluten-associated conditions: celiac disease and gluten sensitivity. *BMC Med.* 9:23.

Sawada, N., Murata, M., Kikuchi, K., Osanai, M., Tobioka, H., & Kojima, T. (2003). Tight junctions and human diseases. *Med Electron Microsc.* 36:147-56.

Schulzke, JD., Ploeger, S., Amasheh, M., Fromm, A., Zeissig, S., & Troeger, H. (2009). Epithelial tight junctions in intestinal inflammation. *Ann N Y Acad Sci.* 1165:294-300.

Schulzke, JD. (2000). Epithelial transport and barrier function: pathomechanisms in gastrointestinal disorders. Proceedings of a conference. March 26-27, 1999. Berlin, Germany. *Ann N Y Acad Sci.* 915:1-375.

Sellitto, M., Bai, G., Serena, G., Fricke, WF., Sturgeon, C., Gajer, P., White, JR., Koenig, SS., Sakamoto, J., Boothe, D., Gicquelais, R., Kryszak, D., Puppa, E., Catassi, C., Ravel, J., Fasano, A. (2012) Proof of concept of microbiome-metabolome analysis and delayed gluten exposure on celiac disease autoimmunity in genetically at-risk infants. *PLoS One.* 7(3):e33387.

Smedley, JG., Saputo, J., Parker, JC., Fernandez-Miyakawa, ME., Robertson, SL., McClane, BA., & Uzal, FA. (2008). Noncytotoxic Clostridium perfringens enterotoxin variants localize CPE intestinal binding and demonstrate a relationship between CPE-induced cytotoxicity and enterotoxicity. *Infection and immunity.* 76:3793-3800.

Staehelin, LA. (1974). Structure and function of intercellular junctions. *Int Rev Cytol.* 39:191-283.

Steed, E., Balda, MS., & Matter, K. (2010). Dynamics and functions of tight junctions. *Trends Cell Biol.* 20:142-9.

Stevenson, BR., Anderson, JM., & Bullivant, S. (1988). The epithelial tight junction: structure, function and preliminary biochemical characterization. *Mol Cell Biochem*. 83:129-45.

Sung, CO., Han, SY., & Kim, SH. (2011). Low expression of claudin-4 is associated with poor prognosis in esophageal squamous cell carcinoma. *Ann Surg Oncol*. 18:273-81.

Szakal, DN., Gyorffy, H., Arato, A., Cseh, A., Molnár, K., Papp, M., Dezsofi, A., & Veres, G. (2010). Mucosal expression of claudins 2, 3 and 4 in proximal and distal part of duodenum in children with coeliac disease. *Virchows Arch*. 456:245-50.

Thijs, WJ., van Baarlen, J., & Kleibeuker, JH. (2004). Duodenal versus jejunal biopsies in suspected celiac disease. *Endoscopy*. 36:993-6.

Thompson, JJ., Zinsser, KR., & Enterline, HT. (1983). Barrett's metaplasia and adenocarcinoma of the esophagus and gastroesophageal junction. *Hum Pathol*. 14:42-61

Tobioka, H., Isomura, H., & Kokai, Y. (2002). Polarized distribution of carcinoembryonic antigen is associated with a tight junction molecule in human colorectal adenocarcinoma. *J Pathol*. 198:207-12.

Ueda, J., Semba, S., Chiba, H., Sawada, N., Seo, Y., Kasuga, M., & Yokozaki, H. (2007). Heterogeneous expression of claudin-4 in human colorectal cancer: decreased claudin-4 expression at the invasive front correlates cancer invasion and metastasis. *Pathobiology*. 74:32-41.

Visser, J., Rozing, J., & Sapone, A. (2009). Tight junctions, intestinal permeability, and autoimmunity: celiac disease and type 1 diabetes paradigms. *Ann N Y Acad Sci*. 1165:195-205.

Weber, CR., Nalle, SC., Tretiakova, M., Rubin, DT., & Turner, JR. (2008). Claudin-1 and claudin-2 expression is elevated in inflammatory bowel disease and may contribute to early neoplastic transformation. *Lab Invest*. 88:1110-20.

Weber, CR., Raleigh, DR., Su, L., Shen, L., Sullivan, EA., Wang, Y., & Turner, JR. (2010). Epithelial myosin light chain kinase activation induces mucosal interleukin-13 expression to alter tight junction ion selectivity. *J Biol Chem*. 285:12037-46.

Yu, LC., Wang, JT., Wei, SC., Ni, YH. (2012). Host-microbial interactions and regulation of intestinal epithelial barrier function: From physiology to pathology. *World J Gastrointest Pathophysiol*. 3(1):27-43.

Zavala-Zendejas, VE., Torres-Martinez, AC., Salas-Morales, B., Fortoul, TI., Montaño, LF., & Rendon-Huerta, EP. (2011). Claudin-6, 7, or 9 overexpression in the human gastric adenocarcinoma cell line AGS increases its invasiveness, migration, and proliferation rate. *Cancer Invest*. 29:1-11.

2

Heat Shock Proteins in Coeliac Disease

Erna Sziksz[1,2], Leonóra Himer[1,2], Gábor Veres[2], Beáta Szebeni[1,2], András Arató[2], Tivadar Tulassay[1,2] and Ádám Vannay[1,2]

[1]*Research Group for Paediatrics and Nephrology, Semmelweis University and Hungarian Academy of Sciences, Budapest,*
[2]*First Department of Paediatrics, Semmelweis University, Budapest, Hungary*

1. Introduction

Coeliac disease is a complex inflammatory disorder of the small intestine with autoimmune features in genetically predisposed individuals and triggered by chronic exposure to gluten of wheat, barley and/or rye (Trynka et al., 2010). The aim of the recent chapter is to introduce and characterize a family of proteins, called heat shock proteins (HSPs), which are known to be key molecules during stress responses (Polla & Cossarizza, 1996). We will discuss the potential involvement of HSPs in the pathomechanism of coeliac disease based on recent scientific results. We will also refer to some future directions and potential therapeutic intervention.

1.1 What is coeliac disease?

Coeliac disease also known as gluten-sensitive enteropathy or nontropical sprue is a digestive disease occurring in genetically susceptible individuals, triggered by dietary gluten and related prolamins, which damage small intestine and interfere with absorption of nutrients (Setty et al., 2008). Gluten and prolamins are present in wheat, rye and barley, but also in some products such as stamp and envelope adhesive, medicines, and vitamins (Rodrigo, 2009). The genetic predisposition has been associated with the major histocompatibility complex region on chromosome 6p21. More than 90% of coeliac disease patients express the antigen-presenting molecules human leukocyte antigen-DQ2 and the remaining coeliac patients express DQ8 (Silano et al., 2010; Schuppan et al., 2005). Approximately 1% of the population is affected by coeliac disease (it remains mostly undiagnosed) (Green, 2005). It is not clear, why the prevalence of coeliac disease increased over the last decades, but similarly to other immune mediated diseases — such as allergy or asthma — this tendency suggests the importance of environmental stress factors besides the genetic predisposition (Rubio-Tapia & Murray, 2010). In addition, novel and trustful diagnostic marker (tissue transglutaminase) could help to uncover previously undiagnosed cases. Coeliac disease was traditionally considered to be a childhood disease, however, most patients are diagnosed in adulthood (Virta et al., 2009). Coeliac disease often becomes active for the first time after surgery, pregnancy, childbirth, viral infection, emotional or other stress situations (Baldassarre et al., 2008). Concepts/hypothesis such as the hygiene hypothesis, perhaps changes in wheat or other cereals may lead to the increased prevalence of coeliac disease. The disease leads to intestinal inflammation, villous atrophy, and crypt hyperplasia of the small intestine (Kaukinen et al, 2010). Furthermore coeliac disease may be associated with various extra-intestinal complications, including isolated iron deficiency anemia (Doganci & Bozkurt, 2004), bone and skin disease (Maniar et al., 2010; Reunala, 2001), infertility, endocrine and neurologic disorders (Gupta & Kohli, 2010). Presumed disease is mainly detected by serologic screening for the presence of tissue transglutaminase specific immunglobulin A antibodies, and this should be followed by taking biopsy samples from the small intestine mucosa to establish a definite diagnosis (Rostom et al., 2005). In the pathomechanism of coeliac disease both the adaptive and innate immunity may be involved. The importance of the adaptive immune response to gluten has been well established, but recent observations also suggest the central role for the gluten-induced innate stress response in the pathogenesis of coeliac disease (Jabri & Sollid, 2006). It is characterized by the presence of lymphocytic infiltration in the epithelial membrane and the lamina propria, and expression of multiple cytokines and signaling proteins (Briani et al., 2008). Recently gluten-free diet is the most effective mode to treat coeliac disease (Fric et al., 2011).

1.2 How is stress involved in the development and pathomechanism of coeliac disease?

As mentioned above there is a broad spectrum of environmental, genetic and immunologic factors, which may be involved in the development of coeliac disease. Here we focus on the common effects of different stress factors in the pathogenesis of coeliac disease. Stress is an acute menace to the homeostasis of an organism that may have both a short- and long-term influence on the function of the organs. Stress evokes adaptive responses that serve to defend the stability of the internal environment and to ensure the survival of the organism (Bhatia & Tandon, 2005). There are several types of stress circumstances: intrinsic, such as genetic and endoplasmic reticulum stress; extrinsic/environmental including heat-, toxin-, radiation-, infection- and injury-induced stress, mechanical and regenerative stress; metabolic stress such as hypoxia-induced, osmotic and oxidative stress. Under normal circumstances the epithelial cells are connected to each other with tight junctions and adherent junctions in the small intestine and in the large bowel as well. These structures of the epithelial cells serve as a barrier and inhibit the transcellular and paracellular permeation of molecules (Turner, 2009). Mechanical, chemical or oxidative stress can impair mucosal integrity (Lewis, 2009), modulate gut motility, epithelial barrier function (John et al., 2011) and inflammatory states (Lyte et al., 2011) and in genetically susceptible persons may lead to the development of coeliac disease (Szaflarska-Poplawska et al., 2011), because incompletely digested peptides of wheat gluten (gliadin and glutenins) and related proteins, as dietary antigens, can be transported across the epithelium and enter into the lamina propria of the small intestine (Alaedini & Green, 2005). The major processes of the pathogenesis of coeliac disease are shown on Figure 1.

Tissue transglutaminase 2 enzymes, which are the components of endomysium, become activated in the intestinal mucosa (lamina propria) (Schuppan et al., 2009). Transglutaminase 2 is a calcium-dependent enzyme which catalyzes protein cross-linking, polyamination or deamidation at selective glutamine residues (Caccamo et al., 2010) and

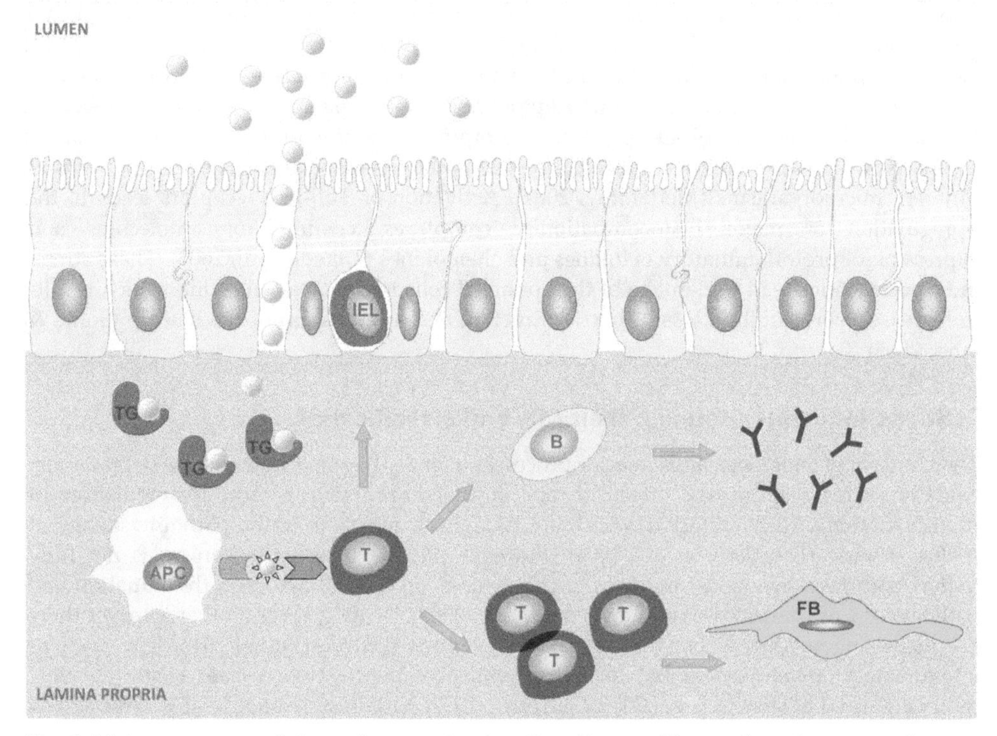

Fig. 1. Major processes of the pathogenesis of coeliac disease. (For explanation see text) Abbreviations: TG: transglutaminase; APC: antigen presenting cell; T: T lymphocyte; B: B lymphocyte; Fb: fibroblast; IEL: intraepithelial lymphocyte

may be involved in different pathological conditions, such as neurodegenerative disorders (Malorni et al., 2008), tumour progression (Chhabra et al., 2009), autoimmune and inflammatory diseases (Elli et al., 2009). Due to its activity neutral glutamine residues of the gluten protein will be deamidated and can be converted into negatively charged glutamic acids, creating epitopes with increased immunostimulatory potential (Briani et al., 2008). Some of the deamidated gliadins may cross-link to transglutaminase and form covalently linked complexes (Alaedini & Green, 2008; Fleckenstein et al, 2004). Antigen presenting immune cells such as macrophages, dendritic cells and B lymphocytes present the deamidated peptides or complexes through their disease associated human leukocyte antigen-DQ2 and human leukocyte antigen-DQ8 molecules to $CD4^+$ T helper cells in the lamina propria (Qiao et al, 2009). Activated T cells promote B cell maturation, isotype switch, and differentiation into plasma cells producing anti-gluten and anti-transglutaminase 2 antibodies (Sollid, 2000). Furthermore activated T cells express proinflammatory cytokines, such as tumor necrosis factor alpha and interferon gamma, which trigger the release of matrix metalloproteinases by fibroblasts causing epithelial cell damage, degradation of the mucosal matrix and tissue remodeling (Schuppan et al., 2009). Interleukin-15 secreted by epithelial cells in response to gluten exposure activates intraepithelial $CD8^+$ T lymphocytes called cytotoxic T cells, which can destroy epithelial cells, that express stress-induced non-classical major histocompatibility complex class I ligands and human leukocyte antigen E molecules (Briani et al., 2008; Jabri et al., 2005). Gliadin peptides can also directly elicit innate immune responses in macrophages and dendritic cells via pattern recognition receptors such as Toll-like receptor 2 and 4 (Szebeni et al., 2007). Mammalian Toll-like receptors comprise a family of type I transmembrane receptors, which originally recognize conserved pathogen-associated molecular patterns of different microorganisms (Medzhitov, 2001). Activation of Toll-like receptors leads to the upregulation of major histocompatibility complexes, costimulatory molecules and expression of proinflammatory cytokines and chemokines (Takeda et al, 2003). These stress-induced reactions lead to damage of the epithelial cells in the small intestine, which results in increased permeability, loss of barrier function and aggravation of the disease (Sollid & Jabri, 2005).

2. Stress inducible proteins: their role and classification

There are some major key molecules or processes, namely basement membrane degradation, oxidative stress, apoptosis, effect of matrix metalloproteinases and dysregulation of proliferation and differentiation, which are thought to play role in the pathophysiology of coeliac disease (Diosdado et al., 2004), however the exact pathomechanism is not fully understood. Here we focus on stress circumstances, as critical factors in the initiation and pathogenesis of coeliac disease (Lewis & McKay, 2009). Among several other diseases there are increasing evidences between stress and various gastrointestinal disorders, such as inflammatory bowel disease, irritable bowel syndrome, peptic ulcer disease, gastrointestinal reflux disease (Levenstein et al., 2000; Gué et al., 1997). Organisms must be able to sense and respond rapidly to changes in their environment in order to maintain homeostasis and survive. Therefore as consequence of stress several processes and molecules become activated. Based on the review by Richter K. et al. these proteins can be grouped into classes, namely molecular chaperones (called as HSPs), components of the proteolytic system, RNA/DNA modifying enzymes, metabolic enzymes, regulatory proteins, cell organisatory proteins and transport, detoxifying and membrane-modulating proteins (Richter et al., 2010) (Table 1).

The first discovered stress inducible proteins, called HSPs are recently referred to as "molecular chaperones" (discussed in details later). They are involved in adequate folding of proteins, which means, that these ubiquitous, conserved proteins help other proteins and macromolecules to fold or re-fold and reach their final, native conformation (Papp et al., 2003). Cells are equipped with an efficient surveillance system to selectively eliminate abnormally folded, damaged proteins (Mishra et al., 2009). First with the help of molecular chaperones the cell tries to refold the unfolded proteins (Bukau et al, 2006), but if the refolding is no more possible, the misfolded or irreversibly aggregated proteins will be degraded by the ubiquitin proteasome system (Shang & Taylor, 2011). In the second class of proteins belong the components of the ubiquitin-proteasome pathway, which is the primary cytosolic proteolytic machinery for the selective degradation of various forms of damaged proteins, so it is an important protein quality control mechanism (Dantuma & Lindsten, 2010). Degradation of the target protein by ubiquitin proteasome system is a multistep process consisting of activating, conjugating, and ligating enzymes to ensure covalent attachment of multiple molecules of ubiquitin to the target proteins, which finally leads to

#	Functional protein class name	Function	Examples	Reference
1.	Molecular chaperones (HSPs)	Role in protein folding, decrease the amount of nonnative proteins and unwanted intermolecular interactions	HSP (heat shock protein) 60, HSP70, HSP90	Tiroli-Cepeda & Ramos, 2011
2.	Proteolytic system components	Help to eliminate misfolded and irreversibly aggregated proteins	Lap4 (vacuolar aminopeptidase), Yps6 (aspartic protease)	Maupin-Furlow et al., 2000
3.	DNA/RNA modifying enzymes	Necessary to repair DNA damage and failures, that occur during stress	DNA helicase, RNAse p subunit, topoisomerase	, Jantschitsch & Trautinger, 2003; Biamonti & Caceres, 2009
4.	Metabolic enzymes	Cell energy supply stabilization and reorganization during and after stress	acetyl-CoA hydrolase, NADH ubiquinone oxidoreductase	Malmendal et al., 2006
5.	Regulatory proteins	Transcription factors or kinases to regulate stress responses	CREB, Fas, HSF	Akerfelt et al., 2007
6.	Cell organisatory proteins	Sustain cellular structures such as cytoskeleton	claudin, actin, Las 17 (actin patch protein)	Levitsky et al., 2008
7.	Transport, detoxifying, membrane-modulating proteins	Stabilization of membrane structure and function	MarR (antibiotic resistance), ABC transporters	Vigh et al., 2007

Table 1. Functional classification of proteins induced by heat stress response. For explanations see text. Abbreviations: HSP: heat shock protein; NADH: nicotinamide adenine dinucleotide; CREB: cAMP response element-binding; Fas: FS7-associated cell surface antigen; HSF: heat shock factor; ABC: ATP binding cassette. (Based on review of Richter K. et al., 2010)

degradation of the targeted protein by 26S proteasome complex (Glickman & Ciechanover, 2002). The third functional class of proteins (involved in the response to stress) is the group of DNA/RNA modifying enzymes. They are essential to repair DNA damage that occurs during stress (Jantschitsch & Trautinger, 2003; Biamonti & Caceres, 2009). The fourth class is that of metabolic enzymes, which are involved in cell energy supply stabilization and reorganization during and after stress. Malmendal et al. characterized the metabolomic profile of Drosophila melanogaster after heat stress exposure, and found relatively reduced level of some metabolites following shock compared to controls, which were involved in energy metabolism (Malmendal et al., 2006). They described that following heat stress energy storage were decreased in the form of reduced glycogen and fatty acid-like or lipid-like molecules and glucose levels (Malmendal et al., 2006). During stress response regulating proteins such as transcription factors and kinases play also crucial role. They are involved in further initiation of signaling pathways in response to stress or have role in ribosome biogenesis and assembly (Al Refaii & Alix, 2009). One family of the most important transcription factors involved in stress response is that of heat shock factors (Akerfelt et al., 2007). Heat shock factors play significant role in suppressing protein misfolding in cells by the induction of classical as well as of nonclassical heat shock genes, both of which might be required to maintain protein homeostasis (Fujimoto & Nakai, 2010). Proteins involved in maintenance of cell structure, such as the cytoskeleton, are also significantly induced by stress (Richter et al., 2010). RNA expression and protein levels of the cytoskeletal intermediate filaments, which are essential to the structural integrity of epithelial cells (Sivaramakrishnan et al., 2008), become induced several fold in response to a variety of stress circumstances (Toivola et al., 2010). Initially intermedier filaments were described as molecules, which protect cells and tissues from mechanical stress (Kim & Coulombe, 2007; Pekny & Lane, 2007). Due to their special properties namely that their filaments can stretch 3 times their initial length before breaking, intermedier filaments are unique among cytoskeletal proteins (Wagner et al, 2007). The seventh functional group comprises upregulated transport, detoxifying and membrane-modulating proteins (Richter K. et al., 2010). The major role of these proteins is the stabilization of the membrane and preservation of its original function (Welker et al., 2010). Stress induces alterations in the lipid phase of membranes and lipids are known to influence the distribution of proteins within membranes (Vigh et al., 2007). It was also described, that stress stimuli alter the gene expression of multidrug resistance gene 1, which codes an ATP-dependent membrane-bound transporter called P-glycoprotein (Sharom, 2008). Transporters, such as members of ATP-binding cassette-superfamily are multidrug efflux pumps, play important role in cell protection against harmful chemicals, toxic xenobiotics and endogenous metabolites and they are also involved in the cellular response against stress (Sukhai & Piquette-Miller, 2000). It has been reported a direct correlation between multidrug resistance gene 1 and heat shock response, and basal activity of the multidrug resistance gene 1 promoter requires heat shock factor-mediated transactivation (Kim et al., 1997). Our present study provides an overview about functional groups of proteins potentially involved in stress response. Hereinafter we will focus especially on heat shock proteins commonly referred to as "molecular chaperones"(Ellis et al., 1989).

3. What are heat shock proteins?

Temperatures above the optimum may sensed as heat stress by living organisms, which disturbs cellular homeostasis and can lead to severe retardation in growth and development, and even to death (Baniwal et al., 2004). It has been shown, that cells response to heat stress by increased expression of heat stress proteins (Stetler et al., 2010). HSPs — also referred to as extrinsic chaperones or "molecular chaperones" — are a suite of highly conserved proteins with various molecular weights, which are produced in all organisms, when those are exposed to cellular stress (Welch, 1993). The discovery of HSPs started in the early 1960s (Ritossa, 1962). Ritossa et al. observed different puffing pattern of the chromosomes in Drosophila melanogaster after shifting the incubator temperature (Ritossa, 1996). Later these puffs were found to code proteins, which were identified as HSPs (Moran et al., 1978). When eukaryotic cells were exposed to temperatures 5-15 °C above their optimum for growth, they responded also by induction of HSPs (DiDomenico et al., 1982). These molecules were found also in prokaryotes and other eukaryotes (Lemaux et al., 1978; Carper et al., 1987; Kelley & Schlesinger, 1978; Timperio et al., 2008). HSPs are evolutionally highly conserved proteins indicating that heat shock response may be universal mechanism (Richter et al., 2010). Early on, researchers suggested that HSPs function as molecular chaperones mediating the folding and assembly of polypeptides and their translocation across the intracellular membranes (Burel et al., 1992). HSPs are also involved in protein degradation as essential components of the ubiquitin-dependent degradative pathway

(Morandi et al., 1989). The HSP chaperone machinery may stabilize the target protein to degradation by the ubiquitin-proteasome pathway of proteolysis (Pratt et al., 2004). These functions of HSPs are important during cell repair process after damage. Generally there are two major groups of HSPs, constitutive, which are continually present in the cell, and inducible HSPs (Petrof et al., 2004). HSPs are rapidly induced by a variety of cellular stressors, such as heat, UV light, or cytotoxic agents (Rajaiah & Moudgil, 2009; Aufricht, 2004), ischaemia-reperfusion injury, oxidative stress and nutritional stress (Akerfelt et al, 2010). Recently our knowledge about their roles have been expanded, including their involvement in the modulation of immune responses (Hauet-Broere et al., 2006; Johnson & Fleshner, 2006), autoimmunity (Rajaiah & Moudgil, 2009), cell signaling (Csermely et al., 2007), cell proliferation (Pechan, 1991), and apoptosis (Padmini & Lavanya, 2011). The expression of HSPs has been reported in several tissues and cell types, including heart (Ghayour-Mobarhan, 2009), brain (Stetler, 2010), muscle (Geiger & Gupte, 2011), lung (Wong & Wispé, 1997), kidney (Kelly, 2005), liver (Tashiro, 2009) and intestinum (Asano et al., 2009). It is also known, that HSPs are overexpressed in a wide range of human cancers and are implicated in tumour cell proliferation, differentiation, invasion, metastasis, death, and recognition by the immune system (Ciocca & Calderwood, 2005). HSPs can be classified into five major families, namely HSP60s, HSP70s, HSP90s, HSP100s and small HSPs (Richter et al., 2010; Roberts et al., 2010) based on their molecular weight. There are also some not ubiquitous HSPs, for example redox-regulated chaperon HSP33, which can not be ranked into these classical groups (Graf & Jakob, 2002). Major families of HSPs can be seen on Table 2.

#	HSP family	Subunit molecular mass	Example members	Cellular localization
1.	HSP100	80-110 kDa	HSP100, HSP104	cytoplasm, nucleus, mitochondia, plasma membrane
2.	HSP90	82-96 kDa	HSP90α (inducible), HSP90β	cytoplasm, nucleus, mitochondria, endoplasmic reticulum
3.	HSP70	67-76 kDa	HSP70, HSP72, HSP73, HSP80	cytoplasm, nucleus, mitochondria, endoplasmic reticulum, lysosomes and extracellular compartments
4.	HSP60	58-65 kDa	HSP60, HSP65	mitochondria
5.	small HSPs	8-40 kDa	alphaB-crystallin, HSP25, HSP27, ubiquitin	cytoplasm, nucleus
6.	Others (not ubiquitous)	various	HSP33	various

Table 2. Major families of HSPs. For explanations see text. (Based on review of Roberts et al., 2010 and Otaka et al., 2006)

3.1 HSP100 family

The HSP100 proteins belong to the superfamily of AAA (ATPase associated with various cellular activities) + domain-containing ATPases (Mayer, 2010). They are localized to different subcellular compartments, such as cytoplasm, nucleus, mitochondria and plasma membrane (Singh & Grover, 2010). Interestingly HSP100 proteins and also their homologues are absent in Archaea (Large et al., 2009), but they are found in Bacteria and Eukaryotes (Barends et al, 2010). Main function of HSP100 proteins is that they protect organisms under extreme stress conditions. It was demonstrated on heat-shocked yeast that their survival is significantly reduced in the absence of HSP100 protein (Schirmer et al., 1996). HSP100 molecules function as chaperones in an ATP-dependent fashion leading either to the renaturation or proteolytic degradation of individual proteins (Parsell & Lindquist, 1993; Liang & MacRae, 1997). They are important components of the protein quality control system controlling the intracellular levels of global regulatory proteins (Maurizi & Xia, 2004). It was demonstrated, that HSP104, a member of HSP100 family collaborates with the HSP70 chaperone systems to reactivate stress-denatured proteins from aggregates, which mechanism is crucial for the survival of cells during severe stress (Miot et al., 2011).

3.2 HSP90 family

Members of the 90 kDa heat shock proteins (HSP90) family are expressed in various organisms ranging from prokaryotes to eukaryotes (Pearl & Prodromou, 2006). They are one of the most highly abundant constitutively expressed proteins, comprising 1–2% of cellular proteins. HSP90 proteins are involved in various cellular processes, such as controlling of cell proliferation, differentiation and apoptosis and their expression increases markedly during stress (Sreedhar et al., 2004; Liang & MacRae, 1997). Eukaryotes require a functional cytoplasmic HSP90 for their viability: these proteins have role in the folding of a set of cell regulatory proteins and in the re-folding of stress-denatured polypeptides (Obermann et al., 1998; Borkovich et al., 1989). HSP90 proteins are ATP-dependent chaperones and the chaperone machine is driven by the hydrolysis of ATP and ADP/ATP nucleotide exchange. This ATP hydrolysis is coupled to conformation changes of HSP90s, which facilitate target protein folding and maturation (Hao et al, 2010). Recently several HSP90 members have been identified in mammalian cells, including the two major cytoplasmic homologues, the inducible HSP90-alpha and the constitutive HSP90-beta, the glucose-regulated protein 94 in the endoplasmic reticulum, and tumor necrosis factor receptor-associated protein 1 in the mitochondrial matrix (Stetler et al., 2010). Interestingly the bacterial homologue of HSP90 called HtpG is dispensable under non-heat stress conditions (Thomas & Baneyx, 1998). HSP90s contains nine alpha-helices and eight anti-parallel beta pleated sheets, which combine to form several alpha/beta sandwiches. HSP90 chaperones exist as obligate homodimers, and each monomer consist of an N-terminal regulatory domain, a non-conserved and dispensable charged region, a middle domain, and a C-terminal dimerization domain (Dollins et al., 2007).

A recent study demonstrates that inhibition of HSP90s abrogates the protective effect of bone marrow stromal cells, inhibits angiogenesis and osteoclastogenesis and a HSP90 inhibitor called tanespimycin is able to reduce tumour cell survival in vitro (Richardson et al., 2011). Because HSP90 chaperones play essential housekeeping functions and may be involved in a broad range of processes from signal transduction to immune responses, inhibitors may be promising for novel therapies (Sharp & Workman, 2006).

3.3 HSP70 family

70 kDa heat shock proteins (HSP70s) are the major components of the network of molecular chaperones, which are ubiquitously expressed, highly conserved and may be involved in a wide range of folding processes such as modulating polypeptide folding, degradation and translocation across membranes, as well as protein-protein interactions (Ryan & Pfanner, 2001). The HSP70 family is a most widely studied group of chaperones and comprises at least 13 related proteins expressed constitutively or induced by stress response and exert important cellular housekeeping functions (Daugaard et al., 2007). They can be found in cytoplasm, nucleus, mitochondria, endoplasmic reticulum, lysosomes and extracellular compartments (Stetler et al., 2010). While certain family members, such as HSP73 also known as heat shock cognate 70 is constitutively expressed in the cytosol, transcription of HSP72 is highly responsive to stress (Evans et al., 2010). HSP70 chaperones operate by an ATP dependent manner, namely their polypeptide binding and release capacity is driven by ATP. Various nucleotide exchange factors and co-chaperones (for example the so called DnaJ proteins, which associate with HSP70s and may control their nucleotide turnover (Laufen et al., 1999)) may promote the HSP70 ATPase cycle (Young, 2010). HSP70s may exert important cytoprotective functions in gastric and colonic mucosa (Odashima et al., 2002; 2006).

3.4 HSP60 family

A special group of chaperones and comolecules exist in the organisms, which is involved in mitochondrial protein folding. Such proteins are the members of the HSP60 family also called as chaperonins. HSP60s are essential for the health and maintenance of mitochondrial function, as well as for proper mitochondrial biogenesis (Stetler et al, 2010). Although the majority of HSP60 proteins can be found in the mitochondria, 15–20% of them is located extramitochondrially (in the cytosol, on the cell surface or in the extracellular space) (Soltys & Gupta, 1996; Pfister et al., 2005). In the animal model of transient global ishaemia, HSP60s can be induced during stress (Truettner et al., 2009). Kuwabara et al. also have found that HSP60s are specifically induced in rat colonic mucosa after 5-hydroxytryptamine-induced ischaemia and it may have cytoprotective effects (Kuwabara et al., 1994). HSP60 proteins also have immunomodulatory functions, because they are activator of Toll-like receptor 4 signaling in macrophages and dendritic cells and also regulate the activity of effector T cells and regulatory T cells via innate Toll-like receptor 2 signaling. It is proposed that HSP60s can serve as biomarkers to monitor the immune status of the individual, providing a potential to modulate immunity for therapeutic purposes in diseases such as in rheumatoid arthritis and type I diabetes (Quintana & Cohen, 2011).

3.5 Small HSPs

The family of small HSPs (sHSPs) is the less conserved family of molecular chaperones. Their only common characteristics is the conserved alpha-crystallin or HSP20 core domain (Richter et al., 2010) named according to its discovery in alpha-crystallin, a highly abundant protein in the vertebrate eye lens (Horwitz, 1992). sHPSs have general importance, they are present in Archaea, Bacteria, and Eukarya, but there is a broad variation of primary sequences within the superfamily and different organisms (Kriehuber et al, 2010). sHSPs are ATP-independent chaperones, which forms large oligomers containing often more than 20 monomers (Van Montfort et al., 2001). Recent evidences suggest that sHSPs maintain protein homeostasis by binding proteins in non-native conformations, thereby preventing substrate aggregation (Haslbeck et al., 2005). They are also associated with a variety of severe diseases (e.g., myopathies, dystrophies, cataracts, Alzheimer's or other amyloidal diseases, and diverse cancers) and their expression is enhanced under environmental stress conditions such as elevated temperature or exposure to heavy metals or arsenate (Sun & MacRae, 2005; Haslbeck et al., 2005). Major family members alphaB-crystallin, HSP25 and HSP27 might be involved in the prevention of apoptosis and cell protection against heat shock and oxidative stress, they can stabilize microfilaments (Arrigo, 2007). Modulation of the expression and activities of HSP27 and alphaB-crystallin may have therapeutic potential in the future (Arrigo et al., 2007). Also ubiquitin, a small protein weighting 8 kD, belongs to the family of HSPs and it is involved in nonlysosomal protein degradation, which is an important pathway of proteolysis (Kiang, 2004; Heo &Rutter, 2011; von Mikecz et al., 2008).

4. Regulation of the HSPs

As mentioned above, cellular events, which lead to protein unfolding or denaturation (such as elevated temperature, oxidative stress and metabolic disturbances) can activate heat shock response, which leads to the upregulation of HSPs (Noble et al., 2008). Specific transcription factors play a key role in these processes: transcription factor sigma 32 in prokaryotic cells (Rodriguez et al., 2008) and heat shock factor 1 in eukaryotic cells (Anckar & Sistonen, 2007). However sigma 32 and heat shock factor 1 are not related in their sequence and structure, they share common mechanistic properties leading to HSP overexpression (Richter et al., 2010). In prokaryotes, for example in Escherichia Coli there are a HSP70 and a HSP40 chaperone homologes called DnaK and DnaJ, respectively, which normally form a complex with the transcription factor sigma 32. Thereby the bound sigma 32, which is an alternative subunit of the bacterial RNA polymerase, remains in inactive state and will be degraded by specific AAA (ATPase associated with various cellular activities) proteases called FtsH metalloproteases. Under normal circumstances this mechanism results in reduced intracellular level of transcription factor sigma 32, keeping the heat shock genes untranscribed (Rodriguez et al., 2008). During stress the protein homeostasis is disturbed, the number of unfolded proteins is increased, which then bind to DnaK and DnaJ chaperone molecules. Until these chaperones are in complex with unfolded proteins, they are no more able to bind the sigma 32 transcription factor, which becomes activated. Activated sigma 32 binds to RNA polymerase and replaces the normal regulatory σ70 subunit and stimulates the transcription of heat shock genes. Similarly to sigma 32 in prokaryotes, in eukaryotes the transcription factor heat shock factor 1 forms complex with HSP70 and HSP40 proteins, which keep it in inactive form inhibiting its function. But compared to the prokaryotes the function of the heat shock factor 1 regulatory system is much more complex, because multimerization, phosphorilation and numerous posttranscriptional modifications might be involved in the mechanism (Prahlad & Morimoto, 2009). Under stress circumstances the HSPs, also HSP70 and HSP40 bind to unfolded proteins losing their ability to form complex with heat shock factor 1, which then leads to the release of heat shock factor 1 monomers. After trimerization heat shock factor 1 is transported into the nucleus and becomes hyperphosphorylated by kinases at multiple sites within its regulatory domain (Holmberg et al., 2001). Heat shock factor 1 binds to heat-shock elements found in the promoter regions of its target HSP genes, which finally leads to the transcription of heat shock genes (Figure 2).

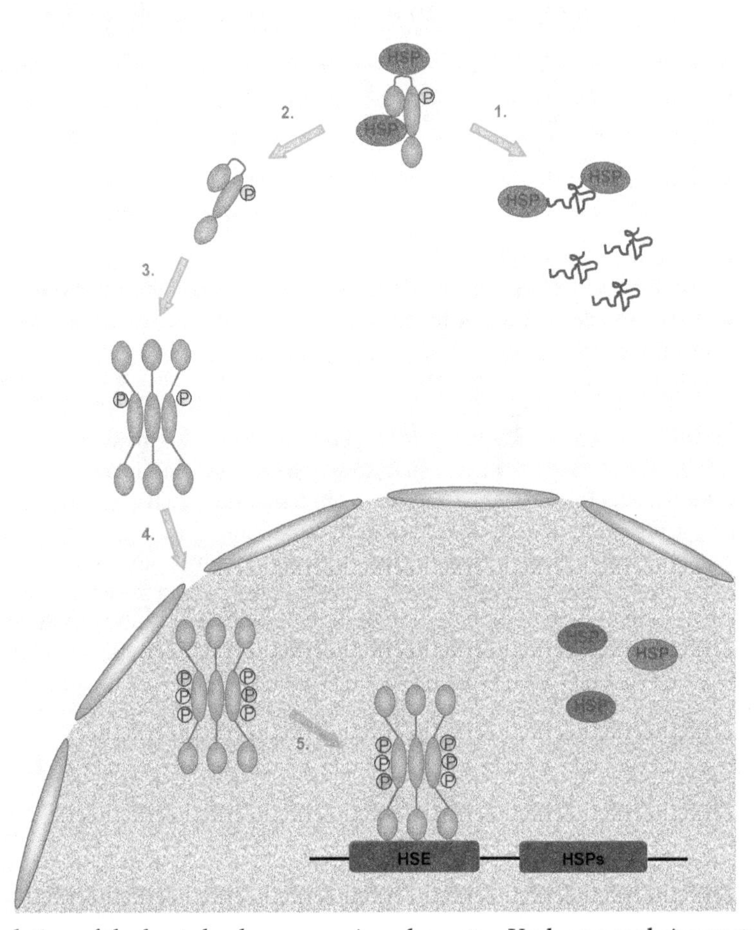

Fig. 2. Regulation of the heat shock response in eukaryotes. Under normal circumstances HSPs are in complex with the transcription factor heat shock factor 1. Under stress HSPs bind to unfolded proteins (1.) losing their ability to form complex with heat shock factor 1, therefore leading to the release of heat shock factor 1 monomers (2.). After trimerization (3.) heat shock factor 1 is transported into the nucleus and becomes hyperphosphorylated (4.). Heat shock factor 1 then binds to the HSE in the promoter regions of target HSP genes (5.). This process leads to the transcription of HSPs. Abbreviations: HSP: heat shock protein; P: phosphorylation; HSF1: heat shock factor 1; HSE: heat-shock elements

On the other hand the formation of HSP-heat shock factor complex suppresses heat shock factor production maintaining a negative feed-back regulatory system. Furthermore heat shock factor 1 may be inducibly acetylated at a specific residue, which regulates negatively its DNA binding activity (Westerheid et al., 2009). Heat shock factor binding protein 1 has been reported to be a negative regulator of the heat shock response, because heat shock factor binding protein 1 binds specifically the active trimeric form of heat shock factor1, thus inhibiting its activity (Liu et al, 2009).

5. Molecular functions of HSPs with special focus on coeliac disease

In this part we introduce the major molecular functions of HSPs in those processes, which may be also involved in the pathogenesis of coeliac disease, such as oxidative stress, immune response and inflammation, apoptosis and mucosal damage.

5.1 Oxidative stress

Different chemical and environmental stressors often act by induction of oxidative damage in the cells (Limón-Pacheco & Gonsebatt, 2009). In this process reactive oxygen species play a key role. Reactive oxygen species are generated continuously during the respiration process, and their level is markedly elevated by a range of different stress conditions causing oxidative deterioration of proteins, lipids and DNA (Avery, 2011). When production of reactive oxygen species exceeds the capacity of cellular antioxidant defenses to remove these toxic species, it is referred as oxidative stress and together with decreased reductive potential it may induce cell damage or death (Rivabene et al., 1999). It has been assumed that oxidative stress plays an important role in the development of celiac disease, because gliadin can induce oxidative stress responses (Diosdado et al., 2005). Gluten peptides could enhance the mRNA expression of the inducible form of nitric oxide synthase in the small intestine, (van Straaten et al., 1999). Increased inducible nitric oxide synthase and nitric oxide levels contribute to subsequent mucosal damage by promoting the generation of peroxynitrite and free-radicals and can play a role in the mechanism leading to villous atrophy in coeliac disease (Murray et al., 2002). Levels and activity of antioxidant enzymes epoxide hydrolases and glutathione peroxidases and other antioxidants, such as a-tocopherol and lipoproteins (cholesterol and apolipoproteins), which major biological role is the protection of the organism from oxidative damage, were reduced in biopsies taken from patients with coeliac disease (Stojiljković et al., 2007; Odetti et al., 1998). In these processes HSPs may be involved in several ways. Oxygen free radicals, such as superoxide can be an inducer of HSPs (Omar & Pappolla, 1993). HSP32, also known as heme oxygenase-1 enzyme participates in the cell defense against oxidative stress by degrading heme to vasoactive carbon monoxide, free iron, and to potent antioxidant biliverdin (Aztatzi-Santillán et al., 2010). HSP60 plays a role in protecting small intestinal mucosal cells from H_2O_2-induced cell injury by enhancing the cytoprotective function of small intestinal epithelial cells (Takada et al., 2010). After hemorrhage the inducible form of HSP70 specifically couples to inducible nitric oxide synthase and its transcription factor called Krueppel-like factor 6, which has been demonstrated using immunoprecipitation and immunoblotting analysis (Kiang, 2004). Bellmann et al. found, that HSP70 overexpressing fibrosarcoma cells produced two to three times more nitric oxide than control cells after treatment with interleukin-1β or a combination of lipopolisacharide and interferon gamma-γ. This HSP70-mediated increase of nitric oxide production was accompanied by an enhanced transcription of the inducible nitric oxide synthase gene and an increased accumulation of inducible nitric oxide synthase mRNA and protein. This phenomenon may be specific to HSP70, because overexpression of other HSPs, such as HSP27 does not elevate the levels of nitric oxide. HSP70 can modulate the cellular response to cytokines by acting on signaling elements upstream of p38, which acts as an enhancing factor in the activation of inducible nitric oxide synthase (Bellmann et al., 2000). Furthermore, induction of HSP70s protects intestinal epithelial cells against oxidant injury by preserving the integrity of the actin cytoskeleton and cell-cell contact (see detailed in part 5.4.) (Musch et al., 1999). HSP90 was reported to form a complex with endothelial nitric oxide synthase to activate it, which resulted in elevated nitric oxide levels of cardiac cells *in vitro*, leading to downregulation of O_2 consumption in heat-shocked cells and to subsequent attenuation of cellular respiration (Ilang et al., 2004). HSP90 also mediates cytoprotection against chemical hypoxia-induced injury via antioxidant and H_2S-induced antiapoptotic effects (Chen et al., 2010).

5.2 Inflammation

Gluten-derived peptides can activate a harmful immune response in the lamina propria of genetically predisposed individuals (Schuppan, 2000). Antigen presentation of gluten-derived peptides to T cells by antigen presenting cells, such as macrophages and dendritic cells, play a pivotal role in the pathogenesis of coeliac disease. Stimulated CD4+ T helper type 1 cells through release of T helper 1-type cytokines activate other immune cells, and therefore they have central role in controlling the immune response to gluten that causes the immunopathology of coeliac disease (Di Sabatino et al., 2007). HSPs (such as HSP60, HSP90), which can bind to peptides, are also able to induce immune response. They play important role in antigen presentation and activation of lymphocytes, macrophages and dendritic cells (Li et al., 2002). If the cell is damaged, the HSP-peptide complexes appear in the extracellular space and bind to certain surface molecules or receptors (such as to Toll-like receptor 2 and Toll-like receptor 4) of antigen presenting cells, which take up these complexes by receptor endocytosis (Binder et al., 2004). This process leads to antigen presentation by major histocompatibility complex molecules to lymphocytes and finally to the activation of T cell pathway (,Suto & Srivastava, 1995; Dudeja et al., 2009). HSPs stimulate the production of inflammatory cytokines such as tumor necrosis factor alpha, interleukin-1, interleukin-6, interleukin-12 and C-C chemokines by monocytes, macrophages and dendritic cells (Tsan & Gao, 2009). These effects are mediated by the CD14/Toll-like receptor 2 and Toll-like receptor 4 complex leading to the activation of mitogen-activated protein kinase signaling pathway and nuclear factor kappa-light-chain-enhancer of activated B cells (Asea et al., 2000). HSP60 induces the maturation of dendritic cells and stimulates their activation more rapidly than lipopolisacharide and elicits a T helper type 1-promoting phenotype (Flohé et al., 2003). Furthermore HSPs contribute to the proliferation and activation of natural killer cells (Multhoff, 2009), which may be involved in coeliac disease due to the interaction between their natural killer group 2 member D activating receptors and major histocompatibility complex class I polypeptide-related sequence A molecules expressed on epithelial cells (Gianfrani et al., 2005). The natural killer group 2 member D/ major histocompatibility complex class I polypeptide-related sequence A interaction may have a pivotal role in the activation of intraepithelial immune cells and development of villous atrophy during coeliac disease (Hüe et al., 2004). Since Toll-like receptors can serve as receptors of HSPs (Tsan & Gao, 2004; Asea, 2008) and their activation leads to elevated expression of proinflammatory cytokines and chemokines, in this manner HSPs may be involved in the pathomechanism of coeliac disease (Takeda et al., 2003). Due to their cytokine-like effects, HSPs may serve as "danger signals" for the immune system at sites of tissue injury (Osterloh & Breloer, 2008).

5.3 Apoptosis

Apoptosis or programmed cell death is essential to the maintenance of the intestinal epithelial functions, because it is involved in the normal enterocyte turnover. Under physiological conditions apoptotic cells of the small bowel are restricted to the tips of the villous and are replaced by equal number of proliferating immature crypt cells (Watson, 1995). Increased apoptosis of enterocytes is one of the major mechanisms responsible for villous atrophy in coeliac disease. Apoptosis in coeliac disease may be caused directly by the toxic domains of gliadin peptides or it is mediated by intraepithelial and lamina propria lymphocytes (Di Sabatino et al., 2001). Digested wheat gliadin peptides induce apoptosis by the FS7-associated cell surface antigen (Fas) mediated apoptotic pathway. The ligand of Fas is a cell surface molecule, which belongs to the tumor necrosis factor family and binds to the Fas receptor and induce apoptosis of Fas-bearing cells (Ehrenschwender & Wajant, 2009). Fas receptor is widely expressed by many cell types, including also enterocytes. Fas was found on most enterocytes isolated from biopsies of patients with coeliac disease, and mononuclear cells of the lamina propria were shown to expressed Fas ligand (Ciccocioppo et al., 2001). Giovanni et al. found increased Fas and Fas ligand mRNA expression in coeliac disease, and this gliadin-induced apoptosis could be blocked by Fas cascade inhibiting agents and neutralizing antibodies (Giovannini et al., 2003). HSPs are also involved in cell death processes, because they may exert anti-apoptotic effects (Dudeja et al, 2009). Fas-Fas ligand ligation induces the binding of heat shock factor 1 to the DNA and increases the production of HSP72 and HSP72-induced chemokines, which than promote cell survival (Choi et al., 2011). HSP70 can inhibit not only the death receptor-mediated extrinsic, but also intrinsic apoptotic pathways, which are initiated by intracellular stress signals and regulated by mitochondrial proteins (Dudeja et al., 2009). During heat-induced apoptosis HSP70 prevents the formation of pores in the mitochondrial membrane by inhibiting the translocation of Bax - a proapoptotic Bcl-2 family member - into the mitochondria and prevents cytochrome c release (Stankiewicz et al., 2005). After inhibition of HSP70, cytochrome c appears in the cytosol released from the mitochondria, which results in the stimulation of caspase-9 and caspase-3 leading to the activation of apoptotic protease cascade and finally to cell death (Li et al., 1997). HSP70 can modulate the calcium signaling, which also has a major role in the regulation of apoptosis (Rizzuto et al., 2003; Creagh et al., 2000). Furthermore, HSP70 has been demonstrated to be a natural inhibitor of cJun N-terminal kinase (Park et al., 2001), which through the induction of Fas ligand promotes an early apoptotic pathway initiated by heat shock (Volloch et al., 2000). Thereby HSP70 may modulate stress-activated signaling, because blocking of cJun N-terminal kinase appears to be involved in the protection against caspase-dependent apoptosis (Gabai et al., 2000). HSP70 also prevent the release of lysosomal enzymes into the cytosol by inhibiting lysosomal membrane permeabilization and therefore stabilizing the lysosomes (Gyrd-Hansen et al., 2004). In contrast to other HSPs, the role of HSP60 during apoptosis is controversial. Recent reports suggest, that HSP60 may have an antiapoptotic effect, but early studies refer to its pro-apoptotic function, because it may facilitate the activation of caspase 3 (Xanthoudakis et al., 1999). However, recently HSP60 has been described as a novel regulator of mitochondrial permeability transition, which contributes to a cytoprotective chaperone network (Ghosh et al., 2010).

5.4 Mucosal damage

A critical function of the intestinal mucosa is to form a barrier that separates luminal contents from the underlying interstitium. Integrity of the intestinal barrier is essential for maintaining health and preventing tissue injury. All the above mentioned processes (such as oxidative stress, inflammation and enhanced epithelial cell apoptosis) lead finally to mucosal damage, loss of epithelial barrier function and therefore increased mucosal permeability (Farhadi et al., 2003). Integrity of the epithelial barrier is determined by an apical junctional complex that is composed of tight junction and adherens junction (Bruewer et al., 2006). In patients with inflammatory bowel disease the level of key tight junction (occludin, junctional adhesion molecule, zonula occludens 1, claudin 1) and adherens junction (E-cadherin, beta-catenin) proteins reduced or disappeared from the intercellular junctions resulting in the loss of barrier function (Ivanov et al., 2004). HSPs were reported to play a pivotal role in the preservation of the intestinal barrier function (Petrof et al., 2004). Dokladny K et al. suggested that the upregulation of occludin expression mediated by HSPs may be an important mechanism involved in the maintenance of intestinal epithelial tight junction barrier function during heat stress (Dokladny et al., 2006). Using Caco2 colonic epithelial cells it was shown that HSP72 can directly bind and stabilize tight junction-associated proteins, such as zonula occludens (Musch et al., 1999). Also HSP25 takes part in the stabilization of cell-cell contact, and epithelial cells transfected with antisense to HSP25 demonstrated reduced interleukin-11-mediated cytoprotection, which refer to the protective role of HSPs (Ropeleski et al., 2003). The connection between other HSPs and tight junction proteins was also demonstrated (Tsapara et al., 2006). Furthermore in the pathomechanism leading to villous atrophy the degradation of the extracellular matrix by matrix metalloproteinases may be also implicated. Matrix metalloproteinases belong to a group of zinc-dependent proteins, which are normally produced at very low concentrations and have a primary role in repairing tissue injury and remodelling (Zitka et al., 2010). In the gut of coeliac disease patients the expression of matrix metalloproteinase-1, matrix metalloproteinase-3 and a tissue inhibitor of metalloproteinases were increased, which suggest the importance of these proteases and protease inhibitors in the pathomechanism of coeliac disease (Daum et al., 1999). Furthermore, the elevated levels of tumor necrosis factor alpha during T cell mediated immune response in the lamina propria, which is also associated with mucosal injury, increased the expression of matrix metalloproteinases promoting mucosal degradation (Pender et al., 1997). A correlation between matrix metalloproteinases and HSPs was also demonstrated by Sims JD et al. Extracellular HSP90α was shown to activate matrix metalloproteinase-2. Cochaperones HSP70 and HSP40 increased the association of HSP90α and matrix metalloproteinase-2 *in vitro* and enhanced the HSP90α-mediated activation of matrix metalloproteinase-2, leading to increased cell migration (Sims et al., 2011). HSP60 may induce tumor necrosis factor alpha and matrix metalloproteinase production by macrophages (Kol et al., 1998). Based on these results HSPs have an important regulatory role in the maintenance of epithelial barrier functions.

6. Recent facts and research results: HSPs and coeliac disease

Recently there are only few data in the literature about the direct connection between HSPs and coeliac disease. Most of our knowledge about the involvement of HSPs in the intestinal tract is based on the results found in other gastrointestinal disorders and gut disease models. Here we summarize the recent research results related to HSPs and coeliac disease based also on findings of our research group. Furthermore we take an outlook to other intestinal abnormalities with specially focus on inflammatory bowel disease because there are similarities between the pathomechanism of inflammatory bowel disease (mainly Crohn's disease) and coeliac disease.

6.1 Localization of the HSPs in the gastrointestinal tract

Studies examining the HSP expression have been shown, that however HSPs are present in all tissues, there are differences in their localization and amount throughout the gastrointestinal tract (Tanguay et al., 1993). Normally high expression of HSPs (such as HSP25 and HSP72) was found in gastric mucosal epithelial cells and in colon epithelial cells. Explanation for this phenomenon may be the fact, that these parts of the gastrointestinal tract are exposed to continuously high acidic pH, mechanical stress or bacterial fermentation, which microenvironment may promote HSP response (Kojima et al., 2003). In contrast, the expression of HSPs in the small intestine is negligible under normal, stress-free circumstances, except the distal part of the ileum, which is exposed to high amounts of enteric bacteria. This luminal microflora and their metabolic products may direct the expression of HSPs in gut epithelial cells (Arvans et al., 2005). Under cellular stress conditions increased expression of HSPs were found also in other parts of the small intestine (Petrof et al., 2004). Generally, HSPs are predominantly localized in the epithelial cells rather than in the underlying lamina propria in the gastrointestinal tract suggesting that HSPs may have crucial role in the protection of epithelial cells preserving their function and structure (Kojima et al., 2003).

6.2 HSPs in coeliac disease: recent research results

Since mechanical, chemical or oxidative stress can impair mucosal integrity (Lewis & McKay, 2009) and has crucial role in the development of coeliac disease, it is important to understand its molecular mechanism. Because HSPs were demonstrated to have mainly cytoprotective function under stress circumstances (Kalmar & Greensmith, 2009), it is very actual to examine the potential involvement of HSPs in the pathogenesis of coeliac disease. Three genes of the HSP70 family are located in the major histocompatibility complex class III region. These genes are of particularly interest since the HSPs seem to be involved in the antigen processing and presentation (Pierce et al., 1991) and are thought to play a role in the pathogenesis in some autoimmune-like systemic disorders (Panchapakesan et al., 1992). In 1993 Partanen et al. examined 19 families with patients suffering from celiac disease and 95 individuals from the normal population and found that gene frequencies in the affected haplotypes of the heat-shock protein 70 gene cluster significantly deviated from those observed in the normal population. Based on their results they suggested, that polymorphism of human leukocyte antigen-linked HSP70 (called HSP70-2) gene may be involved in the pathomechanism of coeliac disease (Partanen et al., 1993). Ramos-Arroyo et al. studied the polymorphisms in the 5' regulatory region of the HSP70-1 gene and performed genomic human leukocyte antigen-DQ and -DR typing in 128 patients with coeliac disease and 94 healthy controls. They found that among coeliac disease patients the frequency of the C allele of HSP70-1 gene was significantly elevated. Furthermore, those individuals, who expressed the classical human leukocyte antigen alleles in coeliac disease and also carried the HSP70-1 CC genotype, were twelve times more likely to develop coeliac disease than the matched controls. The authors concluded that HSP70-1 gene might be a component of the high risk haplotype, playing a role as an additional predisposing gene for coeliac disease (Ramos-Arroyo et al., 2001). Our research group first examined the expression of HSP72, a member of HSP70 family in the duodenal mucosa of children with coeliac disease (Sziksz et al., 2010). We demonstrated increased mRNA expression and protein levels of HSP72 in their duodenal mucosa localized mainly in the villous enterocytes and in the immune cells of the lamina propria. We suggest that HSP72 may have role in the defense against the gliadin-mediated cytotoxicity partly because of its antiapoptotic effects fostering the survival of epithelial cells. Furthermore, earlier we also demonstrated increased Toll-like receptor 2 and Toll-like receptor 4 expressions in the duodenal mucosa of patients with coeliac disease localized in the villous enterocytes and immune cells of the lamina propria (Szebeni et al., 2007) similarly to the tissue distribution of HSP72. Cario et al. showed, that activation of Toll-like receptor 2 can preserve tight junction proteins (such as zonula occludens 1) associated intestinal barrier integrity against stress-induced damage through the promotion of phosphatidylinositol 3-kinase/Akt-mediated signaling pathway (Cario et al., 2007). Since HSPs can serve as ligands of Toll-like receptors (Asea, 2008), our data suggest that HSP72-Toll-like receptor 2/Toll-like receptor 4 signaling may modify the immune response against gluten peptides and may alter the integrity of intestinal barrier. We also analyzed the HSP72 expression in coeliac disease patients maintained on gluten free diet and found markedly decreased levels of HSP72 in their duodenal mucosa compared to untreated children with coeliac disease, but its level remained higher than that in controls. We propose, that HSP72 as a "danger signal" for the immune cells may promote their protection against damage in coeliac disease. Since intact protein absorption is thought to be a causative factor in celiac disease, Yang et al. examined transepithelial electric resistance and permeability after performing heat stress *in vitro* using T84 human intestinal epithelial cells. Heat stress significantly increased protein transport across the intestinal epithelial monolayer and this heat stress-induced T84 monolayer barrier disruption was inhibited by pretreatment with HSP70 suggesting the intestinal barrier protective role of HSP70 (Yang et al., 2007). Examining the involvement of other HSPs in coeliac disease, Iltanen et al. analyzed jejunal biopsies of seventy-eight children with clinical suspicion of coeliac disease. They found increased expression of mitochondrial HSP65 in the epithelial cells in 80% of patients suffering from coeliac disease, but in only 7% of control individuals. Moreover, enhanced HSP65 levels were associated with higher gammadelta+ T cell densities and serum Immunglobulin A-class endomysial autoantibodies. They concluded that enhanced expression of epithelial cell stress proteins might be indicators also in some patients, which were excluded for the disease on biopsy (Iltanen et al., 1999). Yeboah et al. investigated the involvement of alphaB-crystallin, a small HSP in the pathomechanism of coeliac disease. Biopsy specimens of 12 celiac patients and 10 control individuals were investigated by immunoperoxidase screening. The intestinal epithelial cells of patients with coeliac disease stained more intensively for the sHSP alphaB-crystallin than that of controls. The amount and intracellular distribution of alphaB-crystallin in the duodenal mucosa of the patients with coeliac disease were closely related to the degree of villous atrophy, which may indicate its involvement in mucosal damage (Yeboah & White, 2001). In summary, these data suggest that HSPs may be involved in the pathomechanism of coeliac disease, but further studies are needed to clarify their more precise role.

6.3 HSPs in other gastrointestinal disorders

Since stress-induced tissue damage is involved in different gastrointestinal diseases, HSPs were examined also in gastric ulcer (Rokutan, 2000), chronic pancreatitis (Ogata et al., 2000) and inflammatory bowel disease, that means Crohn's disease and ulcerative colitis (Rodolico et al., 2010). Similarly to coeliac disease, inflammatory bowel disease is an inflammatory disease of the intestinal tract and there are relevant overlaps in their pathology. In both diseases the inflammation leads to the damage of the intestinal mucosa resulting in enhanced permeability and impaired function of the epithelial barrier in genetically susceptible individuals (Festen et al., 2009). Increased HSP70 (Ludwig et al., 1999), HSP60 and HSP10 (Rodolico et al., 2010) expression was observed in the colon mucosa of patients with inflammatory bowel disease. HSPs localized mainly within the epithelial cells and in lesser extent in the lamina propria (Rodolico et al., 2010). Protective functions of HSPs were demonstrated in inflammatory gastrointestinal diseases (Otaka et al., 2010). Using heat shock factor 1-null mice and HSP70 overexpressing transgenic mice HSP70 seems to have a protective role against colitis: various mechanisms may be involved in this process, such as the suppression of proinflammatory cytokines and cell adhesion molecules expression or the inhibition of programmed cell death (Tanaka & Mizushima, 2009). A correlation between HSPs and probiotics was reported. Advantageous effect of probiotics was demonstrated in inflammatory bowel disease (Sartor, 2004) and one mechanism responsible for this can be the ability, that probiotics may induce the expression of HSPs (Dotan & Rachmilewitz, 2005). Tao et al. found that treatment of intestinal epithelial cells with the probiotic Lactobacillus GG strain induces HSP72 expression, which contributes to the beneficial clinical effects through preservation of cytoskeletal integrity (Tao et al., 2006). Using Caco-2 colonic epithelial cells Musch et al. demonstrated that HSP72 can bind and stabilize key cytoskeleton-associated proteins, such as alpha-actinin, or tight junction-associated proteins, such as zonula occludens 1 (Musch et al., 1999). In summary, cytoprotective effects of HSPs were suggested in different gastrointestinal diseases.

7. Future directions

Based on these beneficial effects of HSPs they can be potential therapeutic targets in the future. Using transgenic mice Mizushima et al. reported that a non-toxic HSP-inducer called geranylgeranylacetone, which is basically an anti-ulcer drug, achieves its anti-ulcer effect through induction of HSPs, which are protective against irritant-induced gastric lesions (Mizushima, 2010). Furthermore they reported that geranylgeranylacetone has protective effects against inflammatory bowel disease-related colitis and prevents lesions of the small intestine by the induction of HSPs. These findings predict the possibility, that HSPs may have therapeutic potential also in coeliac disease. Recently there are investigations to find HSP based therapies in other disorders, for instance the development of HSP-based vaccines to treat cancer with promising opportunities, because tumor derived HSP-peptide complexes are able to induce immunity against several malignancies as shown in preclinical studies (di Pietro et al., 2009). In conclusion, in the future it will be important to understand the precise role of HSPs in the pathomechanism of coeliac disease, because due to their protective effects HSPs could be regarded as potential therapeutic agents to treat several gastrointestinal diseases, maybe also coeliac disease.

8. Acknowledgments

Ádam Vannay and Gábor Veres are holders of the János Bolyai Research grant; this book chapter was supported by the János Bolyai Research Scholarschip of the Hungarian Academy of Sciences and by OTKA-K81117, -84087/2010, -T-71730 grants.

9. References

Akerfelt, M.; Morimoto, RI. & Sistonen L. (2010). Heat shock factors: integrators of cell stress, development and lifespan. *Nat Rev Mol Cell Biol.* 11(8):545-55.

Akerfelt, M. ; Trouillet, D. ; Mezger, V. & Sistonen, L. (2007). Heat shock factors at a crossroad between stress and development. *Ann N Y Acad Sci.* 1113:15-27.

Al Refaii, A. & Alix, JH. (2009). Ribosome biogenesis is temperature-dependent and delayed in Escherichia coli lacking the chaperones DnaK or DnaJ. *Mol Microbiol.* 71(3):748-62.

Alaedini, A. & Green, PH. (2008). Autoantibodies in celiac disease. *Autoimmunity.* 41(1):19-26.

Alaedini, A. & Green, PH. (2005). Narrative review: celiac disease: understanding a complex autoimmune disorder. *Ann Intern Med.* 142(4):289-98.

Anckar, J. & Sistonen, L. (2007). Heat shock factor 1 as a coordinator of stress and developmental pathways. *Adv Exp Med Biol.* 594:78-88.

Arrigo, AP., Simon, S., Gibert, B., Kretz-Remy, C., Nivon, M., Czekalla, A., Guillet, D., Moulin, M., Diaz-Latoud, C. & Vicart, P. (2007). Hsp27 (HspB1) and alphaB-crystallin (HspB5) as therapeutic targets. *FEBS Lett.* 581(19):3665-74.

Arrigo, AP (2007). The cellular "networking" of mammalian Hsp27 and its functions in the control of protein folding, redox state and apoptosis. *Adv Exp Med Biol.* 594:14-26.

Arvans, DL., Vavricka, SR., Ren, H., Musch, MW., Kang, L., Rocha, FG., Lucioni, A., Turner, JR., Alverdy, J. & Chang, EB. (2005). Luminal bacterial flora determines physiological expression of intestinal epithelial cytoprotective heat shock proteins 25 and 72. *Am J Physiol Gastrointest Liver Physiol.* 288(4):G696-704.

Asano, T., Tanaka, K., Yamakawa, N., Adachi, H., Sobue, G., Goto, H., Takeuchi, K. & Mizushima, T.(2009). HSP70 confers protection against indomethacin-induced lesions of the small intestine. *J Pharmacol Exp Ther.* 330(2):458-67.

Asea, A., Kraeft, SK., Kurt-Jones, EA., Stevenson, MA., Chen, LB., Finberg, RW., Koo, GC. & Calderwood, SK. (2000). HSP70 stimulates cytokine production through a coeliac disease14-dependant pathway, demonstrating its dual role as a chaperone and cytokine. *Nat Med.* 6(4):435-42.

Asea, A. (2008). Heat shock proteins and toll-like receptors. *Handb Exp Pharmacol.* (183):111-27.

Aufricht, C. (2004). HSP: helper, suppressor, protector. *Kidney Int.* 65(2):739-40.

Avery, SV. (2011) . Molecular targets of oxidative stress. *Biochem J.* 434(2):201-10.

Aztatzi-Santillán E, Nares-López FE, Márquez-Valadez B, Aguilera P, Chánez-Cárdenas ME. The protective role of heme oxygenase-1 in cerebral ischemia. Cent Nerv Syst Agents Med Chem. 2010 Dec 1;10(4):310-6.

Baldassarre, M., Laneve, AM., Grosso, R. & Laforgia, N. (2008). Celiac disease: pathogenesis and novel therapeutic strategies. *Endocr Metab Immune Disord Drug Targets.* 8(3):152-8.

Baniwal, SK., Bharti, K., Chan, KY., Fauth, M., Ganguli, A., Kotak, S., Mishra, SK., Nover, L., Port, M., Scharf, KD., Tripp, J., Weber, C., Zielinski, D., & von Koskull-Döring, P. (2004). Heat stress response in plants: a complex game with chaperones and more than twenty heat stress transcription factors. *J Biosci.* 29(4):471-87.

Barends, TR., Werbeck, ND. & Reinstein, J. (2010). Disaggregases in 4 dimensions. *Curr Opin Struct Biol.* 20(1):46-53.

Bellmann, K., Burkart, V., Bruckhoff, J., Kolb, H. & Landry, J. (2000) p38-dependent enhancement of cytokine-induced nitric-oxide synthase gene expression by heat shock protein 70. J Biol Chem. 275(24):18172-9.

Bhatia, V. & Tandon, RK. (2005). Stress and the gastrointestinal tract. *J Gastroenterol Hepatol.* 20(3):332-9.

Biamonti, G. & Caceres, JF. (2009). Cellular stress and RNA splicing. *Trends Biochem Sci.* 34(3):146-53.

Binder, RJ., Vatner, R. & Srivastava P. (2004). The heat-shock protein receptors: some answers and more questions. *Tissue Antigens.* 64(4):442-51.

Borkovich, KA., Farrelly, FW., Finkelstein, DB., Taulien, J. & Lindquist, S. (1989) Hsp82 is an essential protein that is required in higher concentrations for growth of cells at higher temperatures. *Mol Cell Biol.* 9(9):3919-30.

Briani, C., Samaroo, D. & Alaedini, A. (2008). Celiac disease: from gluten to autoimmunity. *Autoimmun Rev.* 7(8):644-50.

Bruewer, M., Samarin, S. & Nusrat A. (2006). Inflammatory bowel disease and the apical junctional complex. *Ann N Y Acad Sci.* 1072:242-52.

Bukau, B., Weissman, J. & Horwich, A. (2006). Molecular chaperones and protein quality control. *Cell.* 125(3):443-51.

Burel, C., Mezger, V., Pinto, M., Rallu, M., Trigon, S. & Morange, M. (1992). Mammalian heat shock protein families. Expression and functions. *Experientia.* 48(7):629-34.

Caccamo, D., Currò, M. & Ientile, R. (2010). Potential of transglutaminase 2 as a therapeutic target. *Expert Opin Ther Targets.* 14(9):989-1003.

Cario, E., Gerken, G. & Podolsky, DK. (2007). Toll-like receptor 2 controls mucosal inflammation by regulating epithelial barrier function. *Gastroenterology.* 132(4):1359-74.

Carper, SW., Duffy, JJ. & Gerner, EW. (1987). Heat shock proteins in thermotolerance and other cellular processes. *Cancer Res.* 47(20):5249-55.

Chen, SL., Yang, CT., Yang, ZL., Guo, RX., Meng, JL., Cui, Y., Lan, AP., Chen, PX. & Feng, JQ. (2010). Hydrogen sulphide protects H9c2 cells against chemical hypoxia-induced injury. *Clin Exp Pharmacol Physiol.* 37(3):316-21.

Chhabra, A., Verma, A. & Mehta, K. (2009). Tissue transglutaminase promotes or suppresses tumors depending on cell context. *Anticancer Res.* 29(6):1909-19.

Choi, K., Ni, L. & Jonakait, GM. (2011). Fas ligation and tumor necrosis factor α activation of murine astrocytes promote heat shock factor-1 activation and heat shock protein expression leading to chemokine induction and cell survival. *J Neurochem.* 116(3):438-48.

Ciccocioppo, R., Di Sabatino, A., Parroni, R., Muzi, P., D'Alò, S., Ventura, T., Pistoia, MA., Cifone, MG. & Corazza, GR. (2001). Increased enterocyte apoptosis and Fas-Fas ligand system in celiac disease. *Am J Clin Pathol.* 115(4):494-503.

Ciocca, DR. & Calderwood SK. (2005). Heat shock proteins in cancer: diagnostic, prognostic, predictive, and treatment implications. *Cell Stress Chaperones.* 10(2):86-103.

Creagh, EM., Carmody, RJ. & Cotter, TG. (2000). Heat shock protein 70 inhibits caspase-dependent and -independent apoptosis in Jurkat T cells. *Exp Cell Res.* 257(1):58-66.

Csermely, P., Söti, C. & Blatch GL. (2007). Chaperones as parts of cellular networks. *Adv Exp Med Biol.* 594:55-63.

Dantuma, NP. & Lindsten, K. (2010). Stressing the ubiquitin-proteasome system. *Cardiovasc Res.* 85(2):263-71.

Daugaard, M., Kirkegaard-Sørensen, T., Ostenfeld, MS., Aaboe, M., Høyer-Hansen, M., Orntoft, TF., Rohde, M. & Jäättelä M. (2007). Lens epithelium-derived growth factor is an Hsp70-2 regulated guardian of lysosomal stability in human cancer. *Cancer Res.* 67(6):2559-67.

Daum, S., Bauer, U., Foss, HD., Schuppan, D., Stein, H., Riecken, EO. & Ullrich, R. (1999). Increased expression of mRNA for matrix metalloproteinases-1 and -3 and tissue inhibitor of metalloproteinases-1 in intestinal biopsy specimens from patients with coeliac disease. *Gut.* 44(1):17-25.

di Pietro, A., Tosti, G., Ferrucci, PF. & Testori A. (2009). Heat shock protein peptide complex 96-based vaccines in melanoma: How far we are, how far we can get. *Hum Vaccin.* 5(11).

Di Sabatino, A., Ciccocioppo, R., D'Alò, S., Parroni, R., Millimaggi, D., Cifone, MG. & Corazza, GR. (2001). Intraepithelial and lamina propria lymphocytes show distinct patterns of apoptosis whereas both populations are active in Fas based cytotoxicity in coeliac disease. *Gut.* 49(3):380-6.

Di Sabatino, A., Pickard, KM., Gordon, JN., Salvati, V., Mazzarella, G., Beattie, RM., Vossenkaemper, A., Rovedatti, L., Leakey, NA., Croft, NM., Troncone, R., Corazza, GR., Stagg, AJ., Monteleone, G. & MacDonald, TT. (2007). Evidence for the role of interferon-alfa production by dendritic cells in the Th1 response in celiac disease. *Gastroenterology.* 133(4):1175-87.

DiDomenico, BJ., Bugaisky, GE. & Lindquist S. (1982). Heat shock and recovery are mediated by different translational mechanisms. *Proc Natl Acad Sci U S A.* 79(20):6181-5.

Diosdado, B., van Oort, E. & Wijmenga, C. (2005). "Coelionomics": towards understanding the molecular pathology of coeliac disease. *Clin Chem Lab Med.* 43(7):685-95.

Doganci, T. & Bozkurt, S. (2004). Celiac disease with various presentations. *Pediatr Int.* 46(6):693-6.

Dokladny, K., Moseley, PL. & Ma, TY. (2006). Physiologically relevant increase in temperature causes an increase in intestinal epithelial tight junction permeability. *Am J Physiol Gastrointest Liver Physiol.* 290(2):G204-12.

Dollins, DE., Warren, JJ., Immormino, RM. & Gewirth, DT. (2007). Structures of GRP94-nucleotide complexes reveal mechanistic differences between the hsp90 chaperones. *Mol Cell.* 28(1):41-56.

Dotan, I. & Rachmilewitz D. (2005). Probiotics in inflammatory bowel disease: possible mechanisms of action. *Curr Opin Gastroenterol.* 21(4):426-30.

Dudeja, V., Mujumdar, N., Phillips, P., Chugh, R., Borja-Cacho, D., Dawra, RK., Vickers, SM. & Saluja AK. (2009). Heat shock protein 70 inhibits apoptosis in cancer cells through simultaneous and independent mechanisms. *Gastroenterology.* 136(5):1772-82.

Dudeja, V., Vickers, SM. & Saluja AK. (2009). The role of heat shock proteins in gastrointestinal diseases.*Gut.* 58(7):1000-9.

Ehrenschwender, M. & Wajant, H. (2009). The role of FasL and Fas in health and disease. *Adv Exp Med Biol.* 647:64-93.

Elli, L., Bergamini, CM., Bardella, MT. & Schuppan, D. (2009). Transglutaminases in inflammation and fibrosis of the gastrointestinal tract and the liver. *Dig Liver Dis.* 41(8):541-50.

Ellis, RJ., van der Vies, SM., & Hemmingsen, SM. (1989). The molecular chaperone concept. *Biochem Soc Symp.* 55:145-53.

Evans, CG., Chang, L. & Gestwicki, JE. (2010). Heat shock protein 70 (hsp70) as an emerging drug target. *J Med Chem.* 53(12):4585-602.

Farhadi, A., Banan, A., Fields, J. & Keshavarzian, A. (2003). Intestinal barrier: an interface between health and disease. *J Gastroenterol Hepatol.* 18(5):479-97.

Festen, EA., Szperl, AM., Weersma, RK., Wijmenga, C. & Wapenaar, MC. (2009). Inflammatory bowel disease and celiac disease: overlaps in the pathology and genetics, and their potential drug targets. *Endocr Metab Immune Disord Drug Targets.* 9(2):199-218.

Fleckenstein, B., Qiao, SW., Larsen, MR., Jung, G., Roepstorff, P. & Sollid, LM. (2004). Molecular characterization of covalent complexes between tissue transglutaminase and gliadin peptides. *J Biol Chem.* 279(17):17607-16.

Flohé, SB., Brüggemann, J., Lendemans, S., Nikulina, M., Meierhoff, G., Flohé, S. & Kolb H. (2003). Human heat shock protein 60 induces maturation of dendritic cells versus a Th1-promoting phenotype. *J Immunol.* 170(5):2340-8

Fric, P., Gabrovska, D. & Nevoral, J. (2011). Celiac disease, gluten-free diet, and oats. *Nutr Rev.* 69(2):107-15.

Fujimoto, M. & Nakai, A. (2010). The heat shock factor family and adaptation to proteotoxic stress. *FEBS J.* 277(20):4112-25.

Gabai, VL., Yaglom, JA., Volloch, V., Meriin, AB., Force, T., Koutroumanis, M., Massie, B., Mosser, DD., Sherman, MY. (2000). Hsp72-mediated suppression of c-Jun N-terminal kinase is implicated in development of tolerance to caspase-independent cell death. *Mol Cell Biol.* 20(18):6826-36.

Geiger, PC. & Gupte, AA. (2011). Heat shock proteins are important mediators of skeletal muscle insulin sensitivity. *Exerc Sport Sci Rev.* 39(1):34-42

Ghayour-Mobarhan, M., Rahsepar, AA., Tavallaie, S., Rahsepar, S. & Ferns GA. (2009). The potential role of heat shock proteins in cardiovascular disease: evidence from in vitro and in vivo studies. *Adv Clin Chem.* 48:27-72.

Ghosh, JC., Siegelin, MD., Dohi, T. & Altieri, DC. (2010). Heat shock protein 60 regulation of the mitochondrial permeability transition pore in tumor cells. *Cancer Res.* 70(22):8988-93.

Gianfrani, C., Auricchio, S. & Troncone, R. (2005). Adaptive and innate immune responses in celiac disease. *Immunol Lett.* 99(2):141-5.

Giovannini, C., Matarrese, P., Scazzocchio, B., Varí, R., D'Archivio, M., Straface, E., Masella, R., Malorni, W. & De Vincenzi M. (2003). Wheat gliadin induces apoptosis of intestinal cells via an autocrine mechanism involving Fas-Fas ligand pathway. *FEBS Lett.* 540(1-3):117-24.

Glickman, MH. & Ciechanover, A. (2002). The ubiquitin-proteasome proteolytic pathway: destruction for the sake of construction. *Physiol Rev.* 82(2):373-428.

Graf, PC. & Jakob, U. (2002). Redox-regulated molecular chaperones. *Cell Mol Life Sci.* 59(10):1624-31.

Green, PH. (2005). The many faces of celiac disease: clinical presentation of celiac disease in the adult population. *Gastroenterology*. 128(4 Suppl 1):S74-8.

Gué, M., Bonbonne, C., Fioramonti, J., Moré, J., Del Rio-Lachèze, C., Coméra, C. & Buéno, L. (1997). Stress-induced enhancement of colitis in rats: CRF and arginine vasopressin are not involved. *Am J Physiol*. 272(1 Pt 1):G84-91.

Gupta, V. & Kohli A. (2010). Celiac disease associated with recurrent Guillain Barre syndrome. *Indian Pediatr*. 47(9):797-8.

Gyrd-Hansen, M., Nylandsted, J. & Jäättelä, M. (2004). Heat shock protein 70 promotes cancer cell viability by safeguarding lysosomal integrity. Cell Cycle. 3(12):1484-5.

Hao, H., Naomoto, Y., Bao, X., Watanabe, N., Sakurama, K., Noma, K., Motoki, T., Tomono, Y., Fukazawa, T., Shirakawa, Y., Yamatsuji, T., Matsuoka, J. & Takaoka M. (2010). HSP90 and its inhibitors. *Oncol Rep*. 23(6):1483-92.

Haslbeck, M., Franzmann, T., Weinfurtner, D. & Buchner J. (2005). Some like it hot: the structure and function of small heat-shock proteins. *Nat Struct Mol Biol*. 2005 Oct;12(10):842-6.

Hauet-Broere, F., Wieten, L., Guichelaar, T., Berlo, S., van der Zee, R. & Van Eden W. (2006). Heat shock proteins induce T cell regulation of chronic inflammation. *Ann Rheum Dis*. 65 Suppl 3:iii65-8

Heo, JM. & Rutter, J. (2011). Ubiquitin-dependent mitochondrial protein degradation. (2011). Int J Biochem Cell Biol. 2011 Jun 12. Epub ahead of print.

Holmberg, CI., Hietakangas, V., Mikhailov, A., Rantanen, JO., Kallio, M., Meinander, A., Hellman, J., Morrice, N., MacKintosh, C., Morimoto, RI., Eriksson, JE. & Sistonen, L. (2001). Phosphorylation of serine 230 promotes inducible transcriptional activity of heat shock factor 1. *EMBO J*. 20(14):3800-10.

Horwitz, J. (1992). Alpha-crystallin can function as a molecular chaperone. *Proc Natl Acad Sci U S A*. 89(21):10449-53.

Hüe, S., Mention, JJ., Monteiro, RC., Zhang, S., Cellier, C., Schmitz, J., Verkarre, V., Fodil, N., Bahram, S., Cerf-Bensussan, N. & Caillat-Zucman, S. (2004). A direct role for NKG2D/MICA interaction in villous atrophy during celiac disease. *Immunity*. 21(3):367-77.

Ilangovan, G., Osinbowale, S., Bratasz, A., Bonar, M., Cardounel, AJ., Zweier, JL. & Kuppusamy, P. (2004). Heat shock regulates the respiration of cardiac H9c2 cells through upregulation of nitric oxide synthase. *Am J Physiol Cell Physiol*. 287(5):C1472-8

Iltanen, S., Rantala, I., Laippala, P., Holm, K., Partanen, J. & Maki, M. (1999). Expression of HSP-65 in jejunal epithelial cells in patients clinically suspected of coeliac disease. *Autoimmunity*. 31(2):125-32.

Ivanov, AI., Nusrat, A. & Parkos, CA. (2004). The epithelium in inflammatory bowel disease: potential role of endocytosis of junctional proteins in barrier disruption. *Novartis Found Symp*. 263:115-24; discussion 124-32, 211-8.

Jabri, B., Kasarda, DD. & Green, PH. (2005). Innate and adaptive immunity: the yin and yang of celiac disease. *Immunol Rev*. 206:219-31.

Jabri, B. & Sollid, LM. (2006). Mechanisms of disease: immunopathogenesis of celiac disease. *Nat Clin Pract Gastroenterol Hepatol*. 3(9):516-25.

Jantschitsch, C. & Trautinger, F. (2003). Heat shock and UV-B-induced DNA damage and mutagenesis in skin. Photochem Photobiol Sci. 2(9):899-903.

John, LJ., Fromm, M., & Schulzke, JD. (2011). Epithelial Barriers in Intestinal Inflammation. *Antioxid Redox Signal.* 15(5):1255-70.

Johnson, JD. & Fleshner, M. (2006). Releasing signals, secretory pathways, and immune function of endogenous extracellular heat shock protein 72. *J Leukoc Biol.* 79(3):425-34.

Kalmar, B. & Greensmith, L. (2009). Induction of heat shock proteins for protection against oxidative stress. *Adv Drug Deliv Rev.* 61(4):310-8.

Kaukinen, K., Lindfors, K., Collin, P., Koskinen, O. & Mäki, M. (2010). Coeliac disease--a diagnostic and therapeutic challenge. *Clin Chem Lab Med.* 48(9):1205-16.

Kelley, PM. & Schlesinger, MJ. (1978). The effect of amino acid analogues and heat shock on gene expression in chicken embryo fibroblasts. *Cell.* 15(4):1277-86.

Kelly, KJ. (2005). Heat shock (stress response) proteins and renal ischemia/reperfusion injury. *Contrib Nephrol.* 148:86-106.

Kiang, JG. (2004). Inducible heat shock protein 70 kD and inducible nitric oxide synthase in hemorrhage/resuscitation-induced injury. *Cell Res.* 14(6):450-9.

Kim, S. & Coulombe, PA. (2007). Intermediate filament scaffolds fulfill mechanical, organizational, and signaling functions in the cytoplasm. *Genes Dev.* 21(13):1581-97.

Kim, SH., Hur, WY., Kang, CD., Lim, YS., Kim, DW. & Chung, BS. (1997). Involvement of heat shock factor in regulating transcriptional activation of MDR1 gene in multidrug-resistant cells. *Cancer Lett.* 115(1):9-14.

Kojima, K., Musch, MW., Ren, H., Boone, DL., Hendrickson, BA., Ma, A. & Chang, EB. (2003). Enteric flora and lymphocyte-derived cytokines determine expression of heat shock proteins in mouse colonic epithelial cells. *Gastroenterology.* 124(5):1395-407.

Kol, A., Sukhova, GK., Lichtman, AH. & Libby, P. (1998). Chlamydial heat shock protein 60 localizes in human atheroma and regulates macrophage tumor necrosis factor-alpha and matrix metalloproteinase expression. *Circulation.* 98(4):300-7.

Kriehuber, T., Rattei, T., Weinmaier, T., Bepperling, A., Haslbeck, M. & Buchner, J. (2010). Independent evolution of the core domain and its flanking sequences in small heat shock proteins. *FASEB J.* 24(10):3633-42.

Kuwabara, T., Otaka, M., Itoh, H., Zeniya, A., Fujimori, S., Otani, S., Tashima, Y. & Masamune, O. (1994). Regulation of 60-kDa heat shock protein expression by systemic stress and 5-hydroxytryptamine in rat colonic mucosa. *J Gastroenterol.* 29(6):721-6.

Large, AT., Goldberg, MD. & Lund, PA. (2009). Chaperones and protein folding in the archaea. *Biochem Soc Trans.* 37(Pt 1):46-51.

Laufen, T., Mayer, MP., Beisel, C., Klostermeier, D., Mogk, A., Reinstein, J. & Bukau, B. (1999). Mechanism of regulation of hsp70 chaperones by DnaJ cochaperones. *Proc Natl Acad Sci U S A.* 96(10):5452-7.

Lemaux, PG., Herendeen, SL., Bloch, PL. & Neidhardt, FC. (1978). Transient rates of synthesis of individual polypeptides in E. coli following temperature shifts. *Cell.* 13(3):427-34.

Levenstein, S., Prantera, C., Varvo, V., Scribano, ML., Andreoli, A., Luzi, C., Arcà, M., Berto, E., Milite, G. & Marcheggiano, A. (2000). Stress and exacerbation in ulcerative colitis: a prospective study of patients enrolled in remission. *Am J Gastroenterol.* 95(5):1213-20.

Levitsky, DI., Pivovarova, AV., Mikhailova, VV. & Nikolaeva OP. (2008). Thermal unfolding and aggregation of actin. *FEBS J.* 275(17):4280-95.

Lewis, K. & McKay, DM. (2009). Metabolic stress evokes decreases in epithelial barrier function. *Ann N Y Acad Sci.* 1165:327-37.

Li, P., Nijhawan, D., Budihardjo, I., Srinivasula, SM., Ahmad, M., Alnemri, ES & Wang, X. (1997). Cytochrome c and dATP-dependent formation of Apaf-1/caspase-9 complex initiates an apoptotic protease cascade. *Cell.* 91(4):479-89.

Li, Z., Menoret, A. & Srivastava, P. (2002). Roles of heat-shock proteins in antigen presentation and cross-presentation. *Curr Opin Immunol.* 14(1):45-51.

Liang, P. & MacRae, TH. (1997). Molecular chaperones and the cytoskeleton. *J Cell Sci.* 110 (Pt 13):1431-40.

Limón-Pacheco, J. & Gonsebatt, ME. (2009). The role of antioxidants and antioxidant-related enzymes in protective responses to environmentally induced oxidative stress. *Mutat Res.* 674(1-2):137-47.

Liu, X., Xu, L., Liu, Y., Tong, X., Zhu, G., Zhang, XC., Li, X. & Rao, Z. (2009). Crystal structure of the hexamer of human heat shock factor binding protein 1. *Proteins.* 75(1):1-11.

Ludwig, D., Stahl, M., Ibrahim, ET., Wenzel, BE., Drabicki, D., Wecke, A., Fellermann, K. & Stange, EF. (1999). Enhanced intestinal expression of heat shock protein 70 in patients with inflammatory bowel diseases. *Dig Dis Sci.* 44(7):1440-7.

Lyte, M., Vulchanova, L. & Brown, DR. (2011). Stress at the intestinal surface: catecholamines and mucosa-bacteria interactions. *Cell Tissue Res.* 343(1):23-32.

Malmendal, A., Overgaard, J., Bundy, JG., Sørensen, JG., Nielsen, NC., Loeschcke, V., Holmstrup, M. (2006). Metabolomic profiling of heat stress: hardening and recovery of homeostasis in Drosophila. *Am J Physiol Regul Integr Comp Physiol.* 291(1):R205-12.

Malorni, W., Farrace, MG., Rodolfo, C. & Piacentini, M. (2008). Type 2 transglutaminase in neurodegenerative diseases: the mitochondrial connection. *Curr Pharm Des.* 14(3):278-88.

Maniar, VP., Yadav, SS. & Gokhale, YA. (2010). Intractable seizures and metabolic bone disease secondary to celiac disease. *J Assoc Physicians India.* 58:512-5.

Maupin-Furlow, JA., Wilson, HL., Kaczowka, SJ. & Ou, MS. (2000). Proteasomes in the archaea: from structure to function. *Front Biosci.* 5:D837-65.

Maurizi, MR & Xia, D. (2004). Protein binding and disruption by Clp/Hsp100 chaperones. *Structure.* 12(2):175-83.

Mayer, MP. (2010). Gymnastics of molecular chaperones. *Mol Cell.* 39(3):321-31.

Medzhitov, R. (2001). Toll-like receptors and innate immunity. *Nat Rev Immunol.* 1(2):135-45.

Miot, M., Reidy, M., Doyle, SM., Hoskins, JR., Johnston, DM., Genest, O., Vitery, MC., Masison, DC. & Wickner S. (2011). Species-specific collaboration of heat shock proteins (Hsp) 70 and 100 in thermotolerance and protein disaggregation. *Proc Natl Acad Sci U S A.* 108(17):6915-20.

Mishra, A., Godavarthi, SK., Maheshwari, M., Goswami, A. & Jana, NR. (2009). The ubiquitin ligase E6-AP is induced and recruited to aggresomes in response to proteasome inhibition and may be involved in the ubiquitination of Hsp70-bound misfolded proteins. *J Biol Chem.* 284(16):10537-45.

Mizushima, T. (2010). HSP-dependent protection against gastrointestinal diseases. *Curr Pharm Des.* 16(10):1190-6.

Moran, L., Mirault, ME., Arrigo, AP., Goldschmidt-Clermont, M. & Tissières A. (1978). Heat shock of Drosophila melanogaster induces the synthesis of new messenger RNAs and proteins. *Philos Trans R Soc Lond B Biol Sci.* 283(997):391-406.

Morandi, A., Los, B., Osofsky, L., Autilio-Gambetti, L. & Gambetti, P. (1989). Ubiquitin and heat shock proteins in cultured nervous tissue after different stress conditions. *Prog Clin Biol Res.* 317:819-27.

Multhoff, G. (2009). Activation of natural killer cells by heat shock protein 70. *Int J Hyperthermia.* 25(3):169-75.

Murray, IA., Daniels, I., Coupland, K., Smith, JA. & Long RG. (2002). Increased activity and expression of initric oxideS in human duodenal enterocytes from patients with celiac disease. *Am J Physiol Gastrointest Liver Physiol.* 283(2):G319-26.

Musch, MW., Sugi, K., Straus, D. & Chang, EB. (1999). Heat-shock protein 72 protects against oxidant-induced injury of barrier function of human colonic epithelial Caco2/bbe cells. *Gastroenterology.* 117(1):115-22.

Noble, EG., Milne, KJ. & Melling, CW. (2008). Heat shock proteins and exercise: a primer. *Appl Physiol Nutr Metab.* 33(5):1050-65.

Obermann, WM., Sondermann, H., Russo, AA., Pavletich, NP. & Hartl, FU. (1998). In vivo function of Hsp90 is dependent on ATP binding and ATP hydrolysis. *J Cell Biol.* 143(4):901-10.

Odashima, M., Otaka, M., Jin, M., Konishi, N., Sato, T., Kato, S., Matsuhashi, T., Nakamura, C., Watanabe, S. (2002). Induction of a 72-kDa heat-shock protein in cultured rat gastric mucosal cells and rat gastric mucosa by zinc L-carnosine. *Dig Dis Sci.* 47(12):2799-804.

Odashima, M., Otaka, M., Jin, M., Wada, I., Horikawa, Y., Matsuhashi, T., Ohba, R., Hatakeyama, N., Oyake, J. & Watanabe, S. (2006). Zinc L-carnosine protects colonic mucosal injury through induction of heat shock protein 72 and suppression of NF-kappaB activation. *Life Sci.* 79(24):2245-50.

Odetti, P., Valentini, S., Aragno, I., Garibaldi, S., Pronzato, MA., Rolandi, E. & Barreca, T. (1998). Oxidative stress in subjects affected by celiac disease. *Free Radic Res.* 29(1):17-24.

Ogata, M., Naito, Z., Tanaka, S., Moriyama, Y. & Asano, G. (2000). Overexpression and localization of heat shock proteins mRNA in pancreatic carcinoma. *J Nippon Med Sch..* 67(3):177-85.

Omar, R. & Pappolla, M. (1993). Oxygen free radicals as inducers of heat shock protein synthesis in cultured human neuroblastoma cells: relevance to neurodegenerative disease. *Eur Arch Psychiatry Clin Neurosci.* 242(5):262-7.

Osterloh, A. & Breloer, M. (2008). Heat shock proteins: linking danger and pathogen recognition. *Med Microbiol Immunol.* 197(1):1-8.

Otaka, M., Odashima, M. & Watanabe, S. (2006). Role of heat shock proteins (molecular chaperones) in intestinal mucosal protection. *Biochem Biophys Res Commun.* 348(1):1-5.

Padmini, E., Lavanya, S. (2011). HSP70-mediated control of endothelial cell apoptosis during pre-eclampsia. *Eur J Obstet Gynecol Reprod Biol.* 56(2):158-64.

Panchapakesan J, Daglis M, Gatenby P. Antibodies to 65 kDa and 70 kDa heat shock proteins in rheumatoid arthritis and systemic lupus erythematosus. Immunol Cell Biol. 1992 Oct;70 (Pt 5):295-300.

Papp, E., Nardai, G., Söti, C. & Csermely P. (2003). Molecular chaperones, stress proteins and redox homeostasis. *Biofactors.* 17(1-4):249-57.

Park, HS., Lee, JS., Huh, SH., Seo, JS. & Choi, EJ. (2001). Hsp72 functions as a natural inhibitory protein of c-Jun N-terminal kinase. *EMBO J.* 20(3):446-56.

Parsell, DA. & Lindquist, S. (1993). The function of heat-shock proteins in stress tolerance: degradation and reactivation of damaged proteins. *Annu Rev Genet.* 27:437-96.

Partanen, J., Milner, C., Campbell, RD., Mäki, M., Lipsanen, V. & Koskimies, S. (1993). human leukocyte antigen-linked heat-shock protein 70 (HSP70-2) gene polymorphism and celiac disease. *Tissue Antigens.* 41(1):15-9.

Pearl, LH. & Prodromou, C. (2006). Structure and mechanism of the Hsp90 molecular chaperone machinery. *Annu Rev Biochem.* 75:271-94.

Pechan, PM. (1991). Heat shock proteins and cell proliferation. *FEBS Lett.* 280(1):1-4.

Pekny, M., Lane, EB. (2007). Intermediate filaments and stress. *Exp Cell Res.* 313(10):2244-54.

Pender, SL., Tickle, SP., Docherty, AJ., Howie, D., Wathen, NC. & MacDonald, TT. (1997). A major role for matrix metalloproteinases in T cell injury in the gut. *J Immunol.* 158(4):1582-90.

Petrof, EO., Ciancio, MJ. & Chang, EB. (2004). Role and regulation of intestinal epithelial heat shock proteins in health and disease. *Chin J Dig Dis.* 5(2):45-50.

Pfister, G., Stroh, CM., Perschinka, H., Kind, M., Knoflach, M., Hinterdorfer, P. & Wick, G. (2005). Detection of HSP60 on the membrane surface of stressed human endothelial cells by atomic force and confocal microscopy. *J Cell Sci.* 118(Pt 8):1587-94.

Pierce, SK., DeNagel, DC. & VanBuskirk, AM. (1991). A role for heat shock proteins in antigen processing and presentation. *Curr Top Microbiol Immunol.* 167:83-92.

Polla, BS. & Cossarizza, A. (1996). Stress proteins in inflammation. *EXS.* 77:375-91.

Prahlad, V. & Morimoto, RI. (2009). Integrating the stress response: lessons for neurodegenerative diseases from C. elegans. *Trends Cell Biol.* 19(2):52-61.

Pratt, WB., Galigniana, MD., Morishima, Y. & Murphy, PJ. (2004). Role of molecular chaperones in steroid receptor action. *Essays Biochem.* 40:41-58.

Qiao, SW., Sollid, LM. & Blumberg, RS. (2009). Antigen presentation in celiac disease. *Curr Opin Immunol.* 21(1):111-7.

Quintana, FJ. & Cohen, IR. (2011). The HSP60 immune system network. *Trends Immunol.* 32(2):89-95.

Rajaiah, R. & Moudgil, KD. (2009). Heat-shock proteins can promote as well as regulate autoimmunity. *Autoimmun Rev.* 8(5):388-93.

Ramos-Arroyo, MA., Feijoó, E., Sánchez-Valverde, F., Aranburu, E., Irisarri, N., Olivera, JE. & Valiente, A. (2001). Heat-shock protein 70-1 and human leukocyte antigen class II gene polymorphisms associated with celiac disease susceptibility in Navarra (Spain). *Hum Immunol.* 62(8):821-5.

Reunala ,TL. (2001). Dermatitis herpetiformis. *Clin Dermatol.* 19(6):728-36.

Richardson, PG., Mitsiades, CS., Laubach, JP., Lonial, S., Chanan-Khan, AA. & Anderson, KC. (2011). Inhibition of heat shock protein 90 (HSP90) as a therapeutic strategy for the treatment of myeloma and other cancers. *Br J Haematol.* 152(4):367-79.

Richter, K., Haslbeck, M. & Buchner, J. (2010). The heat shock response: life on the verge of death. *Mol Cell.* 40(2):253-66.

Ritossa, F. (1967). A new puffing pattern induced by temperature shock and DNP in Drosophila. *Experientia.* 18: 571-573. doi: 10.1007/BF02172188.

Ritossa, F. (1996). Discovery of the heat shock response. *Cell Stress Chaperones.* 1(2):97-8.

Rivabene, R., Mancini, E. & De Vincenzi, M. (1999). In vitro cytotoxic effect of wheat gliadin-derived peptides on the Caco-2 intestinal cell line is associated with intracellular oxidative imbalance: implications for coeliac disease. *Biochim Biophys Acta.* 1453(1):152-60.

Rizzuto, R., Pinton, P., Ferrari, D., Chami, M., Szabadkai, G., Magalhães, PJ., Di Virgilio, F. & Pozzan, T. (2003). Calcium and apoptosis: facts and hypotheses. *Oncogene.* 22(53):8619-27.

Roberts, RJ., Agius, C., Saliba, C., Bossier, P. & Sung, YY. (2010). Heat shock proteins (chaperones) in fish and shellfish and their potential role in relation to fish health: a review. *J Fish Dis.* 33(10):789-801.

Rodolico, V., Tomasello, G., Zerilli, M., Martorana, A., Pitruzzella, A., Gammazza, AM., David, S., Zummo, G., Damiani, P., Accomando, S., Conway de Macario, E., Macario, AJ., Cappello, F. (2010). Hsp60 and Hsp10 increase in colon mucosa of Crohn's disease and ulcerative colitis. *Cell Stress Chaperones.* 15(6):877-84.

Rodrigo,L. (2009). Investigational therapies for celiac disease. *Expert Opin Investig Drugs.* 18(12):1865-73.

Rodriguez, F., Arsène-Ploetze, F., Rist, W., Rüdiger, S., Schneider-Mergener, J., Mayer, MP., Bukau, B. (2008). Molecular basis for regulation of the heat shock transcription factor sigma32 by the DnaK and DnaJ chaperones. *Mol Cell.* 32(3):347-58.

Rokutan, K. (2000). Role of heat shock proteins in gastric mucosal protection. *J Gastroenterol Hepatol.* 15 Suppl:D12-9.

Ropeleski, MJ., Tang, J., Walsh-Reitz, MM., Musch, MW. & Chang, EB. (2003). Interleukin-11-induced heat shock protein 25 confers intestinal epithelial-specific cytoprotection from oxidant stress. *Gastroenterology.* 124(5):1358-68.

Rostom, A., Dubé, C., Cranney, A., Saloojee, N., Sy, R., Garritty, C., Sampson, M., Zhang, L., Yazdi, F., Mamaladze, V., Pan, I., MacNeil, J., Mack, D., Patel, D. & Moher D. (2005). The diagnostic accuracy of serologic tests for celiac disease: a systematic review. *Gastroenterology.* 128(4 Suppl 1):S38-46.

Rubio-Tapia, A. & Murray, JA. (2010). Celiac disease. *Curr Opin Gastroenterol.* 26(2):116-22.

Ryan, MT., Pfanner, N. (2001). Hsp70 proteins in protein translocation. *Adv Protein Chem.* 59:223-42.

Sartor, RB. (2004). Therapeutic manipulation of the enteric microflora in inflammatory bowel diseases: antibiotics, probiotics, and prebiotics. *Gastroenterology.* 126(6):1620-33.

Schirmer, EC., Glover, JR., Singer, MA. & Lindquist S. (1996). HSP100/Clp proteins: a common mechanism explains diverse functions. *Trends Biochem Sci.* 21(8):289-96.

Schuppan, D., Dennis, MD. & Kelly, CP. (2005). Celiac disease: epidemiology, pathogenesis, diagnosis, and nutritional management. *Nutr Clin Care.* 8(2):54-69.

Schuppan, D., Junker, Y. & Barisani, D. (2009). Celiac disease: from pathogenesis to novel therapies. *Gastroenterology.* 137(6):1912-33.

Schuppan, D. (2000). Current concepts of celiac disease pathogenesis. *Gastroenterology.* 119(1):234-42.

Setty, M., Hormaza, L. & Guandalini, S. (2008). Celiac disease: risk assessment, diagnosis, and monitoring. *Mol Diagn Ther.* 12(5):289-98.

Shang, F. & Taylor, A. (2011). Ubiquitin-proteasome pathway and cellular responses to oxidative stress. *Free Radic Biol Med.* 51(1):5-16.

Sharom, FJ. (2008). ABC multidrug transporters: structure, function and role in chemoresistance. Pharmacogenomics. 9(1):105-27.

Sharp, S. & Workman, P. (2006). Inhibitors of the HSP90 molecular chaperone: current status. *Adv Cancer Res.* 95:323-48.

Silano, M., Agostoni, C. & Guandalini, S. (2010). Effect of the timing of gluten introduction on the development of celiac disease. *World J Gastroenterol.* 16(16):1939-42.

Sims, JD., McCready, J. & Jay, DG. (2011). Extracellular heat shock protein (Hsp)70 and Hsp90α assist in matrix metalloproteinase-2 activation and breast cancer cell migration and invasion. *PLoS One.* 6(4):e18848.

Singh, A. & Grover, A. (2010). Plant Hsp100/ClpB-like proteins: poorly-analyzed cousins of yeast ClpB machine. *Plant Mol Biol.* 74(4-5):395-404.

Sivaramakrishnan, S., DeGiulio, JV., Lorand, L., Goldman, RD. & Ridge, KM. (2008). Micromechanical properties of keratin intermediate filament networks. *Proc Natl Acad Sci U S A.* 105(3):889-94.

Sollid, LM., Jabri, B. (2005). Is celiac disease an autoimmune disorder? *Curr Opin Immunol.* 17(6):595-600.

Sollid, LM. (2000). Molecular basis of celiac disease. *Annu Rev Immunol.* 18:53-81.

Soltys, BJ. & Gupta RS. (1996). Immunoelectron microscopic localization of the 60-kDa heat shock chaperonin protein (Hsp60) in mammalian cells. *Exp Cell Res.* 222(1):16-27.

Sreedhar, AS., Kalmár, E., Csermely, P. & Shen, YF. (2004). Hsp90 isoforms: functions, expression and clinical importance. *FEBS Lett.* 562(1-3):11-5.

Stankiewicz, AR., Lachapelle, G., Foo, CP., Radicioni, SM. & Mosser, DD. (2005). Hsp70 inhibits heat-induced apoptosis upstream of mitochondria by preventing Bax translocation. *J Biol Chem.* 280(46):38729-39.

Stetler, RA., Gan, Y., Zhang, W., Liou, AK., Gao, Y., Cao, G. & Chen, J. (2010). Heat shock proteins: cellular and molecular mechanisms in the central nervous system. *Prog Neurobiol.* 92(2):184-211.

Stojiljković, V., Todorović, A., Radlović, N., Pejić, S., Mladenović, M., Kasapović, J. & Pajović, SB. (2007). Antioxidant enzymes, glutathione and lipid peroxidation in peripheral blood of children affected by coeliac disease. *Ann Clin Biochem.* 44(Pt 6):537-43.

Sukhai, M. & Piquette-Miller, M. (2000). Regulation of the multidrug resistance genes by stress signals. *J Pharm Pharm Sci.* 3(2):268-80.

Sun, Y. & MacRae, TH. (2005). The small heat shock proteins and their role in human disease. *FEBS J.* 272(11):2613-27.

Suto, R. & Srivastava, PK. (1995). A mechanism for the specific immunogenicity of heat shock protein-chaperoned peptides. *Science.* 269(5230):1585-8.

Szaflarska-Poplawska, A., Siomek, A., Czerwionka-Szaflarska, M., Gackowski, D., Różalski, R., Guz, J., Szpila, A., Zarakowska, E. & Olinski, R. (2010). Oxidatively damaged

DNA/oxidative stress in children with celiac disease. *Cancer Epidemiol Biomarkers Prev.* 19(8):1960-5.

Szebeni, B., Veres, G., Dezsofi, A., Rusai, K., Vannay, A., Bokodi, G., Vásárhelyi, B., Korponay-Szabó, IR., Tulassay, T. & Arató, A. (2007). Increased mucosal expression of Toll-like receptor (Toll-like receptor)2 and Toll-like receptor4 in coeliac disease. *J Pediatr Gastroenterol Nutr.* 45(2):187-93.

Sziksz, E., Veres, G., Vannay, A., Prókai, A., Gál, K., Onody, A., Korponay-Szabó, IR., Reusz, G., Szabó, A., Tulassay, T., Arató, A. & Szebeni, B. (2010). Increased heat shock protein 72 expression in celiac disease. *J Pediatr Gastroenterol Nutr.* 51(5):573-8.

Takada, M., Otaka, M., Takahashi, T., Izumi, Y., Tamaki, K., Shibuya, T., Sakamoto, N., Osada, T., Yamamoto, S., Ishida, R., Odashima, M., Itoh, H. & Watanabe, S. (2010). Overexpression of a 60-kDa heat shock protein enhances cytoprotective function of small intestinal epithelial cells. *Life Sci.* 86(13-14):499-504.

Takeda, K., Kaisho, T. & Akira, S. (2003). Toll-like receptors. *Annu Rev Immunol.* 21:335-76.

Tanaka, K. & Mizushima, T. (2009). Protective role of heat shock factor1 and HSP70 against gastrointestinal diseases. *Int J Hyperthermia.* 25(8):668-76.

Tanaka, K., Tanaka, Y., Namba, T., Azuma, A. & Mizushima T. (2010). Heat shock protein 70 protects against bleomycin-induced pulmonary fibrosis in mice. *Biochem Pharmacol.* 80(6):920-31.

Tanguay, RM., Wu, Y. & Khandjian, EW. (1993). Tissue-specific expression of heat shock proteins of the mouse in the absence of stress. *Dev Genet.* 14(2):112-8.

Tao, Y., Drabik, KA., Waypa, TS., Musch, MW., Alverdy, JC., Schneewind, O., Chang, EB. & Petrof, EO. (2006). Soluble factors from Lactobacillus GG activate MAPKs and induce cytoprotective heat shock proteins in intestinal epithelial cells. *Am J Physiol Cell Physiol.* 290(4):C1018-30.

Tashiro, S. (2009). Mechanism of liver regeneration after liver resection and portal vein embolization (ligation) is different? *J Hepatobiliary Pancreat Surg.* 16(3):292-9.

Thomas, JG. & Baneyx, F. (1998). Roles of the Escherichia coli small heat shock proteins IbpA and IbpB in thermal stress management: comparison with ClpA, ClpB, and HtpG In vivo. *J Bacteriol*180(19):5165-72.

Timperio, AM., Egidi, MG. & Zolla, L. (2008). Proteomics applied on plant abiotic stresses: role of heat shock proteins (HSP). *J Proteomics.* 71(4):391-411.

Tiroli-Cepeda, AO. & Ramos, CH. (2011). An overview of the role of molecular chaperones in protein homeostasis. *Protein Pept Lett.* 18(2):101-9.

Toivola, DM., Strnad, P., Habtezion, A. & Omary, MB. (2010). Intermediate filaments take the heat as stress proteins. *Trends Cell Biol.* 20(2):79-91.

Truettner, JS., Hu, K., Liu, CL., Dietrich, WD. & Hu, B. (2009). Subcellular stress response and induction of molecular chaperones and folding proteins after transient global ischemia in rats. *Brain Res.* 1249:9-18.

Trynka, G., Wijmenga, C. & van Heel, DA. (2010). A genetic perspective on coeliac disease. *Trends Mol Med.* 16(11):537-50.

Tsan, MF. & Gao, B. (2004). Endogenous ligands of Toll-like receptors. *J Leukoc Biol.* 76(3):514-9.

Tsan, MF. & Gao, B. (2009). Heat shock proteins and immune system. *J Leukoc Biol.* 85(6):905-10.

Tsapara, A., Matter, K. & Balda, MS. (2006). The heat-shock protein Apg-2 binds to the tight junction protein ZO-1 and regulates transcriptional activity of ZONAB. *Mol Biol Cell.* 17(3):1322-30.

Turner, JR. (2009). Intestinal mucosal barrier function in health and disease. *Nat Rev Immunol.* 9(11):799-809.

Van Montfort, R., Slingsby, C. & Vierling, E. (2001). Structure and function of the small heat shock protein/alpha-crystallin family of molecular chaperones. *Adv Protein Chem.* 59:105-56.

van Straaten, EA., Koster-Kamphuis, L., Bovee-Oudenhoven, IM., van der Meer, R. & Forget, PP. (1999). Increased urinary nitric oxide oxidation products in children with active coeliac disease. *Acta Paediatr.* 88(5):528-31.

Vigh, L., Nakamoto, H., Landry, J., Gomez-Munoz, A., Harwood, JL. & Horvath, I. (2007). Membrane regulation of the stress response from prokaryotic models to mammalian cells. *Ann N Y Acad Sci.* 1113:40-51. Epub 2007 Jul 26.

Virta, LJ., Kaukinen, K. & Collin, P. (2009). Incidence and prevalence of diagnosed coeliac disease in Finland: Results of effective case finding in adults. *Scand J Gastroenterol.* 44(8):933-8.

Volloch, V., Gabai, VL., Rits, S., Force, T. & Sherman, MY. (2000). HSP72 can protect cells from heat-induced apoptosis by accelerating the inactivation of stress kinase JNK. *Cell Stress Chaperones.* 5(2):139-47.

von Mikecz, A., Chen, M., Rockel, T. & Scharf, A. (2008). The nuclear ubiquitin-proteasome system: visualization of proteasomes, protein aggregates, and proteolysis in the cell nucleus. *Methods Mol Biol.* 463:191-202.

Wagner, OI., Rammensee, S., Korde, N., Wen, Q., Leterrier, JF. & Janmey, PA. (2007). Softness, strength and self-repair in intermediate filament networks. *Exp Cell Res.* 313(10):2228-35.

Watson, AJ. (1995). Necrosis and apoptosis in the gastrointestinal tract. *Gut.* 37(2):165-7.

Welker, S., Rudolph, B., Frenzel, E., Hagn, F., Liebisch, G., Schmitz, G., Scheuring, J., Kerth, A., Blume, A. & Weinkauf, S., Haslbeck, M., Kessler, H. & Buchner, J. (2010). Hsp12 is an intrinsically unstructured stress protein that folds upon membrane association and modulates membrane function. *Mol Cell.* 39(4):507-20.

Westerheide, SD., Anckar, J., Stevens, SM Jr., Sistonen, L. & Morimoto, RI. (2009). Stress-inducible regulation of heat shock factor 1 by the deacetylase SIRT1. *Science.* 323(5917):1063-6.

Wong, HR. & Wispé, JR. (1997). The stress response and the lung. *Am J Physiol.* 273(1 Pt 1):L1-9.

Xanthoudakis, S., Roy, S., Rasper, D., Hennessey, T., Aubin, Y., Cassady, R., Tawa, P., Ruel, R., Rosen, A. & Nicholson, DW. (1999). Hsp60 accelerates the maturation of pro-caspase-3 by upstream activator proteases during apoptosis. *EMBO J.* 18(8):2049-56.

Yang, PC., He, SH. & Zheng, PY. (2007). Investigation into the signal transduction pathway via which heat stress impairs intestinal epithelial barrier function. *J Gastroenterol Hepatol.* 22(11):1823-31.

Yeboah, FA. & White, D. (2001). AlphaB-crystallin expression in celiac disease - a preliminary study. *Croat Med J.* 42(5):523-6.

Young, JC. (2010). Mechanisms of the Hsp70 chaperone system. *Biochem Cell Biol.* 88(2):291-300.

Zitka, O., Kukacka, J., Krizkova, S., Huska, D., Adam, V., Masarik, M., Prusa, R. & Kizek, R. (2010). Matrix metalloproteinases. Curr Med Chem. 17(31):3751-68.

3

Antioxidant Status of the Celiac Mucosa: Implications for Disease Pathogenesis

Vesna Stojiljković[1], Jelena Kasapović[1], Snežana Pejić[1], Ljubica Gavrilović[1], Nedeljko Radlović[2], Zorica S. Saičić[3] and Snežana B. Pajović[1]
[1]Laboratory of Molecular Biology and Endocrinology, "Vinča" Institute of Nuclear Sciences, University of Belgrade, Belgrade, Serbia
[2]Department of Gastroenterology and Nutrition, University Children's Hospital, Belgrade, Serbia
[3]Department of Physiology, Institute of Biological Research "Siniša Stanković", University of Belgrade, Belgrade, Serbia

1. Introduction

Aerobic organisms require ground state oxygen to live. However, the use of oxygen during normal metabolism produces reactive oxygen species (ROS), some of which are highly toxic and deleterious to cells and tissues because of the ability to react with and alter all principal molecules of the cell, including lipids, proteins, carbohydrates and nucleic acids. It has been estimated that a human cell is affected by 1.5×10^5 oxidative strokes per day (Beckman & Ames, 1997). Under normal conditions, damage by oxygen radicals is kept in check by an efficient array of antioxidant (AO) mechanisms, such as AO enzymes superoxide dismutase (SOD), catalase (CAT), glutathione peroxidase (GPx) and glutathione reductase (GR), as well as nonenzymatic scavengers. Although potentially deleterious, ROS also have important beneficial functions as a part of protective mechanism against microorganisms and serving as cell signaling molecules.

1.1 Reactive oxygen species (ROS)

The term "reactive oxygen species" is used for a group o f chemical species that contain oxygen and are characterized by a high reactivity towards inorganic molecules, as well as biomolecules. ROS are:

- molecules, such as hydrogen peroxide (H_2O_2),
- ions, such as hypochlorite anion (OCl^-),
- free radicals, like hydroxyl radical ($OH.$),
- superoxide anion radical, which is an anion and a radical ($O_2.^-$).

Free radicals are molecules that contain one or more unpaired electrons in outer orbit (Halliwell & Gutteridge, 1989). The presence of the unpaired electron makes them highly reactive, which means that they can react with the majority of surrounding molecules including proteins, lipids, carbohydrates and nucleic acids. Tending to obtain a stable state, they "attack" the nearest stable molecule "stealing" an electron. When the "attacked" molecule loses an electron, it becomes a free radical itself, beginning a chain reaction that may end with the destruction of a living cell. The most important free radicals in biological systems are $O_2^{\cdot-}$, OH·, nitric oxide (NO·), lipid peroxyl radical (ROO·) and alkoxyl radical (RO·).

1.1.1 The activation of oxygen

Atmospheric oxygen in its basic state is unique among other gaseous elements, because it is a biradical, which means that in its outer orbit it has two unpaired electrons with parallel spins (a "triplet state" $^3O_2$). Due to this feature oxygen can hardly react with organic molecules, unless it is previously activated (Elstner, 1987). If a biradical form of oxygen absorbs energy sufficient to change the spin of one of the unpaired electrons, a "singlet state" ($^1O_2^*$) is generated, having two electrons with opposite spins. The oxygen thus activated can participate in reactions involving simultaneous transfer of two electrons (divalent reduction). Since paired electrons are usual in organic molecules, singlet oxygen is more reactive towards organic molecules than oxygen in the basic state. The other mechanism of activation is a gradual monovalent reduction of oxygen, generating $O_2^{\cdot-}$, H_2O_2, OH· and in the end H_2O.

1.1.2 Sources of ROS

Free radicals and ROS can originate via action of various endogenous and exogenous factors. Endogenous sources of ROS are autoxidation of different organic and inorganic molecules, enzymatically catalyzed oxidation and the "respiratory burst". Superoxide anion radical is the most common oxidant produced by normal cell metabolism. The main sources of $O_2^{\cdot-}$ are electron transport systems in membranes of mitochondria and other organelles (endoplasmic reticulum, chloroplasts). Apart from the mitochondrial respiratory chain, an array of nonenzymatic and enzymatic reactions can be the source of ROS. Autoxidation of various cell molecules (quinones, thiols, flavines, catecholamines, hemoglobin, myoglobin) produce $O_2^{\cdot-}$. Ferrous ions are also subjected to autoxidation followed by ROS production. ROS may be a direct product of enzymatic reactions. Myeloperoxidase in neutrophils in the presence of chloride produces OCl^- from H_2O_2. Xanthine oxidase (XO) catalyzes oxidation of hypoxanthine to xanthine and xanthine to uric acid, producing $O_2^{\cdot-}$ and H_2O_2 (Valko et al., 2004). Certain cells of the immune system (neutrophils, eosinophils, mononuclear phagocytes, B lymphocytes) during phagocytosis produce ROS (OCl^-, OH·, $^1O_2^*$ or chloramines) as microbicidal agents. A precursor of more reactive oxidants is $O_2^{\cdot-}$, whose production is associated with increased oxygen consumption in these cells sometimes even up to 50 times and this metabolic process is known as the "respiratory burst" (Babior, 1984).

Exogenous sources of ROS are drugs, radiation and smoking. Certain drugs such as some antibiotics and antineoplastic agents (anthracyclines, methotrexate) may increase ROS production under hyperoxic conditions (Gressier et al., 1994). In addition, components of some drugs may deplete AO reserves, enhancing effects of lipid peroxidation (Grisham et al., 1992). Radiotherapy can cause free radical production. Electromagnetic and particle irradiation produce primary radicals transferring their energy to the cell molecules. Tobacco smoke contains a great amount of oxidants. It has been suggested that 10^{14} different oxidants such as aldehydes, epoxides, peroxides, quinones, hydroquinones, NO· etc., are being imported in organism by just one breath of cigarette smoke (Church & Pryor, 1985).

1.1.3 Effects of ROS

One of the most important effects of ROS is oxidative damage of polyunsaturated fatty acids (PUFA) in cell membrane lipids. This process is known as lipid peroxidation (LPO). It is a chain reaction that provokes changes in the membrane phospholipid bilayer structure and modifies membrane proteins, causing loss of membrane elasticity and selective permeability and disruption of its other functions (Spiteller, 2007). The damage provoked by LPO can be prevented by chain-breaking antioxidants (β-carotene, lycopene, vitamins A, C, E). Strong oxidants, such as OH· can react with all components of the DNA molecule, causing single- or double-strand breaks and an increased rate of mutations (Egler et al., 2005). Permanent modifications of the genetic material represent the first step towards mutagenesis, carcinogenesis and aging. Proteins can also be oxidized by strong oxidants. Amino acids containing sulfur, especially the thiol group (-SH), are particularly susceptible to ROS. Oxidants can activate or inactivate proteins by oxidizing -SH groups and modifying amino acids (Davies, 1987). As a consequence of the deleterious effects of ROS, necrotic cell death may ensue. In addition, ROS and changes in cellular redox state may play a crucial role in the regulation and initiation of processes associated with apoptosis (Kroemer et al., 1998; Mignotte & Vayssiere, 1998).

Although a great importance is given to the negative effects of ROS, they also have beneficial physiological functions in the cell. Their role in the defense against microorganisms is indispensible. During phagocytosis activated inflammatory cells produce ROS to kill microbes. ROS can also have a critical role in signal transduction and redox regulation of gene expression (Thannickal & Fanburg, 2000) and the regulation of cell growth and proliferation (Burdon, 1996).

1.2 Antioxidant defense system

Detoxification of ROS is a sine qua non of aerobic life, hence a complex AO system has evolved due to evolutionary pressures. Antioxidants are agents which scavenge ROS, inhibit their production and/or repair the damage they have caused (Halliwell, 1991). The AO system involve AO enzymes (SOD, CAT, GPx), nonenzymatic antioxidants (glutathione (GSH), vitamin C, vitamin E, β-carotene, flavonoids), auxiliary enzymes that regenerate active forms of antioxidants (GR, glutathione-S-transferase (GST), glucose-6-phosphate dehydrogenase (G6PDH)), as well as metal binding proteins (transferrin, cerruloplasmin, albumin).

SOD catalyzes dismutation of $O_2^{\cdot -}$ to H_2O_2 and oxygen. This reaction is 10^4 times faster than spontaneous dismutation. In humans three different forms of this enzyme exist: cytosolic or copper, zinc SOD (CuZnSOD), mitochondrial or manganese SOD (MnSOD) and extracellular SOD (ECSOD). Catalase catalyzes decomposition of H_2O_2 to water and oxygen.

The glutathione redox cycle is a key mechanism for protection of cell membranes from damage by LPO. This cycle involves enzymes GPx, which uses GSH to reduce organic peroxides and hydrogen peroxide and GR, which reduces the oxidized form of glutathione (GSSG) with concomitant oxidation of NADPH. In a wider sense this cycle also includes the enzymes that synthesize GSH (γ-glutamylcysteine synthetase and GSH synthetase), G6PDH, which regenerates NADPH, as well as GST. GSH is a potent antioxidant, antitoxin and enzymatic cofactor. It can directly react with free radicals. GSH has also an important role in regenerating active forms of other antioxidants such as vitamins E and C and carotenoids (Jones et al., 2000).

1.3 The role of oxidative stress in the pathogenesis of gastrointestinal diseases

The oxidant versus AO balance may be altered in various pathological conditions, primarily or secondarily. If ROS production overwhelms the AO defense capacity of a cell, oxidative damage occurs and the condition is known as oxidative stress. Oxidative stress plays an important role in the pathogenesis of many diseases including various gastrointestinal disorders. It has been shown that the concentration of ROS is elevated in patients with various liver diseases such as alcoholic hepatitis and cirrhosis, while antioxidant therapy has protective effects in animal models of these disorders (Dryden et al., 2005). Colon cancer, as well as acute and chronic pancreatitis, have also been associated with oxidative stress (Dryden et al., 2005; Opara, 2003). It has been suggested that oxidative stress may have an important role in the pathogenesis of acquired megacolon, since decreased AO levels provoke changes in the intestinal levels of inhibitory neurotransmitters in patients affected by the disease (Koch et al., 1996). Necrotizing enterocolitis, a severe disorder found in infants, is another disease whose pathogenesis is attributed to oxidative stress (Otamiri & Sjödahl, 1991). *Helicobacter pylori* infection, an important factor in the pathogenesis of gastric cancer, is also followed by an increased production of ROS (Farinati et al., 2003).

The role of oxidative stress in pathological changes in gastrointestinal tract has mostly been studied in inflammatory bowel disease (IBD) such as ulcerative colitis and Crohn's disease. It has been suggested that oxidative stress plays an important role in the initiation, as well as progression of IBD and antioxidant therapy, for e.g. use of green tea polyphenols or SOD, significantly attenuates the disorder (Dryden et al., 2005). IBD is characterized by elevation in mucosal inflammatory cells, leading to disruption of the epithelial barrier. This allows highly immunogenic bacterial antigens, present in the intestinal lumen in high concentrations, to enter the normally sterile subepithelial layers, activating a cascade of destructive immunologic responses (Rezaie et al., 2007). Various theories regarding the initiation of the inflammatory response in the intestinal mucosa have been proposed, but none of them is universally accepted (Hendrickson et al., 2002). Many studies have reported the increased concentrations of oxidized biomolecules and the decreased concentrations of various antioxidants in patients affected by IBD, not only in the intestinal mucosa, but also in other parts of the gastrointestinal tract, as well as in the blood and respiratory system (Rezaie et al. 2006). It is known that oxidizing agents can induce clinical and histological alterations characteristic of IBD (Bilotta & Waye, 1989; Meyer et al. 1981). ROS may damage intestinal mucosa and increase its permeability (Rao et al., 1997; Riedle & Kerjaschki, 1997). In addition, it has been shown that patients affected by Crohn's disease in latent phase, as well as their first-degree relatives, have increased intestinal permeability without inflammation. The fact that oxidative stress is present in the bowel before the beginning of the inflammatory cascade suggests that ROS are not collateral products of the inflammatory process, but play an important role in the pathogenesis of the disease (Buhner et al. 2006; Fries et al., 2005).

1.4 Oxidative stress and antioxidant status of patients with celiac disease

There is a growing body of evidence indicating that oxidative stress and the cellular redox status are also implicated in the pathogenesis of celiac disease. The results of various investigations suggest that gliadin disturbs the pro-oxidant-antioxidant balance in small intestinal mucosa of affected persons through overproduction of ROS (Boda et al., 1999; Dugas et al., 2003). Several in vitro studies have also reported redox imbalance and increased levels of free radicals after exposure of cells to gliadin (Dolfini et al., 2002; Maiuri et al., 2003; Rivabene, 1999; Tucková et al., 2002).

Data concerning the AO status of celiac patients are scarce. The results of a few investigations indicate that the AO capacity of celiac patients is diminished. Odetti et al. (1998) found a lowered level of vitamin E and increased levels of markers of oxidized lipids and proteins in the plasma of celiac patients subjected to gluten free diet, while Ståhlberg et al. have reported decreased GSH concentrations and GPx activity in erythrocytes and the small intestinal mucosa of children affected by celiac disease (Ståhlberg et al., 1988; Ståhlberg & Hietanen, 1991). In our previous papers (Stojiljković et al., 2007; Stojiljković et al., 2009) we showed that oxidative stress is strongly associated with CD and that the AO capacity of celiac patients is weakened by a depletion of GSH and reduced activities of GSH-dependent AO enzymes GPx and GR. In this study we describe the results of our investigation regarding the AO status of celiac patients with different degrees of severity of the mucosal lesion. The activities of AO enzymes MnSOD, CuZnSOD, CAT, GPx and GR, as well as the concentrations of GSH and lipid hydroperoxides (LOOH) were examined.

2. Materials and methods

2.1 Subjects

The study involved small intestinal biopsies from 55 children affected by celiac disease (24 boys, 31 girls; median age 8 years; range 1.5-16 years) who were attended at the University Children's Hospital, Belgrade, Serbia, between September 2003 and December 2006. Clinical characteristics of the patients are described in Table 1. Twenty six children were diagnosed in early childhood and by the time of sampling, they had been subjected to gluten-free diet (GFD) for 2-4 years. In the other 29 children, who were using gluten containing diet, the diagnosis was made at the time of the study. Among them, 18 children had active form of the disease with typical symptoms (chronic diarrhea, fatigue, failure to thrive or weight loss), while 11 children were asymptomatic. Typical villous atrophy was found on examination of intestinal biopsy specimens in all children on the gluten containing diet. The diagnosis of celiac disease was based on the revised criteria of the European Society for Paediatric Gastroenterology, Hepatology and Nutrition (Walker-Smith, 1990). The Ethical Committee of the Faculty of Medicine, University of Belgrade, approved the study. The parents of all patients included in the study gave written informed consent.

Histological evaluation was performed according to the modified Oberhuber-Marsh classification (Oberhuber et al., 1999). Patients were divided in 4 groups. In the Marsh 0 group, the mucosa was normal with no signs of inflammation (n = 17, all on GFD). In the Marsh 1+2 group, the mucosa was characterized by intraepithelial lymphocytosis (Marsh 1) or intraepithelial lymphocytosis accompanied by crypt hyperplasia (Marsh 2) (n = 9, six Marsh 1 and three Marsh 2, all on GFD). In the Marsh 3a group (n=20, seven asymptomatic and 13 with active celiac disease) partial villous atrophy was present, while in the Marsh 3b group (n=9, four asymptomatic and five with active form of the disease) subtotal villous atrophy was found.

	Patients		
	active	asymptomatic	GFD
Number	18	11	26
Gender			
Male	6	6	12
Female	12	5	14
Age (years)			
Range	1,5-15	1,5-16	5-16
Median	4,63±1,19	8,34±1,36	8,78±1,24
Body mass index			
<15th percentile	10	3	5
15-75th percentile	7	8	13
>75th percentile	1	-	8
Hemoglobin (g/L)[1]	102.8±3.6	119.2±4.0 **	133.3±4.1*** #
Mean cell volume (fL)[2]	70.1±2.6	73.8±3.5	76.7±1.6*
serum iron (□mol/L)[3]	5.5±0.7	10.9±2.6**	17.6±3.5*** #

[1]Normal value: 120-170 g/L
[2]Normal value: 86-98 fL
[3]Normal value: 10-22 μmol/L

Table 1. Clinical characteristics of patients affected by celiac disease. Hemoglobin, mean cell volume and serum iron are means ± SEM. Statistical significance: *** $P < 0.001$, ** $P < 0.01$, * $P < 0.05$, significantly different from active patients; # $P < 0.05$ significantly different from asymptomatic patients. GFD, patients on gluten-free diet.

2.2 Sample preparation

From each patient 6-8 proximal small intestinal biopsy specimens were obtained. Some of them were used for histopathological analysis and others were washed in ice-cold saline and frozen at -70 °C for SOD, CAT, GPx, GR, GSH and LOOH assays. One biopsy specimen from each patient was kept on -70 °C for the GSH assay, while others were thawed within a week and homogenized in 20 volumes of cold sucrose buffer pH 7.4. Homogenates were vortexed 3 times for 15 seconds and then kept at -70 °C. Thawed homogenates were centrifuged (Eppendorf centrifuge 5417R, Eppendorf-Netheler-Hinz GmbH, Hamburg, Germany) at 8600 g, 4 °C, for 10 minutes. Supernatants were stored at -70 °C.

2.3 Assays

All assays were performed using the Perkin Elmer Lambda 25 Spectrophotometer (Perkin Elmer Instruments, Norwalk, CT, USA). The specific enzyme activities of SODs and CAT were expressed as units per milligram of protein (U/mg) and of GPx and GR as milliunits per milligram of protein (mU/mg). The GSH and LOOH concentrations were expressed in micromoles per liter (μmol/l).

SOD assay. Total SOD activity was measured using the Oxis Bioxytech® SOD-525™ Assay (Oxis International, Inc., Portland, OR, USA). The method is based on the SOD-mediated increase in the rate of autoxidation of reagent 1 (5,6,6a,11b-tetrahydro-3,9,10-trihydroxybenzo[c]fluorene,

R1) in aqueous alkaline solution, yielding a chromophore with maximum absorbance at 525 nm. The kinetic measurement of the change in absorbance at 525 nm is performed. One SOD-525 activity unit is defined as the activity that doubles the autoxidation rate of the control blank. CuZnSOD activity was measured as described above, after pretreating samples with ethanol-chloroform reagent (5/3 vol/vol), which inactivates MnSOD. MnSOD activity was then calculated by subtracting CuZnSOD activity from total SOD activity.

CAT assay. CAT activity was measured by the method of Beutler (1982), which is based on the measurement of the rate of H_2O_2 decomposition by catalase from the examined samples. The decomposition of H_2O_2 was demonstrated by a decrease in absorbance at 230 nm as a function of time. One CAT activity unit is defined as 1 □mol of H_2O_2 decomposed per minute under the assay conditions.

GPx assay. Gpx activity was determined by the Oxis Bioxytech® GPx-340™ Assay (Oxis International, Inc., Portland, OR, USA). Upon reduction of organic peroxide by GPx, oxidized glutathione (GSSG) is produced and its recycling to GSH by GR is accompanied by oxidation of nicotinamide adenine dinucleotide phosphate (NADPH) to $NADP^+$. The rate of NADPH oxidation, followed by a decrease in absorbance at 340 nm as a function of time, is directly proportional to the GPx activity in the sample. One GPx-340 activity unit is defined as 1 □mol of NADPH consumed per minute under the assay conditions.

GR assay. The activity of GR was measured by the Oxis Bioxytech® GR-340™ Assay (Oxis International, Inc., Portland, OR, USA). The assay is based on the oxidation of NADPH to $NADP^+$ by GR from the sample. The rate of NADPH oxidation was determined by the rate of a decrease in absorbance at 340 nm. One GR-340 unit is defined as 1 □mol of NADPH oxidized per minute under the assay conditions.

GSH assay. The concentration of GSH was determined by the Oxis Bioxytech® GSH-420™ Assay (Oxis International, Inc., Portland, OR, USA). The thawed tissue was homogenized in 20 volumes of precipitating reagent (trichloroacetic acid) and homogenates were centrifuged at 3000 g, 4 °C, 10 minutes. Supernatants were used for GSH assay. The reaction is performed in three steps. The sample was first buffered and treated with the reducing agent (tris(2-carboxyethyl)phosphine) to reduce any oxidized glutathione present in the sample. Then the chromogen (4-chloro-1-methyl-7-trifluoromethylquinolinium methylsulphate) was added forming thioethers with all thiols from the sample. After addition of base to raise the pH over 13, a β-elimination specific to the GSH-thioether results in the chromophoric thione. The absorbance at 420 nm is directly proportional to the GSH concentration.

LOOH assay. The concentration of LOOH was determined by the Oxis Bioxytech® LPO-560™ Assay (Oxis International, Inc., Portland, OR, USA). The assay is based on the oxidation of ferrous to ferric ions by LOOH from the sample under acidic conditions. Ferric ions bind with the indicator dye (xylenol orange) and a stable colored complex is formed. The absorbance at 560 nm is directly proportional to the LOOH concentration. To eliminate H_2O_2 interference the samples were pretreated with catalase.

2.4 Statistics

Differences between the groups were tested by the Kruskal-Wallis test. Multiple comparisons of the groups were performed by the Dunn test. Correlations between AO parameters and the degree of mucosal lesion were evaluated by the Spearman's rank order correlation coefficient r_S. A P value lower than 0.05 was considered significant.

3. Results

All parameters, except CuZnSOD and CAT activity, varied significantly between the analyzed groups: MnSOD: H = 8.79, $P < 0.05$; CuZnSOD: H = 5.23, $P > 0.05$; CAT: H = 5.75, $P > 0.05$; GPx: H = 12.61, $P < 0.01$; GR: H = 9.81, $P < 0.05$; GSH: H = 32.70, $P < 0.001$; LOOH: H = 22.92, $P < 0.001$ (Kruskal-Wallis test).

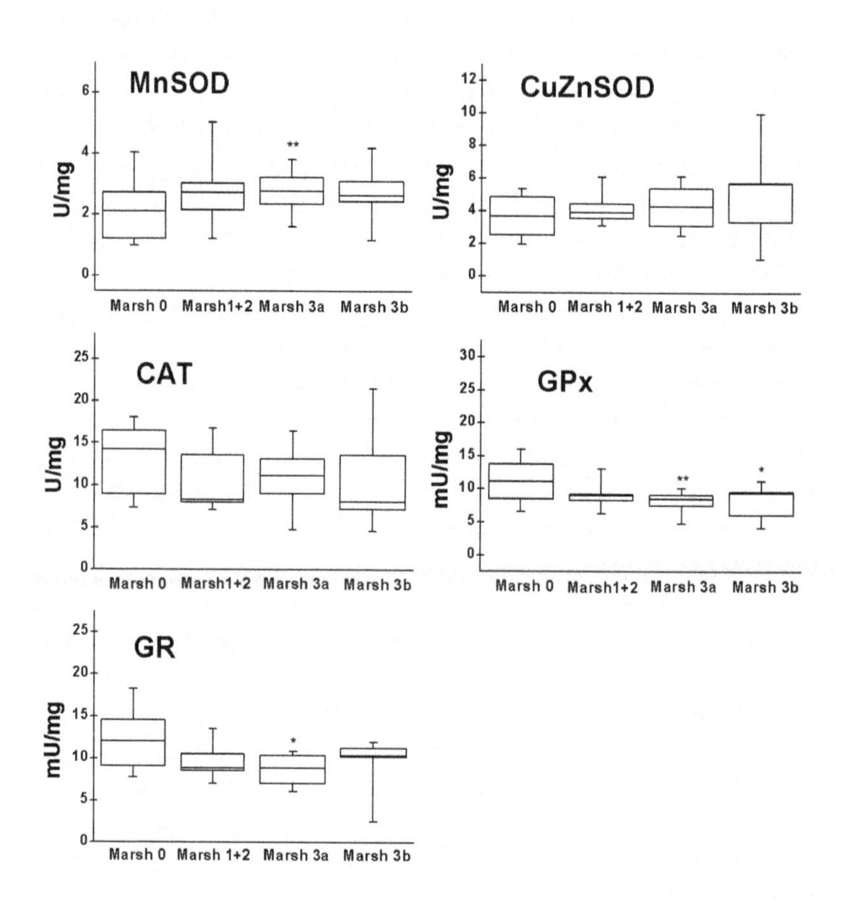

Fig. 1. The activities of manganese superoxide dismutase (MnSOD), copper-zink SOD (CuZnSOD), catalase (CAT), glutathione peroxidase (GPx) and glutathione reductase (GR) in normal intestinal mucosa (Marsh 0), mucosa with intraepithelial lymphocytosis or intraepithelial lymphocytosis accompanied by crypt hyperplasia (Marsh 1+2), mucosa with partial (Marsh 3a) or subtotal villous atrophy (Marsh 3b). Boxes represent values between 25th and 75th percentile. Medians are given inside the boxes. Whiskers extend between min and max values. ** P < 0.01, * P < 0.05, significantly different from Marsh 0 group.

The activities of the AO enzymes are represented in Figure 1. In comparison to Marsh 0 group, the MnSOD activity was significantly elevated in Marsh 3a group ($P < 0.01$). GPx activity was significantly lower in Marsh 3a ($P < 0.01$) and Marsh 3b groups ($P < 0.05$) than in Marsh 0. GR activity was also reduced in Marsh 3a ($P < 0.01$) when compared to Marsh 0.

The patients with villous atrophy (Marsh 3a and 3b) had significantly reduced GSH level in comparison to the patients with normal mucosa (Marsh 0, $P < 0.0001$) or milder mucosal lesion (Marsh 1+2, $P < 0.01$). Significant increase in LOOH levels was found in Marsh 1+2 ($P < 0.01$), Marsh 3a and 3b ($P < 0.001$), comparing to the patients with normal mucosa. LOOH concentration was also higher in patients with villous atrophy than in patients with Marsh 1+2 lesions ($P > 0.05$) (Figure 2).

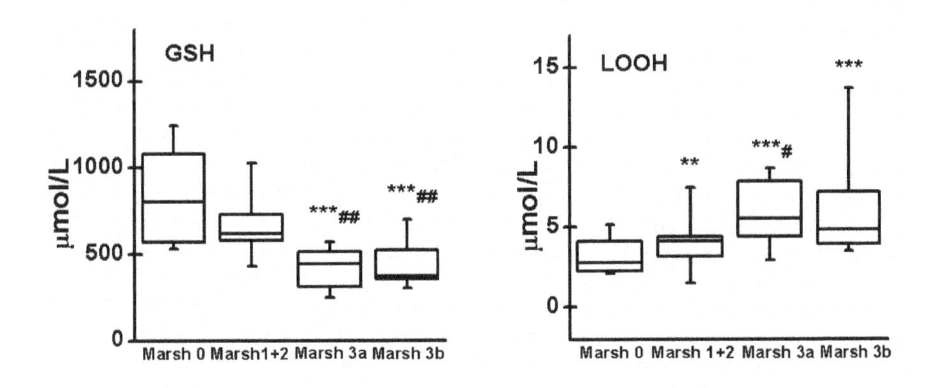

Fig. 2. Concentrations of glutathione (GSH) and lipid hydroperoxides (LOOH) in normal intestinal mucosa (Marsh 0), mucosa with intraepithelial lymphocytosis or intraepithelial lymphocytosis accompanied by crypt hyperplasia (Marsh 1+2), mucosa with partial (Marsh 3a) or subtotal villous atrophy (Marsh 3b). Boxes represent values between 25th and 75th percentile. Medians are given inside the boxes. Whiskers extend between min and max values. *** P < 0.001, ** P < 0.01, significantly different from Marsh 0 group; ## P < 0.01, # P < 0.05, significantly different from Marsh 1+2 group.

All investigated parameters correlated significantly with the degree of mucosal damage (Figure 3). Positive correlations were found between the severity of mucosal lesion and the activities of MnSOD ($r_s = 0.33$, $P < 0.01$), CuZnSOD ($r_s = 0.27$, $P < 0.01$) and CAT ($r_s = 0.25$, $P < 0.05$). On the contrary, GSH concentration as well as the activities of GSH-related enzymes GPx and GR inversely correlated with degree of the mucosal lesion ($r_s = -0.67$, $P < 0.0001$; $r_s = -0.40$, $P < 0.001$; $r_s = -0.27$, $P < 0.05$, respectively). In addition, significant positive correlation was found between the LOOH level and the degree of mucosal damage ($r_s = 0.56$, $P < 0.0001$).

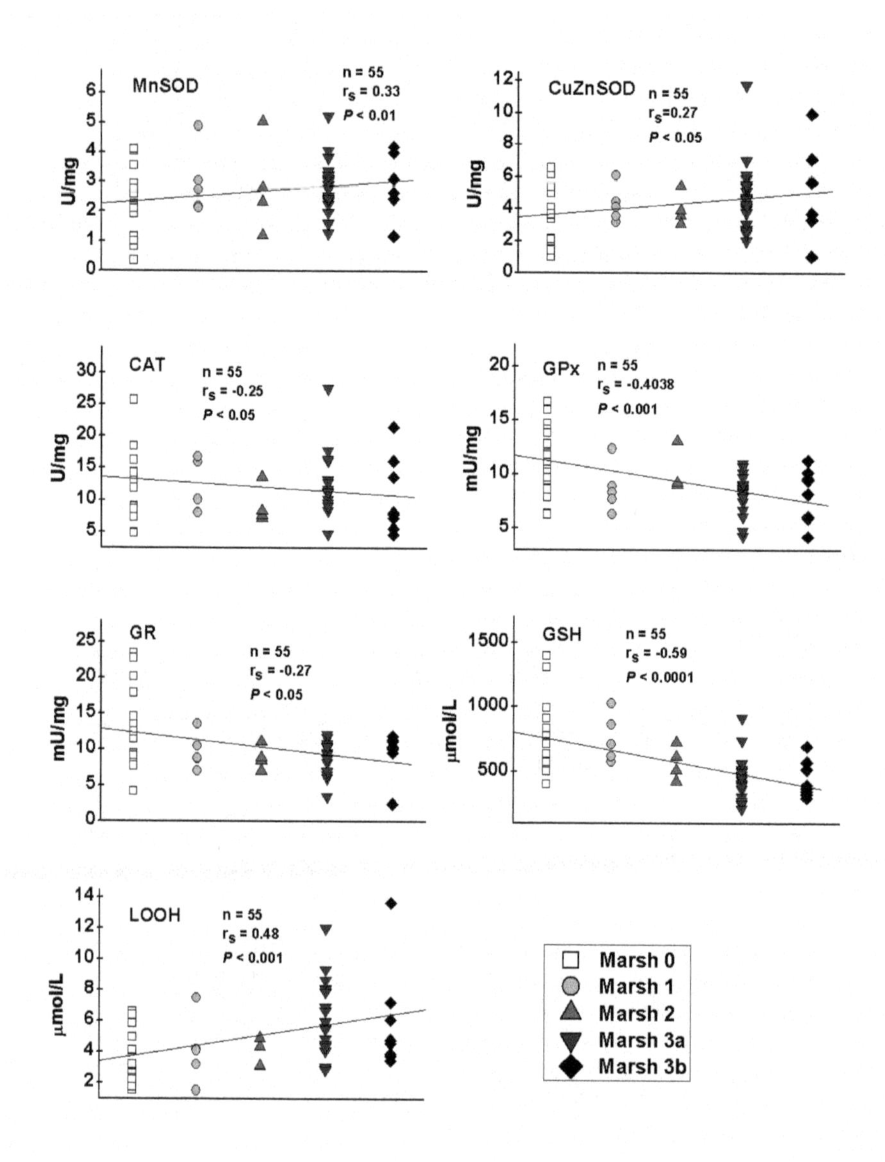

Fig, 3. Data plot and coefficients of Spearman's rank correlation r_s between the parameters of antioxidant status and the severity of mucosal lesion in celiac patients. MnSOD – manganese superoxide dismutase, CuZnSOD - copper-zink superoxid dismutase, CAT - catalase, GPx - glutathione peroxidase, GR - glutathione reductase, GSH – glutathione, LOOH - lipid hydroperoxides; Marsh 0 - normal intestinal mucosa, Marsh 1 - mucosa with intraepithelial lymphocytosis, Marsh 2 - mucosa with intraepithelial lymphocytosis accompanied by crypt hyperplasia, Marsh 3a - mucosa with partial villous atrophy, Marsh 3b - mucosa with subtotal villous atrophy.

4. Discussion

There is a growing body of evidence showing that ROS are involved in the pathology of celiac disease. Pro-oxidant effects of gliadin have also been reported in celiac patients. Activation of XO is one of the mechanisms of free radical and ROS overproduction in the small intestinal mucosa. The xanthine oxidoreductase system is mainly located in the intestinal mucosa and liver (Sarnesto et al., 1996). Distribution of this enzyme in the small bowel is not uniform. Histological studies have shown that the main part of XO is located in the epithelial cells at the top of the intestinal villi, while no XO activity could be detected at the basis of crypts (Pickett et al., 1970). The results of Boda and coworkers (1999) suggest that in patients with active celiac disease, gluten ingestion, along with the resulting inflammation, causes activation of XO in enterocytes, which results in overproduction of ROS and further damage to the mucosa. These pro-oxidant processes are counteracted by AO enzymes MnSOD and CuZnSOD. The activity of MnSOD in our study was elevated in patients with villous atrophy comparing to the Marsh 0 group, while CuZnSOD activity did not vary significantly. However, positive correlations between the activities of both SODs and the degree of mucosal lesion indicate that more severe mucosal damage is associated with increased enzyme activities. This may represent a physiological response to a higher rate of ROS production. On the contrary, the activity of CAT did not vary significantly between the analyzed groups and it correlated inversely with the mucosal lesion. This may be a consequence of the kinetic characteristics of this enzyme. Namely, due to its high Michaelis-Menten constant, CAT is most efficient against high H_2O_2 concentrations. When H_2O_2 concentrations are lower, more effective protection is given by GPx, another H_2O_2 detoxifying enzyme (Eaton, 1991). Since the activity of GPx, the main scavenger of H_2O_2 in gastro-intestinal tissue was significantly decreased in patients with villous atrophy (Marsh 3a and Marsh 3b), the imbalance between H_2O_2 production and scavenging causes pro-oxidant shift, which results in increased LPO and LOOH concentration. In these patients LOOH concentration was ~ 80 % higher than in patients with normal mucosa. Even in some GFD patients (Marsh 1+2) LOOH concentration was elevated ~ 20 % in comparison to the Marsh 0 group. These results are in accordance with the data from an *in vitro* study (Rivabene et al., 1999) where the concentration of LOOH in cell culture was 30-50 % higher after gliadin treatment.

Increased LOOH levels may contribute to the disruption of detoxifying pathways in the bowel and to dysfunction of enterocytes, which may cause various disorders of the digestive tract (Aw, 1998). The intestine differs from other fully differentiated organs by a very high rate of cellular turn over. The lifespan of enterocytes is only 4-6 days (Iatropoulos, 1986). Due to the high cell division rate, the chance of spreading a mutation to the subsequent cell generations is much higher than in cells with a low division rate, which makes the intestine very susceptible to mutagenesis and cancerogenesis. It has been shown that subtoxic concentrations of LOOH can provoke a change in the cellular redox state enough to enhance a mitogenic response in rat enterocytes (Aw, 1999), while more severe oxidative stress activates pro-apoptotic processes (Imai & Nakagawa, 2003). Several in vitro studies have also demonstrated that exposure of human intestinal cells to the subtoxic concentrations of LOOH can induce cell transition from a quiescent to a proliferative state or even growth arrest (Gotoh et al., 2002), while high LOOH levels disturb the intestinal homeostasis to such an extent that pro-apoptotic processes cannot be stopped even after restoration of redox balance (Wang et al., 2000). In addition, LOOH cause damage to intestinal cell membranes in vitro, as well as single- and double-strand DNA breaks and may influence the activity of AO enzymes (Wijeratne & Cuppett, 2006).

Since the intestinal mucosa interfaces with the lumen, which is open to the exterior environment and deeper layers of the intestinal wall, it represents a crucial protective barrier against potential toxic agents. In addition to the nutrients, the intestinal mucosa is constantly exposed to oxidants, mutagens and carcinogens from the diet, as well as to endogenous ROS. Several protective mechanisms preserve cellular integrity and tissue homeostasis: the intestine is able to maintain high concentrations of antioxidants and to up-regulate AO enzymes, while apoptosis is induced to eliminate spent or damaged enterocytes (Aw, 1999). The GSH redox cycle is the key mechanism of LOOH scavenging in the intestine (Aw, 2005). GSH is a powerful antioxidant that acts as a detoxifier of endogenous and exogenous ROS. Published data indicate that epithelial cells of the small and large intestine are highly dependent on GSH. It was demonstrated that in mice treated with L-buthionine SR-sulfoximine (BSO), a specific inhibitor of GSH synthesis, a significant degeneration of enterocytes is induced, as a consequence of GSH deficiency (Mårtensson et al., 1990). High levels of GSH are found in many tissues, including the intestine. Normal concentrations of intracellular GSH are maintained by *de novo* synthesis, regeneration from GSSG or through import via the Na^+-dependent transport system. GSH transport into the cell is demonstrated in several cell types, including enterocytes (Aw, 1994; Mårtensson et al., 1990). The ability of enterocytes to import luminal GSH is important for the intestinal thiol balance, especially in pro-oxidative conditions, since the human diet is extremely various concerning the GSH and LOOH content. In a healthy system, where GSH is not limiting, intracellular metabolism of LOOH is enhanced, decreasing luminal LOOH retention and excretion into lymph. On the contrary, if GSH is insufficient, LOOH catabolism decreases and their luminal retention and lymphatic transport are promoted (LeGrand and Aw, 2001).

In this investigation a significantly lower GSH concentration (~ 40-50 %) was found in the intestinal mucosa with villous atrophy compared to the normal mucosa and mucosa with milder lesions. The decreased GSH concentration is followed by decreased activities of GPx and GR and increased LOOH concentration. Our results are in accordance with the previous data reporting a significant decrease of GPx activity in mucosa of children with severe villous atrophy (Ståhlberg et al., 1988). Similar data have come from in vitro studies investigating the effects of gliadin on intestinal cells in culture (Dolfini et al., 2002; Dolfini et al., 2005). The experiments of Rivabene and coworkers have shown that the antiproliferative effects of gliadin are associated with pro-oxidative changes in the cell, such as elevated LOOH levels, decreased GSH concentration and a loss of SH- groups in proteins; the administration of BSO has demonstrated that the extent of these changes depended on the basal redox state of enterocytes, primarily their GSH content (Rivabene et al., 1999). These results imply that higher GSH concentrations could, at least partly, modify cell susceptibility to the toxic effects of gliadin.

GSH is not only an enzyme cofactor, but can also react directly with free radicals and is involved in recycling of other chain breaking antioxidants, such as vitamin E, whose concentration is reduced in celiac patients on GFD (Odetti et al., 1998). One of the extremely important roles of GSH is detoxification of various endogenous and exogenous toxins by GSH-S-transferases (GST), which use GSH as a cofactor. GSH deficiency should also influence these enzymes. Previous investigations have reported reduced total GST activity, as well as GST α class levels, although GSH concentration was not significantly altered in comparison to the control values (Wahab et al., 2001). In an in vitro study gliadin provoked a reduction in GSH content and gliadin concentration-related decrease in the activity of GPx, GR and GSH-S-transferases (Elli et al., 2003).

Since the activities of GPx and GR in our study were inversely related to GSH concentration, a decrease in these activities in patients with villous atrophy could be a consequence of GSH deficiency. In addition, as Gpx is a selenium-dependent enzyme, low Se levels can also influence its activity. Previous investigations have shown that GPx activity did not change in the conditions of elevated LOOH levels, pointing to the influence of dietary selenium on the glutathione peroxidase system of the gastrointestinal tract in rats (Reddy & Tappel, 1974; Vilas et al., 1976). Selenium deficiency has already been reported in celiac patients (Stazi & Trinti, 2010; Yuce et al., 2004). Several studies have also reported a strong correlation between Gpx activity and Se level in the blood, especially when Se concentration is low ($<$ 80 μg/L) (Lloyd et al., 1989; McKenzie at al., 1978). Aw and coworkers suggested that GPx and GR *per se* are not limited in the catabolism of LOOH in the intestine. The kinetics of these enzymes and the extent of intracellular LOOH degradation depend principally on the availability of cellular reductants (GSH and NADPH) (Aw & Williams, 1992; Aw et al., 1992). It has been shown that a disturbed intestinal GSH/GSSG ratio is involved in the pathogenesis of chronic intestinal inflammation in mice with severe combined immunodeficiency (SCID) reconstituted with $CD4^{+}CD45Rb^{high}$ T-lymphocytes (Aw, 2005). The loss of GSH redox balance preceded tissue hyperplasia, mucosal inflammation and the symptoms of clinical colitis, suggesting that redox imbalance may be a contributor rather than the consequence of disease.

Similar to previous reports, the results of our study indicate that oxidative stress is strongly associated with celiac disease and could be an important factor in disease pathogenesis. The AO status of patients with villous atrophy is severely disturbed. GSH deficiency and decreased activities of GSH-dependent enzymes significantly reduce the AO capacity of these patients, which is reflected in elevated LOOH levels. The AO status of patients with milder mucosal lesions (Marsh 1+2 group) was not significantly altered compared to patients with normal mucosa. However, it should be emphasized that even in this group LOOH concentration was significantly elevated pointing out the incapacity of the GSH redox cycle to efficiently eliminate peroxides. The LOOH challenge may provoke perturbations of normal intestinal cell proliferation, differentiation and apoptotic responses, contributing to the increased risk of malignancy in untreated celiac patients. It is well known that GSH is indispensable for normal function of intestinal epithelium. Since enterocytes are capable of absorbing dietary GSH from the intestinal lumen, it has been demonstrated that oral administration of GSH elevates GSH concentration in small and large intestinal mucosa of mice, protecting the tissue from GSH deficiency provoked by BSO (Mårtensson et al., 1990). We could speculate that the oral administration of GSH would be beneficial for protection of the intestinal epithelium from damage occurring in inflammatory disorders, such as celiac disease, as well as ischemia, chemotherapy or radiation. In addition, as GSH can be regenerated from other antioxidants (Lenton *et al*, 2003), a diet enriched with natural antioxidants, as well as appropriate supplements, could be important complements to the classic GFD. Furthermore, since GPx is more susceptible to the influence of dietary supplements than other AO enzymes (Andersen et al., 1997), administration of antioxidants and Se could enhance GPx activity and promote LOOH scavenging in celiac patients.

Previous data concerning correlations between the activities of AO enzymes and histological changes characteristic of celiac disease are limited. Wahab and coworkers (2001) found decreased levels and activities of GST in small intestinal mucosa of celiac patients in comparison to the healthy individuals, which were proportional to the degree of mucosal damage. Similarly, the activity of uridine 5'-diphospho-glucuronosyltransferase, an enzyme that detoxifies some noxious compounds by catalyzing their addition to glucuronic acid, was also reduced in the intestinal mucosa of patients with celiac disease (Goerres et al., 2006). On the contrary, plasma concentrations of end products of NO metabolism in celiac patients were elevated and correlated with the histological changes of mucosa (Murray et al., 2003; Spencer et al., 2004). The results of our study show that the severity of the mucosal lesion in celiac patients significantly correlated with all analyzed parameters of AO status. Positive correlations were found between severity of histological damage and the activities of both SODs, as well as LOOH concentration. The activities of CAT, GPx and GR and the concentration of GSH inversely correlated with the degree of the mucosal lesion. Concerning the fact that the severity of histological damage is reflective of the AO status in the intestinal mucosa of celiac patients and since similar changes of the AO status in peripheral blood have already been reported (Stojiljković et al., 2007), we suggest that new, noninvasive methods, involving analysis of AO parameters, could be developed for prediction and follow-up of histological changes in patients with celiac disease. In addition, nutritional evaluation should be performed in celiac patients at least annually, to monitor the mucosal damage and the effectiveness of GFD.

5. Conclusions

Our results demonstrate that oxidative stress is implicated in the pathogenesis of celiac disease. A significant disturbance in AO status occurs in patients affected by celiac disease, especially those with the advanced mucosal damage. Changes of AO status significantly correlate with the severity of histological damage. A seriously impaired AO capacity for degradation of lipid hydroperoxides may persist even after several years of GFD. A diet rich in natural antioxidants as well as appropriate dietary supplements could be beneficial for full mucosal healing of celiac patients

6. Acknowledgement

This work received the financial support of the Ministry of Education and Science of the Republic of Serbia (Grants III 41027 and OI 173041).

7. References

Andersen, H.R., Nielsen, J.B., Nielsen, F. & Grandjean, P. (1997). Antioxidative enzyme activities in human erythrocytes. *Clin. Chem.*, Vol. 43, No. 4, (Apr 1997), pp. (562-568)

Aw, T.Y. & Williams, M.W. (1992). Intestinal absorption and lymphatic transport of peroxidized lipids in rats: effect of exogenous GSH. *Am. J. Physiol.*, Vol. 263, No. 5, (Nov 1992), pp. (665-672)

Aw, T.Y. (1994). Biliary glutathione promotes the mucosal metabolism of luminal peroxidized lipids by rat small intestine *in vivo*. *J. Clin. Invest.*, Vol. 94, No. 3, (Sep 1994), pp. (1218-1225)

Aw, T.Y. (1998). Determinants of intestinal detoxication of lipid hydroperoxides. *Free Radic. Res.*, Vol. 128, No. 6, (Jun 1998), pp. (637-646)

Aw, T.Y. (1999). Molecular and cellular responses to oxidative stress and changes in oxidation-reduction imbalance in the intestine. *Am. J. Clin. Nutr.* Vol. 70, No. 4, (Oct 1999), pp. (557-565)

Aw, T.Y. (2005). Intestinal glutathione: determinant of mucosal peroxide transport, metabolism, and oxidative susceptibility. *Toxicol. Appl. Pharmacol.*, Vol. 204, No. 3, (May 2005), pp. (320-328)

Aw, T.Y., Williams, M.W. & Gray, L. (1992). Absorption and lymphatic transport of peroxidized lipids by rat small intestine *in vivo*: role of mucosal GSH. Am. J. Physiol., Vol. 262, No. 1, (Jan 1992), pp. (99-106)

Babior, B.M. (1984). The respiratory burst of phagocytes. *J. Clin. Invest,* Vol. 73, No. 3, (Mar 1984), pp. (599-601)

Beckman, K.B. & Ames, B.N. (1997). Oxidative decay of DNA. *J. Biol. Chem,* Vol. 272, No. 32, (Aug 1997), pp. (19633-19636)

Beutler, E. (1982). Catalase, In: *Red Cell Metabolism, a manual of Biochemical Methods,* Beutler, E. (ed.), pp. (105-106), Grune and Stratton, New York

Bilotta, J.J. & Waye, J.D. (1989). Hydrogen peroxide enteritis: the "snow white" sign. *Gastrointest. Endosc,* Vol. 35, No. 5, (Sep-Oct 1989), pp. (428-430)

Blokhina, O., Virolainen, E. & Fagerstedt, K.V. (2003). Antioxidants, oxidative damage and oxygen deprivation stress: a review. *Ann. Bot,* Vol. 91, Spec No, (Jan 2003), pp. (179-194)

Boda, M., Németh, I. & Boda, D. (1999). The caffeine metabolic ratio as an index of xanthine oxidase activity in clinically active and silent celiac patients. J. Pediatr. Gastroenterol. Nutr, Vol. 29, No. 5, (Nov 1999), pp. (546-550)

Buhner, S., Buning, C., Genschel, J., Kling, K., Herrmann, D., Dignass, A., Kuechler, I., Krueger, S., Schmidt, H.H. & Lochs, H. (2006). Genetic basis for increased intestinal permeability in families with Crohn's disease: role of CARD15 3020insC mutation? *Gut,* Vol. 55, No. 3, (Mar 2006), pp. (342-347)

Burdon, R.H. (1996). Control of cell proliferation by reactive oxygen species. *Biochem. Soc. Trans,* Vol. 24, No. 4, (Nov 1996), pp. (1028-1032)

Davies, K.J. (1987). Protein damage and degradation by oxygen radicals. I. General aspects. *J. Biol. Chem,* Vol. 262, No. 20, (Jul 1987), pp. (9895-9901)

Dolfini, E., Elli, L., Dasdia, T., Bufardeci, B., Colleoni, M.P., Costa, B., Floriani, I., Falini, M.L., Guerrieri, N., Forlani, F. & Bardella, M.T. (2002). *In vitro* cytotoxic effect of bread wheat gliadin on the LoVo human adenocarcinoma cell line. *Toxicol. In Vitro,* Vol. 16, No. 4, (Aug 2002), pp. (331-337)

Dolfini, E., Elli, L., Roncoroni, L., Costa, B., Colleoni, M.P., Lorusso, V., Ramponi, S., Braidotti, P., Ferrero, S., Falini, M.L. & Bardella, M.T. (2005). Damaging effects of gliadin on three-dimensional cell culture model. *World J. Gastroenterol.*, Vol. 11, No. 38, (Oct 2005), pp. (5973-5977)

Dryden, G.W. Jr., Deaciuc, I., Arteel, G. & McClain, CJ. (2005). Clinical implications of oxidative stress and antioxidant therapy. Curr. Gastroenterol. Re, Vol. 7, No. 4, (Aug 2005), pp. (308-316)

Dugas, B., Dugas, N., Conti, M., Calenda, A., Pino, P., Thomas, Y., Mazier, D. & Vouldoukis, I. (2003). Wheat gliadin promotes the interleukin-4-induced IgE production by normal human peripheral mononuclear cells through a redox-dependent mechanism. *Cytokine*, Vol. 21, No. 6, (Mar 2003), pp. (270-280)

Eaton, J.W. (1991). Catalases and peroxidases and glutathione and hydrogen peroxide: mysteries of the bestiary. *J. Lab. Clin. Med.*, Vol. 118, No. 1, (Jul 1991), pp. (3–4)

Egler, R.A., Fernandes, E., Rothermund, K., Sereika, S., de Souza-Pinto, N., Jaruga, P., Dizdaroglu, M. & Prochownik, E.V. (2005). Regulation of reactive oxygen species, DNA damage, and c-Myc function by peroxiredoxin 1. *Oncogene*, Vol. 24, No. 54, (Dec 2005), pp. (8038-8050)

Elli, L., Dolfini, E. & Bardella, M.T. (2003). Gliadin cytotoxicity and in vitro cell cultures. *Toxicol Lett.* Vol. 146, No. 1, (Dec 2003), pp. (1-8)

Elstner, E.F. (1987). Metabolism of activated oxygen species, In: *Biochemistry of plants, Vol. 11,* Davies, D.D. (ed.), pp. (253–315), Academic Press, London

Farinati, F., Cardin, R., Russo, V.M., Busatto, G., Franco, M. & Rugge, M. (2003). Helicobacter pylori CagA status, mucosal oxidative damage and gastritis phenotype: a potential pathway to cancer? *Helicobacter*, Vol. 8, No. 3, (Jun 2003), pp. (227-234)

Fries, W., Renda, M.C., Lo Presti, M.A,, Raso, A., Orlando, A., Oliva, L., Giofré, M.R., Maggio, A., Mattaliano, A., Macaluso, A. & Cottone, M. (2005). Intestinal permeability and genetic determinants in patients, first-degree relatives, and controls in a high-incidence area of Crohn's disease in Southern Italy. *Am. J. Gastroenterol*, Vol. 100, No. 12, (Dec 2005), pp. (2730-2736)

Goerres, M., Roelofs, H.M., Jansen, J.B. & Peters, W.H. (2006). Deficient UDP-glucuronosyltransferase detoxification enzyme activity in the small intestinal mucosa of patients with coeliac disease. Aliment. Pharmacol. Ther., Vol. 23, No. 2, (Jan 2006), pp. (243-246)

Gotoh, Y., Nodam T., Iwakiri, R., Fujimoto, K., Rhoads, C.A. & Aw, T.Y. (2002). Lipid peroxide-induced redox imbalance differentially mediates CaCo-2 cell proliferation and growth arrest. *Cell Prolif.*, Vol. 35, No. 4, (Aug 2002), pp. (221-235)

Gressier, B., Lebegue, S., Brunet, C., Luyckx, M., Dine, T., Cazin, M. & Cazin, J.C.(1994). Pro-oxidant properties of methotrexate: evaluation and prevention by an anti-oxidant drug. *Pharmazie*, Vol. 49, No. 9, (Sep 1994), pp. (679-681)

Grisham, M.B., Ware, K., Marshall, S., Yamada, T. & Sandhu, I.S. (1992). Prooxidant properties of 5-aminosalicylic acid. Possible mechanism for its adverse side effects. *Dig. Dis. Sci*, Vol. 37, No. 9, (Sep 1992), pp. (1383-1389)

Halliwell, B. & Gutteridge, J.M.C. (1989). *Free radicals in Biology and Medicine,* Claredon Press, Oxford

Halliwell, B. (1991). Reactive oxygen species in living systems: source, biochemistry, and role in human disease. *Am. J. Med,* Vol. 91, No. 3C, (Sep 1991), pp. (14-22)

Hendrickson, B.A., Gokhale, R. & Cho, J.H. (2002). Clinical aspects and pathophysiology of inflammatory bowel disease. Clin. Microbiol. Rev, Vol. 15, No. 1, (Jan 2002), pp. (79-94)

Iatropoulos, M.J. (1986). Morphology of the gastrointestinal tract, In: *Gastrointestinal toxicology* , Rozman, K. & Hannenen, O. (Eds.), pp. (246-266), Elsevier, Amsterdam

Imai, H. & Nakagawa, Y. (2003). Biological significance of phospholipid hydroperoxide glutathione peroxidase (PHGPx, GPx4) in mammalian cells. *Free Radic. Biol Med.,* Vol. 34, No. 2, (Jan 2003), pp. (145-169)

Jones, D.P., Carlson, J.L., Mody, V.C., Cai, J., Lynn, M.J. & Sternberg, P. (2000). Redox state of glutathione in human plasma. *Free Radic. Biol. Med,* Vol. 28, No. 4, (Feb 2000), pp. (625-635)

Koch, T.R., Schulte-Bockholt, A., Otterson, M.F., Telford, G.L., Stryker, S.J., Ballard, T. & Opara, E.C. (1996). Decreased vasoactive intestinal peptide levels and glutathione depletion in acquired megacolon. *Dig. Dis. Sci,*Vol. 41, No. 7, (Jul 1996), pp. (1409-1416)

Kroemer, G., Dallaporta, B. & Resche-Rigon, M. 1998: The mitochondrial death/life regulator in apoptosis and necrosis. *Annu. Rev. Physiol,* Vol. 60, (1998), pp. (619-642)

LeGrand, T.S. & Aw, T.Y. (2001). Intestinal absorption of lipid hydroperoxides, In: *Intestinal lipid metabolism,* Mansbach, C., Kuksis, A. & Tso, P. (Eds.), pp. (351-366), Plenum Publishing Corporation, New York

Lenton, K.J., Sané, A.T., Therriault, H., Cantin, A.M., Payette, H. &, Wagner, J.R. (2003). Vitamin C augments lymphocyte glutathione in subjects with ascorbate deficiency. Am. J. Clin. Nutr., Vol. 77, No. 1, (Jan 2003), pp. (189-195)

Lloyd, B., Robson, E., Smith, I. & Clayton, B.E. (1989). Blood selenium concentrations and glutathione peroxidase activity. *Arch. Dis. Child.,* Vol. 64, No. 3, (Mar 1989), (352-356)

Maiuri MC, De Stefano D, Mele G, Iovine B, Bevilacqua MA, Greco L, Auricchio S, Carnuccio, R. (2003). Gliadin increases iNOS gene expression in interferon-gamma-stimulated RAW 264.7 cells through a mechanism involving NF-kappa B. *Naunyn Schmiedebergs Arch. Pharmacol.* Vol. 368, No. 1, (Jul 2003), (63-71)

Marsh, M.N. & Crowe, P.T. (1995). Morphology of the mucosdal lesion in gluten sensitivity. Baillieres Clin. Gastroenterol, Vol. 9, No. 2, (Jun 1995), pp. (273-293)

Mårtensson, J., Jain, A. & Meister, A. (1990). Glutathione is required for intestinal function. *Proc. Natl. Acad. Sci. U S A.,* Vol. 87, No. 5, (Mar 1990), pp. (1715-1719)

McKenzie, R.L., Rea, H.M., Thomson, C.D. & Robinson, M.F. (1978). Selenium concentration and glutathione peroxidase activity in blood of New Zealand infants and children. *Am. J. Clin. Nutr.,* Vol. 31, No. 8, (Aug 1978), pp. (1413-1418)

Meyer, C.T., Brand, M., DeLuca, V.A. & Spiro, H.M. (1981). Hydrogen peroxide colitis: a report of three patients. *J. Clin. Gastroenterol,* Vol. 3, No. 1, (Mar 1981), pp. (31-35)

Mignotte, B. & Vayssiere, J.L. (1998). Mitochondria and apoptosis. *Eur. J. Biochem,* Vol. 252, No. 1, (Feb 1998), pp. (1-15)

Murray, I.A., Bullimore, D.W. & Long, R.G. (2003). Fasting plasma nitric oxide products in coeliac disease. *Eur. J. Gastroenterol. Hepatol.,* Vol. 15, No. 10, (Oct 2003), pp. (1091-1095)

Oberhuber, G., Granditsch, G. & Vogelsang, H. (1999). The histopathology of coeliac disease: time for a standardized report scheme for pathologists. *Eur. J. Gastroenterol. Hepatol,* Vol. 11, No. 10, (Oct 1999), pp. (1185-1194)

Odetti, P., Valentini, S., Aragno, I., Garibaldi, S., Pronzato, M.A., Rolandi, E. & Barreca, T. (1998). Oxidative stress in subjects affected by celiac disease. *Free Radic. Res,* Vol. 29, No. 1, (Jul 1998), pp. (17-24)

Opara, E.C., (2003). Oxidative stress, In: *Colonic Diseases,* Koch, T.R. (ed.), pp. (179-189), Humana Press, Totowa NJ

Otamiri, T. & Sjödahl, R. (1991). Oxygen radicals: their role in selected gastrointestinal disorders. *Dig. Dis,* Vol. 9. No. 3, (n.d. 1991), pp. (133-141)

Pickett, J.P., Pendergrass, R.E., Bradford, W.D. & Elchlepp, J.G. (1970). Localization of xanthine oxidase in rat duodenum; fixation of sections instead of blocks. Stain. Technol. Vol. 45, No. 1, (Jan 1970), pp. (35-36)

Rao, R.K., Baker, R.D., Baker, S.S., Gupta, A. & Holycross, M. (1997). Oxidant-induced disruption of intestinal epithelial barrier function: role of protein tyrosine phosphorylation. *Am. J. Physiol,* Vol. 273, No. 4 Pt 1, (Oct 1997), pp. (812-823)

Reddy, K. & Tappel, A.L. (1974). Effect of dietary selenium and autoxidized lipids on the glutathione peroxidase system of gastrointestinal tract and other tissues in the rat. *J. Nutr.,* Vol. 104, No. 8, (Aug 1974), pp. (1069-1078)

Rezaie, A., Ghorbani, F., Eshghtork, A., Zamani ,M.J., Dehghan, G., Taghavi, B., Nikfar, S., Mohammadirad, A., Daryani, N.E. & Abdollahi, M. (2006). Alterations in salivary antioxidants, nitric oxide, and transforming growth factor-beta 1 in relation to disease activity in Crohn's disease patients. Ann. N. Y. Acad. Sci, No. 1091, (Dec 2006), pp. (110-122)

Rezaie, A., Parker, R.D. & Abdollahi, M. (2007). Oxidative stress and pathogenesis of inflammatory bowel disease: an epiphenomenon or the cause? Dig. Dis. Sci, Vol. 52, No. 9, (Sep 2007), pp. (2015-2021)

Riedle, B. & Kerjaschki, D. (1997). Reactive oxygen species cause direct damage of Engelbreth-Holm-Swarm matrix. Am. J. Pathol, Vol. 151, No. 1, (Jul 1997), pp. (215-231)

Rivabene, R., Mancini, E. & De Vincenzi, M. (1999). *In vitro* cytotoxic effect of wheat gliadin-derived peptides on the Caco-2 intestinal cell line is associated with intracellular oxidative imbalance: implications for coeliac disease. Biochim. Biophys. Acta, Vol. 1453, No. 1, (Jan 1999), pp. (152-160)

Sarnesto, A., Linder, N. & Raivio, K.O. (1996). Organ distribution and molecular forms of human xanthine dehydrogenase/xanthine oxidase protein. *Lab. Invest.* Vol. 74, No. 1, (Jan 1996), pp. (48-56)

Spencer, H.L., Daniels, I., Shortland, J., Long, R.G.& Murray, I.A. (2004). Effect of a gluten-free diet on plasma nitric oxide products in coeliac disease. *Scand. J. Gastroenterol.*, Vol. 39, No. 10, (Oct 2004), (941-945)

Spiteller, G. (2007). The important role of lipid peroxidation processes in aging and age dependent diseases. *Mol. Biotechnol*, Vol. 37, No. 1, (Sep 2007), pp. (5-12)

Ståhlberg, M.R. & Hietanen, E. (1991). Glutathione and glutathione-metabolizing enzymes in the erythrocytes of healthy children and in children with insulin-dependent diabetes mellitus, juvenile rheumatoid arthritis, coeliac disease and acute lymphoblastic leukaemia. *Scand. J. Clin. Lab. Invest*, Vol. 51, No. 2, (Apr 1991), pp. (125-130)

Ståhlberg, M.R., Hietanen, E. & Mäki, M. (1988). Mucosal biotransformation rates in the small intestine of children. *Gut*, Vol. 29, No. 8, (Aug 1988), pp. (1058-1063)

Stazi, A.V. & Trinti, B. (2010). Selenium status and over-expression of interleukin-15 in celiac disease and autoimmune thyroid diseases. *Ann. Ist. Super. Sanita*, Vol. 46, No. 4, (n.d. 2010), pp. (389-399)

Stojiljković, V., Todorović, A., Pejić, S., Kasapović, J., Saičić, Z.S., Radlović, N. & Pajović, S.B. (2009). Antioxidant status and lipid peroxidation in small intestinal mucosa of children with celiac disease. *Clin. Biochem.*, Vol. 42, No. 13-14, (Sep 2009), pp. (1431-1437)

Stojiljković, V., Todorović, A., Radlović, N., Pejić, S., Mladenović, M., Kasapovi, J. & Pajović, S.B. (2007). Antioxidant enzymes, glutathione and lipid peroxidation in peripheral blood of children affected by coeliac disease. *Ann. Clin. Biochem*, Vol. 44, No. Pt 6, (Nov 2007), pp. (537-543)

Thannickal, V.J. & Fanburg, B.L. (2000). Reactive oxygen species in cell signaling. *Am. J. Physiol. Lung Cell Mol. Physiol*, Vol. 279, N0. 6, (Dec 2000), pp. (1005-1028)

Tucková, L., Novotná, J., Novák, P., Flegelová, Z., Kveton, T., Jelínková, L., Zídek, Z., Man, P. & Tlaskalová-Hogenová, H. (2002). Activation of macrophages by gliadin fragments: isolation and characterization of active peptide. J. Leukoc. Biol, Vol. 71, No. 4, (Apr 2002), pp. (625-631)

Valko, M., Izakovic, M., Mazur, M., Rhodes, C.J. & Telser, J. (2004). Role of oxygen radicals in DNA damage and cancer incidence. *Mol. Cell Biochem*, Vol. 266, No. 1-2, (Nov 2004), pp. (37-56)

Vilas, N.N., Bell, R.R. & Draper, H.H. (1976). Influence of dietary peroxides, selenium and vitamin E on glutathione peroxidase of the gastrointestinal tract. J. Nutr,. Vol. 106, No. 5, (May 1976), pp. (589-596)

Wahab, P.J., Peters, W.H., Roelofs, H.M. & Jansen, J.B. (2001). Glutathione S-transferases in small intestinal mucosa of patients with coeliac disease. Jpn. J. Cancer Res., Vol. 92, No. 3, (Mar 2001), pp. (279-284)

Walker-Smith, J.A. (1990). Revised criteria for diagnosis of coeliac disease. Report of Working Group of European Society of Paediatric Gastroenterology and Nutrition. *Arch. Dis Child*, Vol. 65, No. 8, (Aug 1990), pp. (909-911)

Wang, T.G., Gotoh, Y., Jennings, M.H., Rhoads, C.A. & Aw, T.Y. (2000). Lipid hydroperoxide-induced apoptosis in human colonic CaCo-2 cells is associated with an early loss of cellular redox balance. FASEB J., Vol. 14, No. 11, (Aug 2000), pp. (1567-1576)

Wijeratne, S.S. & Cuppett, S.L. (2006). Lipid hydroperoxide induced oxidative stress damage and antioxidant enzyme response in Caco-2 human colon cells. *J. Agric. Food Chem.*, Vol. 54, No. 12, (Jun 2006), pp. (4476-4481)

Yüce, A., Demir, H., Temizel, I.N. & Koçak, N. (2004). Serum carnitine and selenium levels in children with celiac disease. *Indian J. Gastroenterol.*, Vol. 23, No. 3, (May-Jun 2004), pp. (87-88)

Section 2

Clinical Manifestations and Complications of Celiac Disease

4

Hematologic Manifestations of Celiac Disease

Peter Kruzliak[1,2]

[1] 5th Department of Internal Medicine,
University Hospital and Medical Faculty of Comenius University
[2]Department of Physiology and Pathophysiology of the Slovak academy of Sciences
Bratislava,
Slovakia

1. Introduction

Celiac disease is a systemic disease, which is associated with a number of hematologic manifestations. Individuals can present with hematological abnormalities even prior to the diagnosis of celiac disease. Anemia secondary to iron, folic acid and vitamin B12 malabsorption is a common complication of celiac disease. Patients can also present with thrombocytosis, thrombocytopenia, leukopenia, venous thromboembolism, hyposplenism and IgA deficiency. Celiac disease also predisposes to lymphoma development. The highest risk is for enteropathy associated T-cell lymphoma (EATL), an aggressive lymphoma with poor prognosis, however an increased risk for B-cell lymphomas and extraintestinal lymphomas has been described. Strict adherence to a gluten-free diet is known to decrease the risk of lymphomas.

2. Anemia

Anemia is a frequent finding in patients with celiac disease (CD) and may be the presenting feature. It may also be the only abnormality identified. Anemia was particularly common in patients with untreated CD in the past, but it is still frequently encountered in undiagnosed adults.1,2,3,4 The etiology of anemia in celiac disease is multifactorial. The anemia is usually hypoproliferative, reflecting impaired absorption of essential nutrients like iron and various vitamins. In prior studies, the overall prevalence of anemia at the time of diagnosis of celiac disease has been estimated between 12 and 69%. 5,6,7 Anemias caused by hemolysis are very rarely reported in celiac disease patients. Ivanovski et al. reported an 11-year old girl with untreated celiac disease who had hemolytic anemia and suggested that CD should be serologically screened in patient's with Coombs negative "immune" hemolytic anemia. As in this case the anemia improved after initiating a gluten free diet. 8

2.1 Mechanisms of anemia in celiac disease

A number of causative factors deserve consideration for explaining the mechanism of anemia in celiac disease.

2.1.1 Abnormal iron absorption

The most obvious cause of anemia in celiac disease is impaired absorption of iron and other nutrients including folate and cobalamin. Iron is absorbed in the proximal small intestine and the absorption is dependent upon several factors, including an intact mucosal surface and intestinal acidity.9 Villous atrophy of the intestinal mucosa is an important cause of abnormal iron absorption, which is reflected as laboratory evidence of iron deficiency anemia (IDA) in most anemic patients with celiac diasease. Abnormal iron absorption is also supported by the failure to increase serum iron levels following oral iron loading and refractoriness to oral iron treatment. 1,2,3

2.1.2 Increased blood loss

Occult gastrointestinal blood loss was detected in about half the patients with celiac disease in one study, and this finding appeared to correlate with the severity of villous atrophy. 16 An important limitation of that study was the use of an indirect (guaiac) test for detecting bleeding. In a subsequent study employing 51 Cr radiolabeled red blood cells, a daily blood loss exceeding 1.5 mL was detected in only one of 18 subjects studied. Others have also found that the rate of positive occult blood tests in celiac disease is low and does not exceed that in the general population. Thus, the evidence supporting increased fecal blood loss in celiac disease remains controversial, and although abnormal intestinal bleeding may occur in some celiac patients, it does not appear to play a significant role in the causation of anemia. 1,16

2.1.3 Abnormal vitamin absorption

The anemia seen in celiac disease can also result from malabsorption of various micronutrients necessary for normal hematopoiesis. Sideropenia, vitamine B12 and folat acide deficiency has been described in patients with celiac disease. 1, 39, 52 Copper deficiency has been described in adults and children with CD and may result in anemia and thrombocytopenia. 17, 18 Deficiencies in vitamin B6, pantothenic acid, and riboflavin have also been suggested as etiologic factors in patients with CD but recent data are lacking.1

2.1.4 Inflammation

Pro-inflammatory cytokines play an essential role in the inflammatory and cytotoxic mechanisms involved in the pathogenesis of celiac disease. Such cytokines, in particular interferon- γ (IFN-γ), and IL6, are powerful mediators of hypoferremia in inflammation inducing the synthesis of the iron regulatory hormone hepcidin.15, 19, 20, 22 Increased hepcidin synthesis in turn is responsible for increased ferroportin degradation and the inhibition of iron release from macrophages and enterocytes leading to the well known abnormalities in iron homeostasis associated with anemia of chronic disease (ACD). 19

2.2 Iron-deficiency anemia

Iron-deficiency anemia (IDA) is the most commonly encountered anemia in humans and is usually due to either increased iron loss or impaired absorption of iron.23 Iron-deficiency anemia is frequently seen in patients with celiac disease and can be found even in the absence of diarrhea or steatorrhea. IDA has been reported in up to 46% of cases of subclinical CD, with a higher prevalence in adults than children.3, 9 Iron deficiency has also been reported in patients with dermatitis herpetiformis. 10 IDA usually manifests as microcytic, hypochromic anemia and patients characteristically have low serum iron levels, elevated total iron-binding capacity, and low ferritin levels. 9, 11 Measurements of soluble transferrin receptors (sTfRs) can also be valuable in the evaluation of IDA, and the ratio of sTfR to ferritin may indicate CD in children with refractory IDA.12 Iron deficiency that is refractory to therapy can be the sole manifestation of CD, especially in pediatric patients and the prevalence of CD in patients with refractory IDA may be as high as 20%13, 14, 15. Fayed et al. reported that refractory IDA may be due to clinically unapparent CD in children. They recommended treatment with a gluten-free diet rich in iron and suggested that early detection and treatment of IDA with prophylactic iron and folic acid supplementation would go a long way in preserving good mental and psychological functions. 35 Patients with anemia had low levels of erythropoietin for the degree of anemia and increased serum interferon-gamma.This study supported the hypothesis that anemia in celiac disease is multifactorial in etiology and suppression of intestinal inflammatory changes as a result of a gluten-free diet improves anemia by correcting iron and vitamin malabsorption as well as mechanisms contributing to anemia of chronic disease. 19, 20

The prevalence of celiac disease in patients presenting with iron-deficiency anemia ranges from 0 to 8.7%. 23, 24, 25, 26, 27, 28 In a study conducted in Italy, anemic patients were screened for celiac disease using antigliadin and antiendomysial antibodies. 14 Jejunal biopsies were obtained from patients with positive serology. The prevalence of celiac disease was 5% in all patients with anemia and 8.5% in those with iron-deficiency anemia. 23 In a study conducted in the United Kingdom, 115 patients with iron deficiency anemia were assessed with esophagogastroduodenoscopy, flexible sigmoidoscopy, and barium enema; 2.6% of these patients had celiac disease. However, fewer than half of the patients underwent a small bowel biopsy, and hence the true prevalence of celiac disease might have been underestimated. Of interest, however, the three patients with celiac disease had normal appearing mucosa on small bowel endoscopy. 25 In two studies, biopsies were performed on the patients with positive serology, and the prevalence of biopsy-proven CD was 2.3% to 4.7%. 25, 27 Iron deficiency in celiac disease primarily results from impaired absorption of iron but there may also be occult blood loss in the gastrointestinal (GI) tract. 31, 32 Occult gastrointestinal bleeding was detected in 25% to 54% of patients with CD, depending on the degree of villous atrophy, in 1 study. 16 Occult GI blood loss was seen in 26.7% of children with CD that appeared to respond to treatment with a gluten-free diet (GFD), according to another study. 33 More-recent studies have, however, suggested that occult GI bleeding in patients with CD may be much less common. 34, 35 Biopsy-proven CD was reported in 2.6% to 5% of patients. 23, 28 Three other studies included patients with anemia other than IDA but the vast majority in all 3 studies suffered from IDA. 25, 29, 30 Serologic evidence of CD was observed in 2.3% to 10.9% of these anemic patients. In 2 of the studies, biopsies were performed on the patients with positive serology, and the prevalence of biopsy-proven CD was 2.3% to 4.7%. 25, 30 One of the studies suggested that history of chronic diarrhea predicted CD as the cause for the anemia. 36 Clinicians should consider CD as a possible cause of anemia in all subjects with unexplained IDA, including menstruating women. Endoscopic markers of CD in patients with IDA have been shown to lack sensitivity for diagnosis and have limited utility in selecting patients for a small-bowel biopsy. 38 biopsies should be performed even if the duodenal mucosa appears normal to the endoscopist. One recent study has shown that many patients undergoing an endoscopy for anemia do in fact not have a small-bowel biopsy performed.39 In conclusion, IDA is common in CD, and CD is frequently found in patients presenting with IDA. The treatment of IDA associated with CD is primarily a GFD and iron supplementation until the iron stores have been restored.

2.2.1 Folate deficiency

Folic acid is an element essential for amino acid and nucleic acid metabolism. Adequate folic acid is required for normal hematopoiesis and development of the nervous system. 40 Folic acid is primarily absorbed in the jejunum, and malabsorption is frequent in diseases of the small intestine. 40, 41 Deficiency of folic acid usually presents as macrocytic or megaloblastic anemia, but abnormalities of other cell lineages are common. Concomitant iron deficiency as seen in CD can result in atypical findings on the blood smear, and patients with deficiencies of folate and vitamin B12 may not present with the characteristic macrocytosis. Examination of the blood smear may reveal a dimorphic picture reflecting the effects of both deficiencies. Severe folic-acid deficiency can result in a decrease in both leukocytes and platelets and even manifest as severe pancytopenia. The diagnosis is usually made by measuring serum folate and red-cell folate levels. Serum folate is highly dependent on folate intake and is frequently increased in patients with deficiency of vitamin B12. Red-cell folate is not specific for folate deficiency, as it can be decreased in patients with vitamin B12 deficiency, but red-cell folate is less subject to transient changes secondary to variations in folate intake. 41 Elevated serum homocysteine levels can be helpful in diagnosing folate deficiency but the sensitivity of serum homocysteine is somewhat less for vitamin B12 deficiency. 43, 44 Previous studies have shown that many untreated patients with CD are folate deficient. 45Two small studies found that folate deficiency is a common finding in children, but it does not usually result in anemia. 46, 47 More-recent studies have confirmed that folic-acid deficiency continues to be a frequent finding in subjects with newly diagnosed CD and can be observed even in adolescents and young adults with CD detected by screening. 30, 48, 49 Folate deficiency has also been reported in association with dermatitis herpetiformis. 50, 51 Homocysteine levels are commonly elevated in CD patients at the time of diagnosis and may serve as a diagnostic clue. 52

2.2.2 Vitamin B12 deficiency

Vitamin B12 is an essential cofactor and a coenzyme in multiple biochemical pathways, including the pathways of DNA and methionine synthesis. While the main site of vitamin B12 absorption is the distal ileum (where it is absorbed bound to intrinsic factor), a small proportion is also absorbed passively along the entire small bowel. 53 Although celiac disease has been considered a disorder of the proximal small bowel, associated vitamin B12 deficiency has been reported. Deficiency of vitamin B12 is common in CD and frequently results in anemia. Malabsorption of vitamin B12 resulting in anemia has also been described in patients with dermatitis herpetiformis (DH). 54 Dickey et al. in their study reported, that of 159 patients, 13 had low serum B12 at diagnosis. A further six had been receiving B12 replacement therapy for 3-37 years before diagnosis, giving an overall prevalence of 12% (19 patients). Only 2 of 19 patients had gastric corpus atrophy, one with intrinsic factor antibodies and the other with hypergastrinaemia. There was no relationship between low B12 levels and clinical characteristics. 55 The cause of vitamin B12 deficiency in CD is unclear. It may include decreased gastric acid, bacterial overgrowth, autoimmune gastritis, decreased efficiency of mixing with transfer factors in the intestine, or perhaps dysfunction (inflammation) of the distal small intestine. 56, 57 Recent studies suggested that 8% to 41% of previously untreated subjects with CD were deficient in vitamin B12. 58, 59 Bode et al. In their study reported an 11% incidence of vitamin B12 deficiency in 50 consecutively diagnosed patients with CD. 60

Measurements of vitamin B12 levels can be misleading and difficult to interpret, especially if the results fall within the lower range of normal or if there is a coexisting deficiency of folic acid. 61 Patients with vitamin B12 deficiency should receive therapy with parenteral vitamin B12. Even though studies have suggested that oral vitamin B12 may be as effective as parenteral vitamin B12, no such studies have been performed in patients with vitamin B12 deficiency secondary to CD. 62

2.2.3 Anemia of chronic disease

In a study focusing on the clinical features of anemia in celiac disease, Harper et al. noted that although serum ferritin levels were indicative of iron deficiency in the majority of anemic subjects, unexpectedly, in 13% of patients ferritin levels were increased. Because a gluten-free diet resulted in increased serum ferritin in iron-deficient patients, but decreased ferritin levels in those with previously high ferritins, they concluded that nutritional deficiencies alone do not explain anemia in all cases, and that inflammation appears to contribute in some individuals, as evidenced by the presence of anemia of chronic disease (ACD). In a recent study, Bergamaschi et al. decided to focus on the role of anemia of chronic disease in the development of anemia among patients with celiac disease. A peculiar feature in the design of this study was the use of refined precision instruments to identify anemia of inflammation. At the outset, and in a follow-up period of one year on a gluten-free diet, they collected data on serum iron, transferrin, serum ferritin, soluble transferrin receptor (sTfRc), endogenous erythropoietin (Epo) and IFN-γ. Among 65 anemic celiac patients, 45 had uncomplicated iron deficiency anemia, and 2 had cobalamin or folate deficiency. In 11 subjects, anemia of chronic disease alone or in combination with iron deficiency was identified, a prevalence of 17%. To increase the sensitivity and specificity of these blood tests, Bergamaschi et al. employed not only primary data but a combination of findings: (a) the sTfRc/log (ferritin) ratio that increases in iron deficiency and decreases in ACD, (b) the ferritin/transferrin ratio that decreases in iron deficiency and increases in ACD, and (c) the log(Epo) O/P ratio that describes the increase in endogenous serum EPO in proportion to the severity of anemia, a response known to be normal in iron deficiency anemia but blunted in the anemia of chronic disease. Compared with a group of 30 non-anemic celiac subjects, 45 of the celiac patients had findings typical of iron deficiency anemia. However, in 11 the findings indicated anemia of chronic disease with decreased sTfRc/log(ferritin), increased ferritin/transferrin ratio, and a decreased log(Epo) O/P ratio implying a blunted EPO response. Remarkably, serum IFN-γ levels in ACD were 12-fold higher than controls, but even in the iron deficient group they were increased 3-fold, indicating that some degree of inflammation might have been present in all anemic celiac patients. Hepcidin is an important indicator of ACD. By contrast, correlation of iron status with hepcidin is limited. The use of a pro-hepcidin assay instead of direct hepcidin measurements could explain the failure to demonstrate significant differences in prohepcidin levels among the three groups in the above study. In the Bergamaschi et al. study the response to a gluten free diet after one year was favorable in both, the IDA and ACD subjects, indicating that the suppression of intestinal inflammation by a gluten-free diet can improve anemia both by correcting iron and vitamin malabsorption as well as by abolishing the mechanisms responsible for anemia attributable to inflammation. 15, 19, 20, 22

3. Leukopenia

Fisgin et al. reported leukopenia and anemia in a few children with celiac disease as the first sign of disease. 63 Deficiencies of both folate and copper have been implicated as the possible etiology of leukopenia. The data on treatment of these patients are extremely limited but initiating a GFD and dietary supplementation with oral copper sulfate if there is evidence of copper deficiency, can improve the white blood count. 64, 65, 66

4. Thrombocytopenia and thrombocytosis

Thrombocytopenia has rarely been reported in patients with CD and it may have an autoimmune etiology. It has been reported in case reports in association with with keratoconjunctivitis and choroidopathy, suggesting an autoimmune pathophysiology. 67 Therapy for thrombocytopenia in association with CD is unclear, but GFD may result in normalization of the platelet count in some cases. 67-69 Thrombocytosis in association with CD appears to be more common than thrombocytopenia, occurring in up to 60% ofpatients. 70-72 The etiology of thrombocytosis associated with celiac disease is unknown, but it may be secondary to elevations in inflammatory mediators, autoimmune processes or, in some cases, secondary to iron-deficiency anemia or functional hyposplenism. 71, 72 Dupond et al. reported that in 14 of 23 patients with celiac disease thrombocytosis was present and it was unrelated to iron deficiency or an inflammatory syndrome. Among patients with thrombocytosis, 6 had an associated autoimmune disease, but this association was absent in patients without thrombocytosis. 73

Thrombocytosis might probably be useful in the assessment of patients with celiac disease and reflect enhanced disease activity. Moreover, the presence of thrombocytes in these patients' blood may indicate an associated autoimmune disease. Thrombocytosis may resolve after institution of a GFD. 71, 74 Caroccio et al., described an elderly woman hospitalized for extreme thrombocytosis associated with severe anaemia who was diagnosed with celiac disease. 72 They suggested, that celiac disease should be considered in addition to myeloproliferative disorders or other neoplastic conditions in an elderly patient when extreme thrombocytosis and severe anaemia is detected.

5. Venous and arterial thromboembolism

Ramagopalan et al. postulated in their study that men with celiac disease have a higher risk of thromboembolism. 82 Ludvigsson et al. in their study found a significant association between celiac disease and venous thromboembolism and they reported that venous thromboembolism may be the first clinical sign of celiac disease 83 Though celiac disease is not classically thought to predispose to thrombosis, there are several pathophysiological mechanisms that have been noted in celiac disease that may contribute to the development of a potentially prothrombotic state. 83 Cassela et al. in their study showed that hyperhomocysteinemia is relatively frequent in patients with CD, being present in about 20% of the patients in their series. 84 Hyperhomocysteinemia might represent a link between undiagnosed celiac disease and thromboembolism. Hyperhomocysteinemia may be due to genetic factors, with cystathionine beta synthetasis deficiency being considered the most common genetic cause, or from acquired folate and vitamine B12 deficiencies (83, 84). Homozygous deficiency of N5-N10-methyl tetrahydrofolate reductase, the vitamin B12 dependent enzyme required for remethylation of homocysteine to methionine, may cause hyperhomocysteinemia, and this condition is more problematic to manage compared to cystathionine beta synthetasis deficiency, as there is currently no effective therapy 81. Moreover, treatment with a gluten-free diet and folic acid in patients with celiac disease and N5-N10-methyl tetrahydrofolate reductase variants does not consistently improve hyperhomocysteinemia. Thus, celiac disease might lead to increased cardiovascular events due to secondary hyperhomocysteinemia, further aggravated by the possible presence of genetic abnormalities responsible for hyperhomocysteinemia. 81, 84 Hypofibrinolysis has been proposed as another possible cause of thrombosis in patients with celiac disease. Thrombin-activatable fibrinolysis inhibitor (TAFI) is a major inhibitor of fibrinolysis. Increased plasma TAFI levels are associated with a risk for venous thromboembolism. TAFI plasma levels are increased in patients with celiac disease and might contribute to the risk of thromboembolism in these patients. 75, 76, 78, 80 Decreased levels of the K vitamin-dependent anticoagulant proteins, protein S and C, have recently been suggested as a causative factor of thrombosis associated with celiac disease too. 77 Antiphospholipid syndrome is characterized by arterial and venous thrombosis, and its association with celiac disease has been described in a few cases. 85 The clinical spectrum of thromboembolism observed in patients with celiac disease is variable, but most cases appear to involve the venous circulation and resulting in deep vein thrombosis, pulmonary embolism, Budd-Chiari syndrome or splenic thrombosis. 79, 80, 81 Only a few case reports have described patients with arterial thrombosis, and in those cases the role of CD in predisposing to thrombosis is uncertain. 86, 87, 88 Moutawakil et al. Reported a case of a young male lacking typical gastrointestinal symptoms who presented with neurologic signs suggestive of an ischemic stroke. The mechanisms of vascular damage involving the CNS in celiac disease are controversial. The most widely incriminated factor is autoimmune vasculitis due to autoantibodies targeting tissue transglutaminase. Other mechanisms for e.g. vitamin deficiency are still debated,. 89

6. Coagulopathy

Untreated celiac disease may induce malabsorption of many nutrients, which may also induce vitamin K deficiency. CD can be associated with abnormalities in coagulation factors resulting in a bleeding diathesis. A decrease in K vitamin-dependent coagulation factors results in prolongation of coagulation assays or parameters such as the prothrombin time (PT), international normalized ratio (INR), and the activated partial thromboplastin time (aPTT). 90, 91 Cavalloro et al. found that the prevalence of prolonged PT is about 20% in a large series of untreated adult celiac patients, but a prolonged prothrombin time was only found in a few patients with subclinical celiac disease (0.9%). Symptomatic patients were also more likely to present with a prolonged PT. 92 Patients with CD occasionally present with a hemorrhagic disorder as their first symptom. The resulting hemorrhage can be minimal to severe. 95 Granel et al. described an interesting case of bilateral adrenal haemorrage in a patient with an hypocoagulable state due to untreated celiac disease. 93 Therapy is initially with parenteral vitamin K, but occasionally plasma products may be needed in actively bleeding patients. Malabsorption of vitamin K is uncommon in CD patients who do not have evidence of malabsorption of other nutrients. The treatment primarily consists of initiating a GFD and correcting the vitamin K deficiency. 90, 92, 94

7. IgA deficiency

Selective IgA deficiency, as defined by the total or severe deficiency of the IgA class of immunoglobulins in serum and secretions, is the most common immunodeficiency disorder. Studies suggest that 1 in every 500 people may have selective IgA deficiency. Even though a large number of individuals with selective IgA deficiency are relatively healthy, there are many affected with variety of disorders. These include recurrent sinopulmonary and gastronintestinal infections, allergies, and autoimmune disorders. 97, 99 The prevalence of IgA deficiency in patients with CD is 10 to 15 times higher than that in the general population. Approximately 2% to 3% of CD patients have IgA deficiency, and up to 8% of IgA-deficient individuals may have CD. 96, 97, 98 Patients with selective immunoglobulin (Ig) A deficiency have a 10- to 20-fold increased risk of celiac disease 99. Cataldo et al. reported that the clinical presentation of CD patients with selective IgA deficiency is different from that of patients with CD who have normal IgA levels, demonstrating a greater incidence of the silent form in the former. Because of the mild form of clinical presentation in IgA-deficient patients with CD, there may be a delay in recognizing such cases before appropriate GFD therapy can be instituted.96 The serum antibody markers that are currently used in the diagnosis of celiac disease are anti-AGA, ARA, EMA, and tTG antibodies. These serologic markers are highly sensitive and specific markers for CD, especially for IgA-based antibody tests. Because of the high prevalence of IgA deficiency in patients with CD, attention has been focused on the problem of diagnosing such individuals and the optimal testing strategy. IgA deficiency can lead to false-negative serology, as most of the existing serologic methods detect only IgA antibodies. The basic serologic test that can detect IgG antibodies related to CD is the AGA test. However, as the AGA IgG antibody test has limited specificity (76-80%), this test alone may not reliably establish a definitive diagnosis 99. Evaluating EMA IgG antibodies and anti-transglutaminase antibodies can be helpful for diagnosis of celiac disease with IgA deficiency. 99, 100, 101 Celiac disease patients with IgA-deficiency are prone to other enteric conditions such as inflammatory bowel disease or chronic parasitic infections, especially giardiasis, which could mimic CD. Secondly, patients with IgA deficiency are also at risk of developing anaphylactic transfusion reactions that may be life threatening if the recipient has anti-IgA antibodies. 96, 97, 99

8. Lymphoma

The association of CD and intestinal lymphoma is well known. 102 This association was first described in 1937 by Fairley and Mackie.116 Initially it was thought that the enteropathy and malabsorption that occurred was secondary to the lymphoma itself, a concept that persisted for many decades until it became apparent that CD often preceded the development of lymphoma. Later reports suggested that lymphomas involving the GI tract were relatively more common in CD patients and were a major cause of death. 100-105 Multiple studies now support the association of CD and lymphomas. 106-118

Patients with celiac disease have a 50- to a 100-fold increased risk of developing lymphoma compared with the general population Catassi et al. in their study found that celiac disease was diagnosed in 6 (0.92%) of 653 patients with lymphoma. The odds ratio (adjusted for age and sex) for non-Hodgkin lymphoma of any primary site associated with celiac disease was 3.1 for gut lymphoma, and 19.2 for T-cell lymphoma, respectively. The risk for non-Hodgkin lymphoma in this study was 0.63%. 102 The risk of developing an NHL as a complication of CD is not fully known, but recent epidemiologic studies suggest a relative risk ranging from 2.1 to 6.6.112, 113, 116, 117, 132, 133 The risk of contracting lymphoma in the setting of DH appears to be increased to a similar degree. 133, 134 Other studies have indicated that there may be a much higher risk, ranging from a 15-fold up to 100-fold increase. A recently published 30-year population-based study from Finland followed 1147 patients diagnosed with celiac disease or DH at a single medical center over 17 245 person-years. This study reported an standarized incidence ratio of 3.2 and 6.0 for developing NHL in patients diagnosed with CD or DH, respectively. This study provided further support to the theory that compliance with a GFD protects against the development of lymphoma in patients with CD. 131 Smedby et al. reported that celiac disease is associated with a doubled risk of NHL overall that was mainly attributed to a nearly 20-fold increased risk for T-cell lymphoma and to a nearly 3-fold increased risk for diffuse large B-cell lymphoma. There was a substantial and statistically significant, increased risk of gastrointestinal NHL and there was weak evidence for an increased risk for nongastrointestinal lymphoma. 116 A large population-based case-control study undertaken in both Denmark and Sweden assessed the risk of NHL in patients with a variety of autoimmune disorders, including CD. Participants including 3055 patients with NHL identified through a national hospital and tumor registries and 3187 matched controls were surveyed regarding a history of autoimmune disorders. Nineteen patients with NHL and 9 controls reported a previous diagnosis of CD. CD was associated with a doubled risk of NHL with an OR of 2.1. The odds ratio (OR) for diffuse large B-cell lymphoma (DLBCL) was 2.8 in contrast to an OR of 17 for T-cell lymphoma. Ten lymphomas were extranodal, including 5 involving the GI tract. The OR for gastrointestinal NHL was estimated to be 12 in comparison with an OR of 1.7 for non-gastrointestinal NHL.116 Many studies suggest that there may be a reduction of risk with long-term adherence to a GFD.106,107,110,111,113, 115 A GFD may also reduce the risk in patients with DH.135, 136 The benefit of a GFD may be slow in accruing in those who are diagnosed later in life.

In a study by Holmes et al. a two-fold relative risk (RR) of cancer was found, including an increased risk of cancer of the mouth and pharynx, oesophagus, and of non-Hodgkin lymphoma. 110 The risk was increased, however, in those taking a gluten containing diet and when celiac disease was diagnosed late in adulthood. A significant decreasing trend in the excess morbidity rate over increasing use of a gluten freed diet and early diagnosis was found. The findings of Holmes et al. are suggestive of a protective role for a GFD against malignancy in coeliac disease and give further support for advising all patients to adhere to a strict GFD for life. 110

8.1 Enteropathy-associated T-cell lymphoma

The association between CD and a specific type of intestinal T-cell non-Hodgkin lymphoma (NHL), called enteropathy-associated T-cell lymphoma (EATL), appears to be particularly strong, but overall these aggressive lymphomas are rare. EATLs are rare lymphomas accounting for less than 1% of all NHL.153 EATL appears to be more frequent in Europe, where it represents 9.4% of all peripheral T cell lymphomas. An sssociation between EATL and celiac disease is consistently demonstrated in only 30% of patients. The global incidence of this lymphoma is rare, being about 0.5 to 1 per million 119. EATL frequently presents as multifocal lymphoma with ulcerative lesions and commonly results in bowel perforation or other abdominal emergencies. 119, 120, 121 The neoplastic cells of EATL are thought to derive from clonal proliferations of phenotypically abnormal intraepithelial lymphocytes (IELs). 122, 123 In gluten-sensitive individuals with EATL, 68% are homozygotes for the DQB1*02 allele. Constant over-stimulation of intraepithelial T-cells eventually results in neoplastic growth. 129 Loss of CD8 expression by IELs is characteristic for early EATL also refereed to as refractory celiac disease type II. Cellier et al. reported that an immunophenotypically aberrant clonal intraepithelial T-cell population, similar to that observed in most cases of enteropathy-associated T-cell lymphoma, can be found in up to 75% of patients with refractory coeliac sprue. They suggested that refractory sprue associated with an aberrant clonal IEL population may be the missing link between celiac disease and EATL. 127 The IELs seen in refractory CD type II have been shown to express cytosolic CD3 (cCD3) and are monoclonal on analysis for T-cell receptor gene-rearrangements. 126, 127 Interleukin-15 is considered an important signaling molecule in driving the expansion of IELs. 128 The apperance of phenotypically aberrant monoclonal IELs seems to be the first step in the pathogenesis of ETL.123 The etiology of this increase in monoclonal IELs remains unknown, but it may be secondary to chromosomal gains or mutations of tumor-suppressor genes. EATL cells typically express CD3, CD7, and CD103, they may also express CD30, but are usually negative for CD4, CD5, and CD8. Sometimes the EATL cells lack CD3 expression. 123, 126 Immunostaining for CD3, CD8, and CD4 may be helpful for initial screening, but molecular-clonality analysis is required for confirmation in the cases suspected to have early, evolving or cryptic EATL.

EATL originates most often in the jejunum. A single or multiple sites within the jejunum may be involved with lymphoma. The large intestine and stomach are affected much less frequently. EATL rarely causes swollen peripheral lymph nodes that patients can feel. Patients will complain of abdominal pain, diarrhea, vomiting and gastronintestinal hemorrhage. Weight loss is also commonly reported. This is due to decreased absorption of nutrients, especially protein, in the small intestine. Fatigue may also be present due to anemia. As many as 40% of patients will present with acute abdominal symptoms, including lymphoma-mediated intestinal obstruction or perforation. This is a potentially life-threatening complication of EATL, requiring immediate surgery. Late in the course of EATL, the disease may spread to the liver, spleen and other organs. 136, 137, 138 Diagnosis of EATL can be complicated, as many more common disorders can cause abdominal symptoms. Most patients will be diagnosed while undergoing exploratory abdominal surgery, with a biopsy of the affected lymph nodes. Once the diagnosis of EATL is established, patients should undergo diagnostic tests to determine the extent of disease. This should include gastrofibroscopy, colonoscopy and enteroscopy, CT scans of the chest, abdomen and pelvis, a complete blood count, serum chemistries (including liver function tests, lactate dehydrogenase (LDH) and serum albumin) and a HIV test. Hepatitis B testing is also recommended due to reports of hepatitis reactivation during chemotherapy. A bone marrow biopsy is optional, as less than 10% of patients with EATL have involvement of this organ, but this may be an underestimate due to failure to recognize minimal disease. It is clear from recent studies, that the neoplastic cells are widespread even in the early stage of disease pathogenesis. 127 Finally, a baseline echocardiogram to evaluate heart function should be done prior to chemotherapy, as some drugs can damage the heart. The essentials for diagnosis of EATL include histopathology and immunochemical staining analysis. Therefore mentioned tests enhance the diagnostic yield and establish the stage of EATL for each patient. 136, 137, 139 Staging of EATL is as follows 139, 141:

- Stage I: One involved lymph node group
- Stage II: Two or more involved lymph node groups on the same side of the diaphragm
- Stage III: Multiple lymph node groups involved on both sides of the diaphragm
- Stage IV: Disseminated involvement of other extra-nodal sites, such as the liver or spleen

Therapy for CD-associated lymphoma is not different from the therapy used in similar lymphomas in patients without CD. However, the presence of CD may raise issues of malnutrition, an increased risk of infection due to concomitant hyposplenism, and increased likelihood of diarrhea or other consequences of CD 143. Combination chemotherapy is most frequently used, and the choice of regimen depends on the lineage of the lymphoma. B-cell lymphomas are usually treated with combinations such as CHOP (cyclophosphamide, doxorubicin, vincristine, and prednisone) with rituximab. T-cell–derived lymphomas have been more challenging to treat. Therapy of ETL currently remains unsatisfactory, with a 5-year survival ranging from 11% to 20% in 2 studies and a 2-year survival of 28% according to another study. 142, 143, 144 Survival of patients with T-cell intestinal lymphoma appears to be inferior to the survival of patients with intestinal B-cell lymphoma and patients with other types of peripheral T-cell lymphomas.140, 141, 142 A recent study reported stem cell transplantation in patients with EATL. Results suggested, that patients with novel therapy with IVE/MTX (ifosfamide, etoposide, epirubicin/methotrexate) and autologous stem cell transplantation had longer survival like patients with standard therapy withou stem cell transplantation. 145

9. References

[1] Hoffbrand AV. Anaemia in adult coeliac disease. Clin Gastroenterol 1974; 3:71-89
[2] Unsworth DJ, Lock FJ, Harvey RF. Iron-deficiency anaemia in premenopausal women. Lancet 1999; 353:1100.
[3] Bottaro G, Cataldo F, Rotolo N, Spina M, Corazza GR. The clinical pattern of subclinical/silent celiac disease: an analysis on 1026 consecutive cases. Am J Gastroenterol 1999; 94:691-696.
[4] Kolho KL, Farkkila MA, Savilahti E. Undiagnosed coeliac disease is common in Finnish adults. Scand J Gastroenterol 1998; 33:1280-1283.
[5] Hin H, Bird G, Fisher P, Mahy N, Jewell D. Coeliac disease in primary care: case finding study. BMJ 1999; 318:164-167.
[6] Gawkrodger DJ, Ferguson A, Barnetson RS. Nutritional status in patients with dermatitis herpetiformis. Am J Clin Nutr 1988; 48:355
[7] Kastrup W, Mobacken H, Stockbrugger R, Swolin B, Westin J. Malabsorption of vitamin B12 in dermatitis herpetiformis and its association with pernicious anaemia. Acta Med Scand; 1986 220:261-268.
[8] Ivanovski P, Nikolić D, Dimitrijević N, Ivanovski I, Perišić V. Erythrocytic transglutaminase inhibition hemolysis at presentation of celiac disease. World J Gastroenterol 2010 Nov 28;16(44):5647-50.
[9] Andrews NC. Disorders of iron metabolism and heme synthesis. In Greer JP, Foerster J, Lukens JN, Rodgers GM, Paraskevas F, Glader B (Eds.). Wintrobe's Clinical Hematology2004; 11th ed Philadelphia, PA Lippincott Williams & Wilkins Vol 1: pp. 979-1009.

[10] Kastrup W, Magnusson B, Mobacken H, Swolin B, Solvell L. Iron absorption in patients with dermatitis herpertiformis. Acta Derm Venereol 1977; 57:407–412.
[11] Cook JD. Diagnosis and management of iron-deficiency anaemia. Best Pract Res Clin Haematol 2005; 18:319–332.
[12] De Caterina M, Grimaldi E, Di Pascale G, et al. The soluble transferrin receptor (sTfR)-ferritin index is a potential predictor of celiac disease in children with refractory iron deficiency anemia. Clin Chem Lab Med 2005; 43:38–42.
[13] Economou M, Karyda S, Gombakis N, Tsatra J, Athanassiou-Metaxa M. Subclinical celiac disease in children: refractory iron deficiency as the sole presentation. J Pediatr Hematol Oncol 2004; 26:153–154
[14] Mody RJ, Brown PI, Wechsler DS. Refractory iron deficiency anemia as the primary clinical manifestation of celiac disease. J Pediatr Hematol Oncol 2003; 25:169–172.
[15] Carroccio A, Iannitto E, Cavataio F, et al. Sideropenic anemia and celiac disease: one study, two points of view. Dig Dis Sci 1998; 43:673–678.
[16] Fine KD. The prevalence of occult gastrointestinal bleeding in celiac sprue. N Engl J Med 1996;334:1163-7.
[17] Goyens P, Brasseur D, Cadranel S. Copper deficiency in infants with active celiac disease. J Pediatr Gastroenterol Nutr 1985; 4:677–680.
[18] Jameson S, Hellsing K, Magnusson S. Copper malabsorption in coeliac disease. Sci Total Environ 1985; 42:29–36.
[19] Weiss G, Goodnough LT. Anemia of chronic disease. N Engl J Med 2005;352:1011-23.
[20] Harper JW, Holleran SF, Ramakrishnan R, Bhagat G, Green PH. Anemia in celiac disease is multifactorial in etiology. Am J Hematol 2007;82:996-1000.
[21] Nemeth E, Rivera S, Gabayan V, Keller C, Taudorf S, Pedersen BK, et al. IL-6 mediates hypoferremia of inflammation by inducing the synthesis of the iron regulatory hormone hepcidin. J Clin Invest 2004 113:1271-6.
[22] Bergamaschi G, Markopoulos K, Albertini R, Di Sabatino A, Biagi F, Ciccocioppo R, et al. Anemia of chronic disease and defective erythropoietin production in patients with celiac disease. Haematologica 2008;93:1785-91
[23] Corazza GR, Valentini RA, Andreani ML, et al. Subclinical coeliac disease is a frequent cause of iron-deficiency anaemia. Scand J Gastroenterol 1995; 30:153–156.
[24] McIntyre AS and Long RG. Prospective survey of investigations in outpatients referred with iron deficiency anaemia. Gut 1993; 34:1102–1107.
[25] Ransford RA, Hayes M, Palmer M, Hall MJ. A controlled, prospective screening study of celiac disease presenting as iron deficiency anemia. J Clin Gastroenterol 2002; 35:228–233.
[26] Kepczyk T and Kadakia SC. Prospective evaluation of gastrointestinal tract in patients with iron-deficiency anemia. Dig Dis Sci 1995; 40:1283–1289.
[27] Bini EJ, Micale PL, Weinshel EH. Evaluation of the gastrointestinal tract in premenopausal women with iron deficiency anemia. Am J Med 1998; 105:281–286.
[28] Unsworth DJ, Lock RJ, Harvey RF. Improving the diagnosis of coeliac disease in anaemic women. Br J Haematol 2000; 111:898–901.
[29] Haslam N, Lock RJ, Unsworth DJ. Coeliac disease, anaemia and pregnancy. Clin Lab 2001; 47:467–469.
[30] Howard MR, Turnbull AJ, Morley P, Hollier P, Webb R, Clarke A. A prospective study of the prevalence of undiagnosed coeliac disease in laboratory defined iron and folate deficiency. J Clin Pathol 2002; 55:754–757.

[31] de Vizia B, Poggi V, Conenna R, Fiorillo A, Scippa L. Iron absorption and iron deficiency in infants and children with gastrointestinal diseases. J Pediatr Gastroenterol Nutr 1992; 14:21-26.
[32] Kosnai I, Kuitunen P, Siimes MA. Iron deficiency in children with coeliac disease on treatment with gluten-free diet: role of intestinal blood loss. Arch Dis Child 1979; 54:375-378.
[33] Shamir R, Levine A, Yalon-Hacohen M, et al. Faecal occult blood in children with coeliac disease. Eur J Pediatr 2000; 159:832-834.
[34] Logan RF, Howarth GF, West J, Shepherd K, Robinson MH, Hardcastle JD. How often is a positive faecal occult blood test the result of coeliac disease? Eur J Gastroenterol Hepatol 2003; 15:1097-1100.
[35] Mant MJ, Bain VG, Maguire CG, Murland K, Yacyshyn BR. Prevalence of occult gastrointestinal bleeding in celiac disease. Clin Gastroenterol Hepatol 2006; 4:451-454.
[36] Mandal AK, Mehdi I, Munshi SK, Lo TC. Value of routine duodenal biopsy in diagnosing coeliac disease in patients with iron deficiency anaemia. Postgrad Med J 2004; 80:475-477.
[37] Fayed SB, Aref MI, Fathy HM, Abd El Dayem SM, Emara NA, Maklof A, Shafik A. Prevalence of celiac disease, Helicobacter pylori and gastroesophageal reflux in patients with refractory iron deficiency anemia. J Trop pediatr. 2008 Feb;54(1):43-53.
[38] Oxentenko AS, Grisolano SW, Murray JA, Burgart LJ, Dierkhising RA, Alexander JA. The insensitivity of endoscopic markers in celiac disease. Am J Gastroenterol 2002; 97:933-938.
[39] Harewood GC, Holub JL, Lieberman DA. Variation in small bowel biopsy performance among diverse endoscopy settings: results from a national endoscopic database. Am J Gastroenterol 2004; 99:1790-1794.
[40] Gregory JF 3rd and Quinlivan EP. In vivo kinetics of folate metabolism. Annu Rev Nutr 2002; 22:199-220.
[41] Pawson R and Mehta A. Review article: the diagnosis and treatment of haematinic deficiency in gastrointestinal disease. Aliment Pharmacol Ther 1998; 12:687-698.
[42] Carmel R. Megaloblastic anemias: disorders of impaired DNA synthesis. In Greer JP, Foerster J, Lukens JN, Rodgers GM, Paraskevas F, Glader B (Eds.). Wintrobe's Clinical Hematology2004;Philadelphia, PA Lippincott Williams & Wilkins Vol 1: pp. 1367-1395.
[43] Savage DG, Lindenbaum J, Stabler SP, Allen RH. Sensitivity of serum methylmalonic acid and total homocysteine determinations for diagnosing cobalamin and folate deficiencies. Am J Med 1994; 96:239-246.
[44] Snow CF. Laboratory diagnosis of vitamin B12 and folate deficiency: a guide for the primary care physician. Arch Intern Med 1999; 159:1289-1298.
[45] Bode S and Gudmand-Hoyer E. Symptoms and haematologic features in consecutive adult coeliac patients. Scand J Gastroenterol 1996; 31:54-60.
[46] Pittschieler K. [Folic acid concentration in the serum and erythrocytes of patients with celiac disease]. Padiatr Padol 1986; 21:363-366.
[47] Stevens D. Nutritional anaemia in childhood coeliac disease [abstract]. Proc Nutr Soc 1979; 38:102A.
[48] Kemppainen TA, Kosma VM, Janatuinen EK, Julkunen RJ, Pikkarainen PH, Uusitupa MI. Nutritional status of newly diagnosed celiac disease patients before and after

the institution of a celiac disease diet: association with the grade of mucosal villous atrophy. Am J Clin Nutr 1998; 67:482–487.
[49] Haapalahti M, Kulmala P, Karttunen TJ, et al. Nutritional status in adolescents and young adults with screen-detected celiac disease. J Pediatr Gastroenterol Nutr 2005; 40:566–570.
[50] Hoffbrand AV, Douglas AP, Fry L, Stewart JS. Malabsorption of dietary folate (Pteroylpolyglutamates) in adult coeliac disease and dermatitis herpetiformis. Br Med J 1970; 4:85–89.
[51] Fry L, Keir P, McMinn RM, Cowan JD, Hoffbrand AV. Small-intestinal structure and function and haematological changes in dermatitis herpetiformis. Lancet 1967; 2:729–733.
[52] Saibeni S, Lecchi A, Meucci G, et al. Prevalence of hyperhomocysteinemia in adult gluten-sensitive enteropathy at diagnosis: role of B12, folate, and genetics. Clin Gastroenterol Hepatol 2005; 3:574–580.
[53] Kuzminski AM, Del Giacco EJ, Allen RH, Stabler SP, Lindenbaum J. Effective treatment of cobalamin deficiency with oral cobalamin. Blood 1998; 92:1191–1198.
[54] Kastrup W, Mobacken H, Stockbrugger R, Swolin B, Westin J. Malabsorption of vitamin B12 in dermatitis herpetiformis and its association with pernicious anaemia. Acta Med Scand 1986; 220:261–268.
[55] Dickey W, Ward M, Whittle CR, Kelly MT, Pentieva K, Horigan G, Patton S, McNulty H. Homocysteine and related B-vitamin status in coeliac disease: Effects of gluten exclusion and histological recovery. Scand J Gastroenterol. 2008;43(6):682-8.
[56] Gillberg R, Kastrup W, Mobacken H, Stockbrugger R, Ahren C. Gastric morphology and function in dermatitis herpetiformis and in coeliac disease. Scand J Gastroenterol 1985; 20:133–140.
[57] Dickey W and Hughes DF. Histology of the terminal ileum in coeliac disease. Scand J Gastroenterol 2004; 39:665–667.
[58] Dahele A and Ghosh S. Vitamin B12 deficiency in untreated celiac disease. Am J Gastroenterol 2001; 96:745–750.
[59] Dickey W. Low serum vitamin B12 is common in coeliac disease and is not due to autoimmune gastritis. Eur J Gastroenterol Hepatol 2002; 14:425–427.
[60] Bode S and Gudmand-Hoyer E. Symptoms and haematologic features in consecutive adult coeliac patients. Scand J Gastroenterol 1996; 31:54–60.
[61] Ward PC. Modern approaches to the investigation of vitamin B12 deficiency. Clin Lab Med 2002; 22:435–445.
[62] Vidal-Alaball J, Butler CC, Cannings-John R, et al. Oral vitamin B12 versus intramuscular vitamin B12 for vitamin B12 deficiency. Cochrane Database Syst Rev 2005; CD004655.
[63] Fisgin T, Yarali N, Duru F, Usta B, Kara A. Hematologic manifestation of childhood celiac disease. Acta Haematol 2004; 111:211–214.
[64] Pittschieler K. Neutropenia, granulocytic hypersegmentation and coeliac disease. Acta Paediatr 1995; 84:705–706.
[65] Jameson S, Hellsing K, Magnusson S. Copper malabsorption in coeliac disease. Sci Total Environ 1985; 42:29–36.
[66] Goyens P, Brasseur D, Cadranel S. Copper deficiency in infants with active celiac disease. J Pediatr Gastroenterol Nutr 1985; 4:677–680.
[67] Fisgin T, Yarali N, Duru F, Usta B, Kara A. Hematologic manifestation of childhood celiac disease. Acta Haematol 2004; 111:211–214.

[68] Mulder CJ, Pena AS, Jansen J, Oosterhuis JA. Celiac disease and geographic (serpiginous) choroidopathy with occurrence of thrombocytopenic purpura. Arch Intern Med 1983; 143:842.
[69] Eliakim R, Heyman S, Kornberg A. Celiac disease and keratoconjunctivitis: occurrence with thrombocytopenic purpura. Arch Intern Med 1982; 142:1037.
[70] Croese J, Harris O, Bain B. Coeliac disease: haematological features, and delay in diagnosis. Med J Aust 1979; 2:335–338.
[71] Nelson EW, Ertan A, Brooks FP, Cerda JJ. Thrombocytosis in patients with celiac sprue. Gastroenterology 1976; 70:1042–1044.
[72] Carroccio A, Giannitrapani L, Di Prima L, Iannitto E, Montalto G, Notarbartolo A. Extreme thrombocytosis as a sign of coeliac disease in the elderly: case report. Eur J Gastroenterol Hepatol 2002; 14:897–900.
[73] Dupond JL, de Waziéres B, Flausse-Parrot F, Fest T, Morin G, Closs F, Vuitton D. Thrombocytosis of celiac disease in adults: a diagnostic and prognostic marker?. Presse Med 1993 2;22(29):1344-6.
[74] Patwari AK, Anand VK, Kapur G, Narayan S. Clinical and nutritional profile of children with celiac disease. Indian Pediatr 2003; 40:337–342.
[75] Saibeni S, Bottasso B, Spina L, et al. Assessment of thrombin-activatable fibrinolysis inhibitor (TAFI) plasma levels in inflammatory bowel diseases. Am J Gastroenterol 2004; 99:1966–1970.
[76] van Tilburg NH, Rosendaal FR, Bertina RM. Thrombin activatable fibrinolysis inhibitor and the risk for deep vein thrombosis. Blood 2000; 95:2855–2859.
[77] Thorburn D, Stanley AJ, Foulis A, Campbell Tait R. Coeliac disease presenting as variceal haemorrhage. Gut 2003; 52:758.
[78] Miehsler W, Reinisch W, Valic E, et al. Is inflammatory bowel disease an independent and disease specific risk factor for thromboembolism? Gut 2004; 53:542–548.
[79] Zenjari T, Boruchowicz A, Desreumaux P, Laberenne E, Cortot A, Colombel JF. Association of coeliac disease and portal venous thrombosis. Gastroenterol Clin Biol 1995; 19:953–954.
[80] Marteau P, Cadranel JF, Messing B, Gargot D, Valla D, Rambaud JC. Association of hepatic vein obstruction and coeliac disease in North African subjects. J Hepatol 1994; 20:650–653.
[81] Grigg AP. Deep venous thrombosis as the presenting feature in a patient with coeliac disease and homocysteinaemia. Aust N Z J Med 1999; 29:566–567.
[82] Ramagopalan SV, Wotton SV, Handel AE, Yeates D, Goldacre MJ. Risk of venous thromboembolism in people admitted to hospital with selected immune-mediated diseases: record-linkage study. BMC Med. 2011; 10;9:1.
[83] Ludvigsson JF, Welander A, Lassila R, Ekbom A, Montgomery SM. Risk of thromboembolism in 14,000 individuals with coeliac disease. Br J Haematol. 2007;139(1):121-7.
[84] Cassela G, Bassotti G, Villanacci V, Di Bella C, Pagni F, Corti GL. Is hyperhomocysteinemia relevant in patients with celiac disease? W J Gastroenterol. 2011, 28; 17(24): 2941-2944
[85] Jorge O, Jorge A, Camus G. Celiac disease associated with antiphospholipid syndrome. Rev Esp Enferm Dig. 2008, 100(2):102-3.
[86] McNeill A, Duthle F, Galloway DJ. Small bowel infarction in a patient with coeliac disease. J Clin Pathol 2006;59:216-218
[87] Morello F, Ronzani G, Cappellari F. Migraine, cortical blindness, multiple cerebral infarctions and hypocoagulopathy in celiac disease. Neurol Sci 2003; 24:85–89.

[88] Lee ES and Pulido JS. Nonischemic central retinal vein occlusion associated with celiac disease. Mayo Clin Proc 2005; 80:157.
[89] El Moutawakil B, Chourkani N, Sibai M, Moutaouakil F, Rafai M, Bourezgui M, Slassi I.Celiac disease and ischemic stroke. Rev Neurol. 2009;165(11):962-6.
[90] Krasinski SD, Russell RM, Furie BC, Kruger SF, Jacques PF, Furie B. The prevalence of vitamin K deficiency in chronic gastrointestinal disorders. Am J Clin Nutr 1985; 41:639-643.
[91] Jacobs P and Wood L. Macronutrients. Dis Mon 2004; 50:46–115.
[92] Cavallaro R, Iovino P, Castiglione F, et al. Prevalence and clinical associations of prolonged prothrombin time in adult untreated coeliac disease. Eur J Gastroenterol Hepatol 2004; 16:219–223.
[93] Granel B, Rossi P, Frances Y, Henry JF. Bilateral massive adrenal haemorrhage revealing coeliac disease. QJM 2005; 98:70–71.
[94] Hussaini SH, Ahmed S, Heatley RV. Celiac disease and hypoprothrombinemia. Nutrition 1999; 15:389–391.
[95] Lubel JS, Burrell LM, Levidiotis V. An unexpected cause of macroscopic haematuria. Med J Aust 2005; 183:321–323.
[96] Cataldo F, Marino V, Ventura A, Bottaro G, Corazza GR. Prevalence and clinical features of selective immunoglobulin A deficiency in coeliac disease: an Italian multicentre study. Italian Society of Paediatric Gastroenterology and Hepatology (SIGEP) and "Club del Tenue" Working Groups on Coeliac Disease. Gut 1998; 42:362–365.
[97] Meini A, Pillan NM, Villanacci V, Monafo V, Ugazio AG, Plebani A. Prevalence and diagnosis of celiac disease in IgA-deficient children. Ann Allergy Asthma Immunol 1996; 77:333–336.
[98] Samolitis NJ, Hull CM, Leiferman KM, Zone JJ. Dermatitis herpetiformis and partial IgA deficiency. J Am Acad Dermatol 2006; 54:S206–S209.
[99] Collin P, Maki M, Keyrilainen O, Hallstrom O, Reunala T, Pasternack A. Selective IgA deficiency and coeliac disease. Scand J Gastroenterol 1992; 27:367–371.
[100] Gillett HR, Gillett PM, Kingstone K, Marshall T, Ferguson A, Letter, J. Pediatr. Gastroenterol. Nutr. 1997; 25:366-367
[101] Lenhardt A, Plebani A, Marchetti F, et al. Role of human-tissue transglutaminase IgG and anti-gliadin IgG antibodies in the diagnosis of coeliac disease in patients with selective immunoglobulin A deficiency. Dig Liver Dis 2004; 36:730–734.
[102] Catassi C, Bearzi I, Holmes GK. Association of celiac disease and intestinal lymphomas and other cancers. Gastroenterology 2005; 128:S79–S86.
[103] Holmes GK, Stokes PL, Sorahan TM, Prior P, Waterhouse JA, Cooke WT. Coeliac disease, gluten-free diet, and malignancy. Gut 1976; 17:612–619.
[104] Harris OD, Cooke WT, Thompson H, Waterhouse JA. Malignancy in adult coeliac disease and idiopathic steatorrhoea. Am J Med 1967; 42:899–912.
[105] Cooper BT, Holmes GK, Ferguson R, Cooke WT. Celiac disease and malignancy. Medicine (Baltimore) 1980; 59:249–261.
[106] Corrao G, Corazza GR, Bagnardi V, et al. Mortality in patients with coeliac disease and their relatives: a cohort study. Lancet 2001; 358:356–361
[107] Logan RF, Rifkind EA, Turner ID, Ferguson A. Mortality in celiac disease. Gastroenterology 1989; 97:265–271.
[108] Cooper BT, Holmes GK, Cooke WT. Lymphoma risk in coeliac disease of later life. Digestion 1982; 23:89–92.

[109] Nielsen OH, Jacobsen O, Pedersen ER, et al. Non-tropical sprue: malignant diseases and mortality rate. Scand J Gastroenterol 1985; 20:13–18.
[110] Holmes GK, Prior P, Lane MR, Pope D, Allan RN. Malignancy in coeliac disease: effect of a gluten free diet. Gut 1989; 30:333–338.
[111] Collin P, Reunala T, Pukkala E, Laippala P, Keyrilainen O, Pasternack A. Coeliac disease: associated disorders and survival. Gut 1994; 35:1215–1218.
[112] Catassi C, Fabiani E, Corrao G, et al. Risk of non-Hodgkin lymphoma in celiac disease. JAMA 2002; 287:1413–1419.
[113] Askling J, Linet M, Gridley G, Halstensen TS, Ekstrom K, Ekbom A. Cancer incidence in a population-based cohort of individuals hospitalized with celiac disease or dermatitis herpetiformis. Gastroenterology 2002; 123:1428–1435.
[114] Peters U, Askling J, Gridley G, Ekbom A, Linet M. Causes of death in patients with celiac disease in a population-based Swedish cohort. Arch Intern Med 2003; 163:1566–1572.
[115] Freeman HJ. Lymphoproliferative and intestinal malignancies in 214 patients with biopsy-defined celiac disease. J Clin Gastroenterol 2004; 38:429–434.
[116] Smedby KE, Akerman M, Hildebrand H, Glimelius B, Ekbom A, Askling J. Malignant lymphomas in coeliac disease: evidence of increased risks for lymphoma types other than enteropathy-type T cell lymphoma. Gut 2005; 54:54–59.
[117] Green PH, Fleischauer AT, Bhagat G, Goyal R, Jabri B, Neugut AI. Risk of malignancy in patients with celiac disease. Am J Med 2003; 115:191–195.
[118] Fairley NH and Mackie FP. The clinical and biochemical syndrome in lymphoma and allied disease involving the mesenteric lymph glands. BMJ 1937; 1:375–380.
[119] A clinical evaluation of the International Lymphoma Study Group classification of non-Hodgkin's lymphoma: the Non-Hodgkin's Lymphoma Classification Project. Blood 1997; 89:3909–3918.
[120] Gale J, Simmonds PD, Mead GM, Sweetenham JW, Wright DH. Enteropathy-type intestinal T-cell lymphoma: clinical features and treatment of 31 patients in a single center. J Clin Oncol 2000; 18:795–803.
[121] Egan LJ, Walsh SV, Stevens FM, Connolly CE, Egan EL, McCarthy CF. Celiac-associated lymphoma: a single institution experience of 30 cases in the combination chemotherapy era. J Clin Gastroenterol 1995; 21:123–129.
[122] Daum S, Weiss D, Hummel M, et al. Frequency of clonal intraepithelial T lymphocyte proliferations in enteropathy-type intestinal T cell lymphoma, coeliac disease, and refractory sprue. Gut 2001; 49:804–812.
[123] Isaacson PG and Du MQ. Gastrointestinal lymphoma: where morphology meets molecular biology. J Pathol 2005; 205:255–274.
[124] Farstad IN, Johansen FE, Vlatkovic L, et al. Heterogeneity of intraepithelial lymphocytes in refractory sprue: potential implications of CD30 expression. Gut 2002; 51:372–378.
[125] Cellier C, Delabesse E, Helmer C, et al. Refractory sprue, coeliac disease, and enteropathy-associated T-cell lymphoma: French Coeliac Disease Study Group. Lancet 2000; 356:203–208.
[126] Bagdi E, Diss TC, Munson P, Isaacson PG. Mucosal intra-epithelial lymphocytes in enteropathy-associated T-cell lymphoma, ulcerative jejunitis, and refractory celiac disease constitute a neoplastic population. Blood 1999; 94:260–264.
[127] Cellier C, Patey N, Mauvieux L, et al. Abnormal intestinal intraepithelial lymphocytes in refractory sprue. Gastroenterology 1998; 114:471–481.

[128] Mention JJ, Ben Ahmed M, Begue B, et al. Interleukin 15: a key to disrupted intraepithelial lymphocyte homeostasis and lymphomagenesis in celiac disease. Gastroenterology 2003; 125:730–745.
[129] Meijer JW, Mulder CJ, Goerres MG, Boot H, Schweizer JJ. Coeliac disease and (extra)intestinal T-cell lymphomas: definition, diagnosis and treatment. Scand J Gastroenterol Suppl 2004; 241:78–84.
[130] Schuppan D. Current concepts of celiac disease pathogenesis. Gastroenterology 2000; 119:234-42.
[131] Viljamaa M, Kaukinen K, Pukkala E, Hervonen K, Reunala T, Collin P. Malignancies and mortality in patients with coeliac disease and dermatitis herpetiformis: 30-year population-based study. Dig Liver Dis 2006; 38:374–380.
[132] Mearin ML, Catassi C, Brousse N, et al. European multi-centre study on coeliac disease and non-Hodgkin lymphoma. Eur J Gastroenterol Hepatol 2006; 18:187–194.
[133] Card TR, West J, Holmes GK. Risk of malignancy in diagnosed coeliac disease: a 24-year prospective, population-based, cohort study. Aliment Pharmacol Ther 2004; 20:769–775.
[134] Collin P, Pukkala E, Reunala T. Malignancy and survival in dermatitis herpetiformis: a comparison with coeliac disease. Gut 1996; 38:528–530.
[135] Lewis HM, Reunala TL, Garioch JJ, et al. Protective effect of gluten-free diet against development of lymphoma in dermatitis herpetiformis. Br J Dermatol 1996; 135:363–367.
[136] Hervonen K, Vornanen M, Kautiainen H, Collin P, Reunala T. Lymphoma in patients with dermatitis herpetiformis and their first-degree relatives. Br J Dermatol 2005; 152:82–86.
[137] Sonet A, Theate I, Delos M, et al. Clinical and pathological features of 14 non-Hodgkin's lymphomas associated with coeliac disease. Acta Clin Belg 2004; 59:143–151.
[138] Kruzliak P, Cicmancova E. Enteropathy-Associated Non-HodgkinT-Lymphoma as a Complication of Late Diagnosis of Celiac Disease in a Geriatric Patient. Czech and Slovak Gastroent and Hepatol 2010; 64(1): 7-11
[139] Howdle PD, Jalal PK, Holmes GK, Houlston RS. Primary small-bowel malignancy in the UK and its association with coeliac disease. QJM 2003; 96:345–353.
[140] Wöhrer S, Chott A, Drach J, et al. Chemotherapy with cyclophosphamide, doxorubicin, etoposide, vincristine and prednisone (CHOEP) is not effective in patients with enteropathy-type intestinal T-cell lymphoma. Ann Oncol 2004; 15:1680–1683.
[141] Savage KJ, Chhanabhai M, Gascoyne RD, Connors JM. Characterization of peripheral T-cell lymphomas in a single North American institution by the WHO classification. Ann Oncol 2004;
[142] Daum S, Ullrich R, Heise W, et al. Intestinal non-Hodgkin's lymphoma: a multicenter prospective clinical study from the German Study Group on Intestinal non-Hodgkin's Lymphoma. J Clin Oncol 2003; 21:2740–2746.
[143] Gale J, Simmonds PD, Mead GM, Sweetenham JW, Wright DH. Enteropathy-type intestinal T-cell lymphoma: clinical features and treatment of 31 patients in a single center. J Clin Oncol 2000; 18:795–803.
[144] Egan LJ, Walsh SV, Stevens FM, Connolly CE, Egan EL, McCarthy CF. Celiac-associated lymphoma: a single institution experience of 30 cases in the combination chemotherapy era. J Clin Gastroenterol 1995; 21:123–129.
[145] Sieniawskil M, Angamuthul N, Boyd K, Chasty R, Davies J, Forsyth P, Jack F, Lyons S, Mounter P, Revell P, Proctor SJ, Lennardl AL. Evaluation of enteropathy-associated T-cell lymphoma comparing standard therapies with a novel regimen including autologous stem cell transplantation. Blood, 2010; 115: 3664-3670

5

Celiac Disease and Diabetes Mellitus Type 1

Mieczysław Szalecki[1,2], Piotr Albrecht[3] and Stefan Kluzek[4]
[1]*Clinic of Endocrinology and Diabetology, Children's Memorial Health Institute, Warsaw,*
[2]*Faculty of Health Sciences, Jan Kochanowski University, Kielce,*
[3]*Department of Pediatric Gastroenterology and Nutrition, Warsaw Medical University,*
[4]*Sport and Exercise Medicine, Oxford Deanery, Nuffield Orthopaedic Centre, Oxford,*
[1,2,3]*Poland*
[4]*UK*

1. Introduction

A significant increase in autoimmune disease morbidity has been observed in recent years, including disorders manifesting in childhood, concurrent with decreased age of patients at the time of diagnosis. Autoimmune diseases can involve almost every organ system but the endocrine, connective tissue and gastrointestinal systems are the most commonly affected [1, 2, 3].

In terms of epidemiology, autoimmune thyroid diseases (AITD) and diabetes type 1 (T1DM) come to the fore among autoimmune diseases related to the endocrine system, whereas among those unrelated to the endocrine system celiac disease (CD) is one of the more common. These diseases, apart from bronchial asthma, are among the most frequent chronic diseases affecting infants and children and often occur together [1, 3, 4].

Autoimmune polyendocrinopathy syndrome (APS) or polyglandular autoimmune diseases (PGAD) concern primary deficits in two or more endocrine glands and manifest themselves, except for Graves' disease, as organ hypofunction. The main autoimmune endocrinopathies are: type 1 diabetes mellitus, autoimmune thyroid diseases, autoimmune adrenal failure (Addison disease), hypergonadotropic hypogonadism (premature ovarian failure), autoimmune hypoparathyroidism, and pituitary defects (lymphocytic hypophysitis) [5, 6, 7]

Those syndromes are often associated with other non-endocrine autoimmune diseases [5, 6, 7].

For descriptive purposes three to four different types of APS or PGAD have been described. Addison disease is a common element of the first two types i.e. APS-1 Blizzard syndrome, APS-2 Schmidt's syndrome (Carpenter's syndrome). APS-3, on the other hand, is characterised by the presence of autoimmune thyroid disease and diabetes type 1 (3a), pernicious anaemia (3b) or vitiligo, alopecia or other organ specific autoimmune disease (3c).

Some authors also distinguish type 4 disease/syndrome, which comprises varied combinations of autoimmune diseases with the exception of those mentioned above as types 1 and 2. A patient with diagnosed T1DM and CD can be included in this group [5, 6, 7].

In 1969, Walker-Smith and Grigo[8] described a child with T1DM and CD for the first time, highlighting the frequent coexistence of these two diseases. What makes CD unique among autoimmune diseases is the fact that the external or initiating factor is known, which is not the case in T1DM or AITD.

2. Pathophysiology

Recent studies have shown that, apart from environmental causes, such as the ingestion of gluten in celiac disease, other less understood factors like in T1DM, and recent advances in our understanding of genetic predisposition factors, many autoimmune disorders are associated with either primary or secondary disturbances in gastrointestinal mucosal permeability.

Gastrointestinal epithelial cells form the largest body surface area interfacing between an organism and its external environment. Thanks to tight junctions (TJ), a healthy intestinal mucosa serves as a barrier against toxic macromolecules. Under physiological conditions, only a few immunologically active antigens can traverse this barrier. Almost 90% of the proteins that penetrate the barrier via the epithelium are reduced to non-immunogenic, short linear peptides due to the action of lysosomal enzymes. Only a few remain unchanged and are transported by M cells or between the enterocytes through TJ. Breaching of the epithelial barrier by these antigens often results in the development of immunological tolerance rather than triggering the immune response or autoimmunisation [9]. An immature or damaged mucosa makes the mucous barrier more permeable, which can result in an allergic or autoimmune reaction in genetically predisposed individuals [9, 10]. Uibo et al. [11] detected the lowest expression of tight junction protein 1 (TJP1) mRNA in small bowel mucosa samples from celiac patients with diabetes mellitus type 1, indicating an increase in intestinal permeability. Furthermore, these samples displayed the highest expression of forkhead box P3 (FoxP3) mRNA, a marker of regulatory T cells, when compared with controls and celiac patients [11]. Antigen presenting cells (APC), which present antigens to T cells of the intestinal mucosa, are vital to the immunological processes. On their surface, they present glycoproteins encoded by major histocompatibility complex (MHC) class I and II antigens [12, 13]. Almost 50 different conditions, including CD and T1DM, are associated with specific MHC class I or II antigen presentation pathways [13]. Apart from genetic predisposition, the disease or disorder develops when the immune system is exposed to the antigen. This process may be enhanced by increased permeability of the mucosa due to damaged TJ. According to Fasano et al. [14, 15, 16, 17] an excessive production of zonulin stimulated by gluten, increases permeability of TJ. In CD, this process is presumed to be mediated by gliadin binding to the chemokine receptor CXCR3 [18].

Gliadin has lately been speculated to be one of the environmental causes of T1DM. Gliadin, which contains relatively high levels of glutamine and proline, is a source of polypeptides that can penetrate the damaged TJ and presented to T cells by dendritic cells. Activated Th1 lymphocytes can be stimulated to secret gamma interferon (INF-γ) and tumor-necrosis factor-alfa (TNF-α), Th2 lymphocytes to secrete Interleukin-4 (IL-4) and Th17 cells to secrete Interleukin-17A (IL-17A). All these cytokines can stimulate a local inflammatory response, which further augments the permeability of the mucosa [19, 20], hence resulting in a vicious circle that perpetuates damage to the intestinal mucosa.

It seems that the development of CD is dependent on the dose, type, timing and method of gluten ingestion. Breastfeeding and small amounts of gluten administered with breast milk are associated with a reduced risk of developing CD [21, 22]. Breastfeeding favours the growth of beneficial bacteria, such as *Bifidobacterium,* and therefore decreases the proliferation of others, including those less beneficial, like *Bacteroides*.

Diet (and gluten intake) related disorders of the intestinal microflora and permeability of the intestinal mucosa appear to play a significant role in the development of T1DM [23]. According to Visser et al. [24], the influence of gluten on the development of T1DM is as follows: a high gluten diet is favourable for *Bacteroides,* while a gluten-free casein diet reduces their number. The predominance of *Bacteroides* over *Bifidobacterium* and *Lactobacillus,* which occurs in breastfed babies, stimulates zonulin release [25]. In CD zonulin release is enhanced by gliadin binding to the chemokine receptor CXCR3 [18]. An excessive concentration of zonulin and its receptor in the enterocyte changes the structure of TJ proteins and increases the passage of antigens from the intestinal lumen to the *lamina propria* where antigens are presented to the T cells by the APC. In conjunction with a genetic predisposition, this may lead to the trafficking and/or activation of autoaggressive T cells, which may provoke autoimmune responses, including destruction of beta cells in T1DM.

A significant role of gliadin in the etiology and pathogenesis of CD and T1DM has also been hypothesized by Barbeau et al [26].

3. Epidemiology

Around 4.5% of children and almost 6% of adults with T1DM have concurrent CD [27]. This correlation between the two diseases seems to become stronger with increasing age and duration of diabetes. The epidemiological data vary depending on population characteristics as well as on diagnostics criteria. Prevalence of CD among Australian children with newly diagnosed T1DM was 1.2% according to Doolan et al.[28]. This prevalence was 2.7% among children with long-standing T1DM and 8.4% among adults.

In similar populations of children in the USA, the prevalence of CD was 5% percent according to Crone et al, and 3.2% according to Sanchez-Albisua et al [29, 30].

CD coexists with T1DM in only 1.4% of young adults in Wales [31], while the rate is 7.7% in children in British Columbia, 2% in adults in the Czech Republic [33], 2.6% in children and teenagers in Brazil [34] and 12.3% in adults in Denmark [35]. In Iraq it is 11.2% [36], and in Serbia 5.79% [37]. Triolo et al. have found tissue transglutaminase antibodies (anti-tTG) in 11.6% of diabetic children, of whom 24.6% had CD [4]. In a large study of 28,671 T1DM patients under the age of 30 from Germany and Austria, Warncke et al. [38] demonstrated the presence of anti-tTG in 10.7% patients, which was associated with the duration of T1DM. In a recent study form Greece, Kakleas et al. [39] found an 8.6% prevalence of anti-tTG IgA positivity among T1DM children associated with younger age and a shorter duration of diabetes. The highest prevalence of 13.8% was documented in Italy by Picarelli et al. [40]. This study also demonstrated the value of analysing IgA and IgG antibody concentrations simultaneously. The prevalence of CD in the patients with T1DM was 6.4% for IgA-EMA-positive, which increased to 13.8% when IgG1-EMA was also used for screening.

The incidence of CD in Polish children with newly diagnosed T1DM was reported to be 5.7% and 9.4% in those with long-standing T1DM by Mysliwiec et al. [41]. There was no significant difference between the positivity for anti-tTG IgA and IgG in those groups. Gorska et al. [42] reported 4.1% of newly diagnosed type 1 diabetic children to have positive antibodies and our study [43] showed this to be twice as high among girls (5.62%) than among boys (2.57%). These data are consistent with other studies i.e. the prevalence of CD is twice as high in females as in males.

Patients with CD also have a greater risk for developing T1DM (around 5%) [44] and diabetes-associated antibodies are more commonly detected in these individuals. Galii-Tsinopoulou et al. [45] detected anti-GAD and IA-2 antibodies in 23% of patients with CD. The same authors suggested that a strict gluten-free diet might protect the pancreatic β-cells and thus postpone the onset of T1DM. Initiation of a gluten-free diet in T1DM children is associated with a significantly reduced risk of autoimmunisation. According to Ludvigsson et al.[46], early diagnosis of CD (before the age of 2) reduces the risk of developing T1DM before the age of 20 when compared to a group diagnosed between the ages of 3 and 20. The differences, however were not statistically significant.

4. Genetic determinants and associations

Most estimates put the prevalence of CD at close to 1% of the general population [47], and recent evidence suggests that serologic prevalence rates have increased fourfold in the past 50 years [48]. The concordance rate for CD in monozygotic twins is 75% and it highlights the role of other factors besides genetic predisposition [49]. The MHC molecules HLA-DQ2 and HLA-DQ8 are risk factors in the disease. Almost 90% of CD patients carry HLA-DQ2 antigens while most of the rest carry HLA-DQ8 [50, 51]. HLA-DQ2 molecule is encoded by the DQA1*0501 and DQB1*0201 genes [52].

T1DM is strongly associated with HLA DR3-DQ2 and DR4-DQ8 MHC molecules, and associated with DQB1*0302, DQB1*0201, DRB1*0401 and HLA-B alleles [53]. Approximately 90% of CD patients share the HLA DR3/DQ2 configuration [54]. The prevalence of tissue transglutaminase antibodies has been reported to be as high as 32% in HLA DQ2 homozygous T1DM patients, compared with 2% in patients without DQ2 or DQ8 [55].

CD and T1DM also share a number of other genetic susceptibility loci. Out of 8 celiac susceptibility loci, 6 are associated with T1DM. On the other hand, out of 17 diabetes-susceptibility loci, 8 are associated with CD [56]. At least 8 loci appear to be common for both conditions (CCR3, CCR5, SH2B3, RGS1, TAGAP, PTPN2, IL18RAP, CTLA4) [57]. It has been suggested that the immune or inflammatory responses associated with many autoimmune diseases overlap with the function of genes specific for certain diseases, such as IL12A in CD and INS in T1DM [57]. Two new CD risk regions were recently identified at chromosomes 6q23.3 (OLIG3-TNFAIP3) and 2p16.1 (REL) [58]. Polymorphisms within the TAGAP gene are also related to another autoimmune disease: rheumatoid arthritis [59].

The coexistence of T1DM and CD could be explained by a common genetic factor in the HLA region [60, 61] or by molecular mimicry by which gliadin or tissue transglutaminase C activates T cells that are cross-reactive with various antigens. During active β-cell destruction, transglutaminase C, which is expressed in pancreatic islets, might be presented in an immunogenic form. Such inflammatory responses may have the capacity to persist in susceptible hosts and lead to chronic organ-specific autoimmune disease [62]. Furthermore, it has been suggested that in the development of autoimmunity in T1DM, the failure to achieve tolerance to autoantigens is attributable to gut related issues [63].

5. Diagnosing CD in diabetic patients

At the time of writing this chapter, duodenal biopsy remains the gold standard for CD diagnosis. The diagnostic criteria devised by ESPGHAN in 1989 [64] and later modified, consist of finding villous atrophy and crypt hyperplasia in a patient who ingests a sufficient amount of gluten (the Marsh classification [65]) and achieves remission after discontinuing gluten from the diet. The diagnosis is further confirmed by positive serology. Highly sensitive and specific IgA and IgG antiendomysial antibodies (EmA) and tissue transglutaminase antibodies (anti-tTG) are most frequently used. Sometimes, deaminated gliadin antibodies (DGP) are also elevated.

When evaluating anti-EmA and anti-tTG antibodies only of the IgA class (which is often preferred due to the lower cost), it is important to note the IgA concentration as well, as the frequency of isolated IgA deficiency in celiac patients is almost 2% and 7.7% of patients with isolated IgA deficiency suffer from CD [66].

The above criteria are about to change. With exceptionally high levels of antiendomysial antibodies and positive genetic testing (HLA-DQ2, DQ8), CD might be diagnosed without histopathologic examination[67]. The use of three PCR reactions and a single electophoretic step for DQA1, DQB1 and DRB1 typing provides distinction of CD associated alleles and their homo- or heterozygous status. This analysis reduces reagent costs, personnel and instrument time, while enabling improved allelic assignment through HLA-DR-DQ haplotype association [68]. In case of doubt, when the levels of antibodies are low, duodenal biopsy is recommended to confirm the diagnosis.

6. Evaluation for celiac disease in diabetes mellitus type 1 patients

T1DM often coexists with CD. However, the latter is often latent, Larsson et al. suggest that T1DM patients should be screened annually [69].

There is no consensus as to whether all diabetic patients should implement a gluten-free diet, nor is it clear how often they should be screened for CD.

The ADA recommends screening diabetic patients for CD and placing all children with a confirmed diagnosis of CD on a gluten-free diet (GFD) [70]. ISPAD suggests that while it seems sensible to put an asymptomatic child on a GFD to avoid the development of disease complications, evidence supporting this is still not sufficient. Therefore, they recommend that children with confirmed CD and T1DM receive support from a paediatric dietician [71].

Classical presentation of CD can occur in T1DM patients, but many patients with CD and T1DM are either asymptomatic (silent CD) or present with only mild symptoms [72, 73]. In a recent study from a North American CD clinic, 71.4% of children with diabetes reported no gastrointestinal symptoms at the time of a positive screen [74]. Some patients are overweight or obese at diagnosis; 11.2% of children with CD had a BMI greater than the 90th percentile in a recent US study [72]. Based on these data, the ISPAD recommendations for the screening of all T1DM patients for CD appear to be adequate. Screening for CD should be carried out at the time of diagnosis, annually for the first five years and every second year thereafter. More frequent assessment is indicated if the clinical situation suggests the possibility of CD or the child has a first-degree relative with CD [71].

It should be emphasised that both adults and children suffering from CD are at an increased risk for sepsis. The risk is highest for pneumococcal sepsis [75]. Therefore it is recommended to vaccinate these patients against pneumococci.

Patients with both CD and T1DM have gastrointestinal symptoms more often than those who suffer from diabetes only. These include stomach pain, bloating, diarrhea, failure to thrive, and decreased appetite. In the study by Naruli et al. [76], this difference was statistically significant ($p<0.0005$). The symptoms subsided after switching onto a gluten-free diet, which goes to show that CD was in fact not asymptomatic. Patients who observed the diet significantly improved their weight SD score ($p=0.008$) and BMI SD score ($p=0.002$) within a year.

In a study by Fröhlich-Reiterer et al. [77], patients with both T1DM and CD (confirmed by a biopsy) were diagnosed with diabetes at a younger age and were of a generally lower height and weight. Those features were statistically significant ($p<0.001$) and they continued for another five and a half years of observation.

According to Pitocco et al. [78], patients with both diseases are at higher risk of developing atherosclerosis compared to those presenting with diabetes or CD only.

Other recognised side effects associated with untreated CD in patients with T1DM include changes in insulin requirements, frequent hypoglycaemia, failure to thrive, delayed puberty, anaemia, osteopenia, osteoporosis and neurologic complications [79, 80, 81, 82].

The most clinically serious, but rare, complication associated with CD (usually the type resistant to treatment) is the development of small intestinal lymphoma[83]. The incidence of this malignancy in patients with both CD and T1DM, however, has not been adequately assessed.

In conclusion, it appears that despite being inconvenient and restrictive, a gluten-free diet should be implemented for all patients suffering from T1DM and CD. There is evidence that this diet might be effective in protecting the pancreatic β-cells and increasing the levels of insulin secretion in newly diagnosed patients [84, 85, 86]. A gluten-free diet is beneficial for diabetic patients. It improves the indicators of physical development, reduces the risk of atherosclerosis and sepsis (especially pneumococcal), and relieves the gastrointestinal symptoms associated with untreated CD.

We strongly suggest that annual screening for CD become part of routine practice in patients with T1DM.

7. References

[1] Anderson MS. Update in endocrine autoimmunity. J Clin Endocrinol Metab. 2008;93(10):3663-70.
[2] Van den Driessche A, Eenkhorn V, Van Gaal L, De Block C. Type 1 diabetes mellitus and autoimmune polyglandular syndrome: a clinical revive. The Netherlands Journal of Medicine. 2009;67:376-385.

[3] Craig M, Hattersley A, Donaghue K. ISPAD Clinical Practice Consensus Guidelines 2009. Pediatric Diabetes 2009(S12);10:3-12.
[4] Triolo TM, Armstrong TK, McFann K, Yu L, Rewers MJ, Klingensmith GJ, Eisenbarth GS, Barker JM. Additional autoimmune diseases in 33% of patients at type 1 diabetes onset. Diabetes Care. 2011;34(5):1211-3.
[5] Betterlre C, Delpra C, Greggio N. Autoimmunity in isolated Addison disease and in polyglandular autoimmune diseases type 1, 2 and 4. Annales Endocrinology. 2001;62:193.
[6] Eisenbarth GS, Gottlieb PA. Autoimmune Polyendocrine Syndromes. New England Journal of Medicine. 2004;350:2068-79.
[7] Brook CGD, Brown RS. Polyglandular Syndromes in. Handbook of Clinical Pediatric Endocrinology. Blackwell Publishing Inc. Massachusetts USA. 2008:164-171.
[8] Walker-Smith JA, Grigor W. Coeliac disease in a diabetic child. Lancet. 1969 17;1(7603):1021.
[9] Mowat AM. Anatomical basis of tolerance and immunity to intestinal antigens. Nat Rev Immunol. 2003;3(4):331-41.
[10] Fasano A. Intestinal zonulin: open sesame! Gut. 2001;49(2):159-62.
[11] Uibo R, Panarina M, Teesalu K, Talja I, Sepp E, Utt M, Mikeelsar M, Heilman K, Uibo O, Vorobjova T. Celiac disease in patient with type 1 diabetes: a condition with distinct changes in intestinal mucosa. Cell Moll Immunol. 2011;8(2):150-6.
[12] Bjorkman PJ, Saper MA, Samraoui B, Bennett WS, Strominger JL, Wiley DC. Structure of the human class I histocompatibility antigen, HLA-A2. Nature. 1987;329(6139):506-12.
[13] Visser J, Rozing J, Sapone A, Lammers K, Fasano A. Tight junctions, intestinal permeability, and autoimmunity: celiac disease and type 1 diabetes paradigms. Ann N Y Acad Sci. 2009;1165:195-205.
[14] Fasano A, Fiorentini C, Donelli G, Uzzau S, Kaper JB, Margaretten K, Ding X, Guandalini S, Comstock L, Goldblum SE. Zonula occludens toxin modulates tight junctions through protein kinase C-dependent actin reorganization, in vitro. J Clin Invest. 1995;96(2):710-20.
[15] Fasano A, Uzzau S, Fiore C, Margaretten K. The enterotoxic effect of zonula occludens toxin on rabbit small intestine involves the paracellular pathway. Gastroenterology. 1997;112(3):839-46.
[16] Wang W, Uzzau S, Goldblum SE, Fasano A. Human zonulin, a potential modulator of intestinal tight junctions. J Cell Sci. 2000;113 Pt 24:4435-40.
[17] Baudry B, Fasano A, Ketley J, Kaper JB. Cloning of a gene (zot) encoding a new toxin produced by *Vibrio cholerae*. Infect Immun. 1992;60(2):428-34.
[18] Lammers KM, Lu R, Brownley J, Lu B, Gerard C, Thomas K, Rallabhandi P, Shea-Donohue T, Tamiz A, Alkan S, Netzel-Arnett S, Antalis T, Vogel SN, Fasano A. Gliadin induces an increase in intestinal permeability and zonulin release by binding to the chemokine receptor CXCR3. Gastroenterology. 2008;135(1):194-204.e3
[19] Knip M. Diet, gut, and type 1 diabetes: role of wheat-derived peptides? Diabetes. 2009;58(8):1723-4.
[20] Mojibian M, Chakir H, Lefebvre DE, Crookshank JA, Sonier B, Keely E, Scott FW. Diabetes-specific HLA-DR-restricted proinflammatory T-cell response to wheat

polypeptides in tissue transglutaminase antibody-negative patients with type 1 diabetes. Diabetes. 2009;58(8):1789-96.
[21] Sollid LM. Breast milk against coeliac disease. Gut. 2002;51(6):767-8.
[22] Ivarsson A, Hernell O, Stenlund H. Breast-feeding protects against celiac disease. Am J Clin Nutr 2002;75:914–21.
[23] Brugman S, Klatter FA, Visser JT, Wildeboer-Veloo AC, Harmsen HJ, Rozing J, Bos NA. Antibiotic treatment partially protects against type 1 diabetes in the Bio-Breeding diabetes-prone rat. Is the gut flora involved in the development of type 1 diabetes? Diabetologia. 2006;49(9):2105-8.
[24] Visser J, Rozing J, Sapone A, Lammers K, Fasano A. Tight junctions, intestinal permeability, and autoimmunity: celiac disease and type 1 diabetes paradigms. Ann N Y Acad Sci. 2009;1165:195-205.
[25] Fasano A, Nataro JP. Intestinal epithelial tight junctions as targets for enteric bacteria-derived toxins. Adv Drug Deliv Rev. 2004;56(6):795-807.
[26] Barbeau WE, Bassaganya-Riera J, Hontecillas R. Putting the pieces of the puzzle together - a series of hypotheses on the etiology and pathogenesis of type 1 diabetes. Med Hypotheses. 2007;68(3):607-19.
[27] Holmes GK. Screening for coeliac disease in type 1 diabetes. Arch Dis Child. 2002;87(6):495-8.
[28] Doolan A, Donaghue K, Fairchild J, Wong M, Williams AJ. Use of HLA typing in diagnosing celiac disease in patients with type 1 diabetes. Diabetes Care. 2005;28(4):806-9.
[29] Crone J, Rami B, Huber WD, Granditsch G, Schober E. Prevalence of celiac disease and follow up to EMA in children with type 1 diabetes mellitus J Pediatr Gastroenterol Nutr. 2003; 37:67-71.
[30] Sanchez-Albisua I, Wolf J, Neu A, Geiger H, Waschler I, Sterm M. Celiac disease in children with Type 1 diabetes mellitus: the effect of the gluten-free diet. Diabet Med. 2005;22:1079-82.
[31] Li Voon Chong JS, Leong KS, Wallymahmed M, Sturgess R, MacFarlane IA. Is coeliac disease more prevalent in young adults with coexisting Type 1 diabetes mellitus and autoimmune thyroid disease compared with those with Type 1 diabetes mellitus alone? Diabet Med. 2002;19(4):334-7.
[32] Giletti PM, Giletti HR, Israel DM. High prevalence of celiac disease in patients with type 1 diabetes mellitus detected by antibodies to endomysium and tissue transglutaminase. Can J Gastroenterol. 2003;15:297-301.
[33] Prazny M, Skrha J, Limanova Z. Screening for associated autoimmunity in type 1 diabetes mellitus with respect to diabetes control. Physiol Res 2005;54:41-48.
[34] Tanure MG, Silva IN, Bahia M, Penna FJ. Prevalence of celiac disease in Brazilian children with type 1 diabetes mellitus. J Pediatr Gastroenterol Nutr. 2006 Feb;42(2):155-9.
[35] Hansen D, Brock-Jacobsen B, Lund E, Bjørn C, Hansen LP, Nielsen C, Fenger C, Lillevang ST, Husby S. Prevalence of celiac disease (CD) in children with type 1 diabetes (T1D). Ugeskr Laeger. 2007;169(21):2029-32.
[36] Mansour AA, Najeeb AA. Celiac disease in Iraqi type 1 diabetic patients. Arab J Gastroenterol. 2011 Jun;12(2):103-5.

[37] Djurić Z, Stamenković H, Stanković T, Milićević R, Branković L, Cirić V, Katić V. Celiac disease prevalence in children and adolescents with type 1 diabetes from Serbia. Pediatr Int. 2010;52(4):579-83.
[38] Warncke K, Frochlich-Reiterer EE, Thon A, Hofer SE, Wiemann D, Holl RW, DPV Initiative of the German Working Group for Pediatric Diabetology. Polyendocrinopathy in children, adolescents, and young adults with type 1 diabetes: a multicenter analysis of 28.671 patients from German/Austrian DPV-Wiss database. Diabetes Care. 2010;33(9):2010-2.
[39] Kakleas K, Karayjanci C, Cristelis E, Papathanasiou A, Petrou V, Fotinou A, Karavanaki K. The prevalence and risk factors for celiac disease among children and adolescents with type 1 diabetes mellitus. Diabetes Res Clin Prac 2010;90(2):202-8.
[40] Picarelli A, Sabbatella L, Di Tola M, Vetrano S, Casale C, Anania MC, Porowska B, Vergari M, Schiaffini R, Gargiulo P. Anti-endomysial antibody of IgG1 isotype detection strongly increases the prevalence of coeliac disease in patients affected by type I diabetes mellitus. Clin Exp Immunol. 2005 Oct;142(1):111-5.
[41] Myśliwiec M, Balcarska A, Stopiński J. Prognostic factors of celiac disease occurrence in type 1 diabetes mellitus in children. Pediatr Endocrinol Diabetes Metab. 2006;16:281-5.
[42] Górska A, Nazim J, Starzyk J. Ocena częstości wystepowania choroby Hashimoto i celiakii wśród dzieci i młodzieży ze świeżo rozpoznaną cukrzycą typu 1 - badanie prospektywne. Endokrynol Ped. 2004;3(S3):38.
[43] Szalecki M, Ziora K, Biernacka-Florczak I, Domagała Z. Występowanie celiakii u dzieci i młodzieży ze świeżo rozpoznaną cukrzycą typu 1. Endokrynologia Pediatryczna 2007;2(19):23-28.
[44] Collin P, Reunala T, Pukkala E, Laippala P, Keyriläinen O, Pasternack A. Coeliac disease--associated disorders and survival. Gut. 1994;35(9):1215-8.
[45] Galli-Tsinopoulou A, Nousia-Arvanitakis S, Dracoulacos D, Xefteri M, Karamouzis M. Autoantibodies predicting diabetes mellitus type 1 in celiac disease. Horm Res. 1999;52(3):119-24
[46] Ludvigsson JF, Ludvigsson J, Ekbom A, Montgomery SM. Celiac disease and risk of subsequent type 1 diabetes: a general population cohort study of children and adolescents. Diabetes Care. 2006;29(11):2483-8.
[47] Mäki M, Mustalahti K, Kokkonen J, Kulmala P, Haapalahti M, Karttunen T, Ilonen J, Laurila K, Dahlbom I, Hansson T, Höpfl P, Knip M. Prevalence of Celiac disease among children in Finland. N Engl J Med. 2003;348(25):2517-24.
[48] Rubio-Tapia A, Kyle RA, Kaplan EL. Increased prevalence and mortality in undiagnosed celiac disease. Gastroenterology. 2009;137(1):88-93.
[49] Nisticò L, Fagnani C, Coto I, Percopo S, Cotichini R, Limongelli MG, Paparo F, D'Alfonso S, Giordano M, Sferlazzas C, Magazzù G, Momigliano-Richiardi P, Greco L., Stazi MA. Concordance, disease progression, and heritability of coeliac disease in Italian twins. Gut. 2006;55(6):803-8.
[50] Sollid LM, Markussen G, Ek J, Gjerde H, Vartdal F, Thorsby E. Evidence for a primary association of celiac disease to a particular HLA-DQ alpha/beta heterodimer. J Exp Med. 1989;169(1):345-50.
[51] Karell K, Louka AS, Moodie SJ, Ascher H, Clot F, Greco L, Ciclitira PJ, Sollid LM., Partanen J; European Genetics Cluster on Celiac Disease. HLA types in celiac

disease patients not carrying the DQA1*05-DQB1*02 (DQ2) heterodimer: results from the European Genetics Cluster on Celiac Disease. Hum Immunol. 2003;64(4):469-77.

[52] van Heel DA, Hunt K, Greco L, Wijmenga C. Genetics in coeliac disease. Best Pract Res Clin Gastroenterol. 2005;19(3):323-39.

[53] Nejentsev S, Howson JM, Walker NM, Szeszko J, Field SF, Stevens HE, Reynolds P, Hardy M, King E, Masters J, Hulme J, Maier LM, Smyth D, Bailey R, Cooper JD, Ribas G, Campbell RD, Clayton DG, Todd JA. Wellcome Trust Case Control Consortium. Localization of type 1 diabetes susceptibility to the MHC class I genes HLA-B and HLA-A. Nature. 2007 Dec 6;450(7171):887-92.

[54] Smyth DJ, Plagnol V, Walker NM, Cooper JD, Downes K, Yang JH, Howson JM, Stevens H, McManus R, Wijmenga C, Heap GA, Dubois PC, Clayton DG, Hunt KA, van Heel DA, Todd JA. Shared and distinct genetic variants in type 1 diabetes and celiac disease. N Engl J Med. 2008;359(26):2767-77.

[55] Sollid LM, Markussen G, Ek J, Gjerde H, Vartdal F, Thorsby E. Evidence for a primary association of celiac disease to a particular HLA-DQ α/βheterodimer. J Exp Med. 1989;169:345-50.

[56] Bao F, Yu L, Babu S. One third of HLA DQ2 homozygous patients with type 1 diamina diabetes express celiac disease-associated transglutaminase antibodies. J Autoimmun. 1999;13:143-8.

[57] Heap GA, van Heel DA. The genetics of chronic inflammatory diseases. Hum Mol Genet. 2009;18(R1):R101-6.

[58] Trynka G, Zhernakova A, Romanos J, Franke L, Hunt KA, Turner G, Bruinenberg M, Heap GA, Platteel M, Ryan AW, de Kovel C, Holmes GK, Howdle PD, Walters JR, Sanders DS, Mulder CJ, Mearin ML, Verbeek WH, Trimble V, Stevens FM, Kelleher D, Barisani D, Bardella MT, McManus R, van Heel DA, Wijmenga C. Coeliac disease-associated risk variants in TNFAIP3 and REL implicate altered NF-kappaB signalling. Gut. 2009;58(8):1078-83.

[59] Eyre S, Hinks A, Bowes J, Flynn E, Martin P, Wilson AG, Morgan AW, Emery P, Steer S, Hocking LJ, Reid DM, Harrison P, Wordsworth P. Yorkshire Early Arthritis Consortium; Biologics in RA Control Consortium, Thomson W, Worthington J, Barton A. Overlapping genetic susceptibility variants between three autoimmune disorders: rheumatoid arthritis, type 1 diabetes and coeliac disease. Arthritis Res Ther. 2010;12(5):R175.

[60] Bilbao JR, Martin-Pagola A, Vitoria JC, Zubillaga P, Ortiz L, Castano L. HLA-DRB1 and MHC class 1 chain-related A haplotypes in Basque families with celiac disease. Tissue Antigens. 2002;60:71-6.

[61] Lopez-Vazquez A, Rodrigo L, Fuentes D. MHC class I chain related gene A (MICA) modulates the development of celiac disease in patients with the high risk heterodimer DQA1*0501/DQB1*0201. Gut. 2002;50:336-40.

[62] Schuppan D. Current concepts of celiac disease pathogenesis. Gastroenterology. 2000;119:234-42.

[63] Paronen J, Klemetti P, Kantele JM. Glutamate decarboxylasereactive peripheral blood lymphocytes from patients with IDDM express gut-specific homing receptor α4β7-integrin. Diabetes. 1997;46:583-8.

[64] Working Group of ESPGAN: Revised criteria for diagnosis of celiac disease. Arch Dis Child 1990; 65:909-911.

[65] Marsh MN. Gluten, major histocompatibility complex, and the small intestine: a molecular and immunobiologic approach to the spectrum of gluten sensitivity ("celiac sprue"). Gastroenterology 1992; 102: 330-354.

[66] Husby S, Koletzko S, Korponay-Szabó IR, Mearin ML, Phillips A, Shamir R, Troncone R, Giersiepen K, Branski D, Catassi C, Lelgeman M, Mäki M, Ribes-Koninckx C, Ventura A, Zimmer KP; ESPGHAN Working Group on Coeliac Disease Diagnosis; ESPGHAN Gastroenterology Committee. European Society for Pediatric Gastroenterology, Hepatology, and Nutrition guidelines for the diagnosis of coeliac disease. J Pediatr Gastroenterol Nutr. 2012 Jan;54(1):136-60.

[67] NIH Consensus Development Conference on Celiac Disease. NIH Consensus State Sci. Statements. 2004,2,21:1-23.

[68] Lavant EH, Agardh, Nisson A, CarlsonJA. A new PCR-SSP method for HLA DR-DQ risk for celiac disease. Clin Chim Acta. 2011;11(412):9-10.

[69] Larsson K, Carlsson A, Cederwall E, Jönsson B, Neiderud J, Jonsson B, Lernmark A, Ivarsson SA. Skåne Study Group. Annual screening detects celiac disease in children with type 1 diabetes. Pediatr Diabetes. 2008;9(4 Pt 2):354-9.

[70] Standards of medical care in diabetes—2009. Diabetes Care. 2009;32(S1):13–61.

[71] Kordonouri O, Maguire AM, Knip M, Schober E, Lorini R, Holl RW, Donaghue KC. ISPAD Clinical Practice Consensus Guidelines 2009. Pediatric Diabetes 2009(S12);10:204-210.

[72] Mahmud FH, Murray JA, Kudva YC. Celiac disease in type 1 diabetes mellitus in a North American community: prevalence, serologic screening, and clinical features. Mayo Clinic Proceedings. 2005;80(11):1429–1434.

[73] Rami B, Sumnik Z, Schober E. Screening detected celiac disease in children with type 1 diabetes mellitus: effect on the clinical course (a case control study). Journal of Pediatric Gastroenterology and Nutrition. 2005;41(3):317–321.

[74] Telega G, Bennet TR, Werlin S. Emerging new clinical patterns in the presentation of celiac disease. Archives of Pediatrics and Adolescent Medicine. 2008;162(2):164–168.

[75] Ludvigsson JF, Olén O, Bell M, Ekbom A, Montgomery SM. Coeliac disease and risk of sepsis. Gut. 2008 ;57(8):1074-80.

[76] Narula P, Porter L, Langton J, Rao V, Davies P, Cummins C, Kirk J, Barrett T, Protheroe S. Gastrointestinal symptoms in children with type 1 diabetes screened for celiac disease. Pediatrics. 2009;124(3):489-95.

[77] Fröhlich-Reiterer EE, Kaspers S, Hofer S, Schober E, Kordonouri O, Pozza SB, Holl RW; Diabetes Patienten Verlaufsdokumentationssystem-Wiss Study Group. Anthropometry, metabolic control, and follow-up in children and adolescents with type 1 diabetes mellitus and biopsy-proven celiac disease. J Pediatr. 2011;158(4):589-593.e2

[78] Pitocco D, Giubilato S, Martini F, Zaccardi F, Pazzano V, Manto A, Cammarota G, Di Stasio E, Pedicino D, Liuzzo G, Crea F, Ghirlanda G. Combined atherogenic effects of celiac disease and type 1 diabetes mellitus. Atherosclerosis. 2011;217(2):531-5.

[79] Binkley N, Bilezikian JP, Kendler DL, Leib ES, Lewiecki EM, Petak SM. Summary of the International Society for Clinical Densitometry 2005 Position Development Conference. Journal of Bone and Mineral Research. 2007;22(5):643–645.
[80] Collin P, Kaukinen K, Valimaki M, Salmi J. Endocrinological disorders and celiac disease. Endocrine Rev. 2002;23(4):464-83.
[81] Green PH, Cellier C. Celiac disease. N Engl J Med. 2007;357:1731-43.
[82] Hoffenberg EJ, Fallstrom SP, Jansson G, Jansson U, Lindberg T. Clinical features of children with screening-identified evidence of celiac disease. Pediatrics. 2004;113:1254-9.
[83] Mention JJ, Ben Ahmed M, Begue B. Interleukin 15: A key to disrupted intraepithelial lymphocyte homeostasis and lymphomagenesis in celiac disease. Gastroenterology 2003; 125(3):730-45.
[84] Hansed D, Brock-Jacobsen D, Lund E. Clinical benefit of gluten free diet in type 1 diabetic children with screening-detected celiac disease a population based screening study with 2 years follow up. Diabetes Care. 2006;29:2452-2456.
[85] Acerini CL, Ahmed MI, Ross KM. Coeliac disease in children and adolescence with type 1 diabetes mellitus: clinical characteristics and response to gluten free diet. Diabet Med. 1998;15:38-44.
[86] Fuchtenbush M, Ziegler AG, Hummel M. Elimination of dietary gluten and development of type 1 diabetes high risk subjects. Rev Diabet Study. 2004;1:39-41.

6

Multiple Sclerosis and Celiac Disease

Carlos Hernández-Lahoz[1] and Luis Rodrigo[2]
Neurology[1] and Gastroenterology[2] Services, Asturias Central University Hospital (HUCA) School of Medicine, University of Oviedo, Oviedo, Spain

1. Introduction

Celiac disease (CD) has traditionally been thought of as a primarily intestinal disorder, and is now considered the most important autoimmune disease related to gluten intolerance (gluten-sensitive enteropathy) *(Freeman et al., 2011)*. It occurs in genetically susceptible individuals through the ingestion of gluten and is more frequent in women, as is also the case for many autoimmune diseases *(Gleicher & Barad, 2007; Invernizzi et al., 2009)*.

Gluten sensitivity (GS) is an immune-mediated disease which appears in individuals intolerant to gluten without the intestinal involvement that characterizes CD. Genetic susceptibility is less clear here than in CD. The immunopathogenesis associated with gluten is supported by the favorable response to gluten-exclusion diet *(Sapone et al., 2012)*.

Neurologic manifestations of gluten-related disorders (GRDs), with enteropathy (celiac disease) or without enteropathy (non-celiac gluten sensitivity), are frequent, their pathogenesis including an immunological attack on the central (CNS) and peripheral nervous system (PNS) leading to inflammatory lesions accompanied by neurodegenerative changes. The clinical manifestations are varied, but the most common syndromes are cerebellar ataxia and peripheral neuropathy, which can improve if they are treated early on with a gluten-free diet (GFD) *(Ford, 2009; Hadjivassiliou et al., 2010)*.

To a varying degree, GRDs are associated with other complex neurological diseases such as multiple sclerosis (MS) and neuromyelitis optica (NMO), both autoimmune demyelinating diseases of the CNS, whose evolution could be unfavorably influenced by gluten intolerance *(Marrie & Horwitz, 2010)*. The early detection of CD or GS associated with neurological manifestations caused by demyelinating diseases and their subsequent treatment with GFD could prove beneficial to the patients who suffer from them (*Hadjivassiliou et al., 2010; Hernández-Lahoz et al., 2011*).

2. Demyelinating diseases of the CNS

The family of CNS inflammatory demyelinating diseases represents a broad spectrum of disorders. MS is the most common of them, affecting more than one million people worldwide *(Hu & Luccinetti, 2009)*.

2.1 Multiple sclerosis

MS is a chronic neurological disease of unknown etiology associated with autoimmunity. Activated, potentially autoimmune, T cells cross the blood-brain barrier and produce inflammatory plaques and axonal damage in the brain, spinal cord or optic nerves. The end result is the accumulation of focal plaques of demyelination and gliosis in the CNS *(Compston & Coles, 2008)*.

MS is the most common disabling disease of the CNS in young adults. It affects about 1 ‰ of the population in western countries and is twice as prevalent in women as in men *(Fromont et al., 2010; Orton et al., 2006)*.

MS generally starts with episodes of acute neurological dysfunction followed by complete or partial remission and a symptom-free interval until the next outbreak. This relapsing-remitting form (RRMS) is the initial disease course in more than 80% of individuals with MS *(Confavreux et al, 1980; Lublin & Reingold, 1996)*.

The first relapse is usually localized in either the CNS or optic nerves. The patient displays an episode of acute neurological dysfunction, generally followed by recovery, which is known as the clinical isolated syndrome (CIS). In most cases, symptomatic, as well as previously silent demyelinating lesions, can be found through magnetic resonance imaging (MRI). After CIS, new recurrent events occur and eventually lead to more permanent neurological disabilities, and new lesions can also be detected by MRI during the asymptomatic intervals *(Miller et al., 2005; Swanton et al., 2007)*.

Some individuals have an MRI scan that is highly suggestive of MS, but have no signs or symptoms. These asymptomatic patients are referred to as having a radiological isolated syndrome (RIS) and are at risk of developing CIS and full blown MS *(Okuda et al., 2009, 2011; Ramagopalan et al., 2010; Sellner et al., 2010)*.

The diagnosis of MS requires that the symptoms and signs of CNS white-matter involvement are disseminated in time and space, as well as supportive evidence from MRI studies. Detection of oligoclonal bands of immunoglobulin G (IgG) in cerebrospinal fluid (CSF) specimens can be important to support the inflammatory demyelinating nature of CIS, and to predict the future conversion to MS (*Polman et al., 2011*).

Intravenous corticosteroid therapy is commonly the initial treatment for acute attacks of optic neuritis or encephalomyelitis. Using an experimental model of autoimmune encephalitis as a starting point, immunomodulatory and immunosuppressive therapies have proven effective in preventing relapses in RRMS patients, especially when initiated early in the course of disease *(Compston & Coles, 2008)*. Moreover, a new era in the treatment of RRMS, with oral and new parentally administered drugs, is now emerging.

However, the complex etiology of autoimmune diseases not only presents a challenge to the development and testing of new therapies, but also offers a framework that allows the identification of patients who might benefit from particular approaches.

2.2 Neuromyelitis optica

NMO (Devic's disease) is a chronic disease of unknown etiology associated with autoimmunity and is characterized by the presence of inflammatory and demyelinating lesions in the spinal cord and optic nerves. NMO is up to nine times more prevalent in women than in men *(Wingerchuk et al., 2007).*

Initial reports considered NMO to be a variant of MS, but more recent case series have suggested it to be a distinct disorder *(O'Riordan et al., 1996; de Seze et al., 2003).* The combination of clinical, neuroimaging, serologic and pathologic characteristics permit NMO to be distinguished from MS.

NMO is clinically characterized by severe attacks of optic neuritis and myelitis. The attacks in NMO, unlike those in MS, commonly spare the cerebral white matter in the early stages.

MRI of the brain at the onset of NMO is typically normal (except for the optic nerve) in contrast to what happens in MS. MRI findings of the spinal cord in NMO show extensive lesions longitudinally, which characteristically span three or more contiguous vertebral segments. By contrast, in MS the lesions rarely exceed one or two vertebral segments in length.

Prominent CSF pleocytosis is a characteristic of NMO, but is rare in typical MS. Supernumerary oligoclonal bands of IgG in the CSF, signifying synthesis of intrathecal immunoglobulins, are detected in 85% of patients with MS but in only 30% of patients with NMO.

Serologic evidence of B cell autoimmunity has been observed in a high proportion of patients with NMO (*Graber et al., 2008*). The detection of NMO-IgG auto-antibody in the serum of patients is a characteristic finding of this condition and distinguishes it from other demyelinating disorders (*Lennon et al., 2004*). NMO-IgG antibody binds to aquaporin 4, which is the main channel that regulates water homeostasis in the CNS (*Lennon et al., 2005*).

Intravenous corticosteroid therapy is commonly the initial treatment for acute attacks of optic neuritis or myelitis. Plasmapheresis is used to treat patients who do not respond promptly to corticosteroid treatment (*Keegan et al., 2002; Ruprecht et al., 2004*). Maintenance immunosuppressive drugs or alternative treatment with Rituximab, a monoclonal antibody directed against the B cell marker CD20, are generally accepted strategies for reducing relapses of NMO (*Wingerchuk et al., 2005; Bomprezzi et al., 2011*).

3. Association of CD with demyelinating diseases of the CNS

CD is a common condition that affects up to 1% of the population worldwide. The diagnosis is based on the presence of characteristic lesions in small-intestinal biopsy. The genetic basis for gluten intolerance is mainly attributed to the HLA class-II locus located on chromosome 6p21. Serologic tests aid in the diagnosis of disease, although no one test is ideal (*Green & Cellier, 2007; Di Sabatino & Corazza, 2009*).

A high level of IgA anti-tissue transglutaminase-2 (tTG-2) antibody in the serum of the patients is an important serologic marker for diagnosis, and some studies have suggested a correlation with the severity of small intestinal villous atrophy (*Vivas et al., 2009*). Anti-tTG-2 antibody may be negative in the presence of partial villous atrophy or in subjects on a GFD prior to testing (*Sugai et al., 2010*).

Atypical forms of CD, i.e. without prominent gastrointestinal symptoms and with frequent extra-intestinal manifestations, are being increasingly recognized, especially over the past decade, both in adult and pediatric patients (*Roma et al., 2009; Rostami et al., 2009*).

Autoimmune disorders occur 10 times more commonly in CD than in the general population (*Catassi et al., 2010*). The association of autoimmune disorders and CD is considered to be due to a shared genetic tendency. When both occur in a patient, CD is frequently silent, and the patient is initially diagnosed with the autoimmune disease. Several autoimmune diseases may also improve with a GFD (*Green et al., 2005; Green & Cellier, 2007; Freeman et al., 2011*)

CD is around 10 times more frequent than MS. NMO is less frequent than MS, except in East Asians and other nonwhite populations worldwide. The association of CD with autoimmune demyelinating diseases of CNS, such as MS (*Ferro et al., 2008; Frisullo et al., 2008; Pengiran Tengan et al., 2004; Phan-Ba et al., 2011*) and NMO (*Bergamaschi et al., 2009; Jacob et al., 2005; Jarius et al., 2008; Matijaca et al., 2011; McNamara et al., 2011; Meyts et al., 2011*), has been described previously, generally as case reports with a small number of patients and short follow-up.

We have also described (*Hernández-Lahoz et al., 2009*) the case of a 29-year-old woman suffering from RRMS clinically with recurrent relapses of myelitis at different spinal levels, every year for three years. She had typical MS lesions in brain and spinal cord MRI-scan, oligoclonal IgG bands in CSF and delayed spinal conduction in somatosensory-evoked potentials with normal visual evoked potentials. The last relapse appeared associated with symptomatic CD with diarrhea, abdominal pain and loss of weight. She also had high titers of serum IgA anti-tTG-2 antibody, was homozygous for the HLA-DQ2 allele, and exhibited moderate villous atrophy (type 3B of Marsh) in duodenal biopsy. The patient has followed a strict GFD as single treatment for the last seven years. She regained her previous weight and maintained good health all the time. Not only did she not have any digestive disorder, which was expected, but more surprisingly she had no new neurological disorders, staying asymptomatic without suffering any further relapses to date. IgA anti-tTG-2 antibody values, since the first year on GFD, returned to normal. Gastrointestinal (GI) endoscopy, repeated two years after the onset of GFD, showed normal duodenal mucosa, without any inflammation. MRI confirmed a clear reduction of the spinal and brain lesions and probable remyelination. She remains fully asymptomatic and neurologic tests are normal.

4. Prevalence of CD in MS patients

CD and MS are considered T-cell-mediated autoimmune diseases (*Cox et al., 2010; Dørum et al., 2010; Frisullo et al., 2008*). Celiac patients do not tolerate gluten. In the lamina propia, the peptides deamidated by tTG-2 are recognized by CD4+ T cells, facilitating a large cascade of inflammatory processes that damage and eventually destroy the villous architecture of the small intestine (*Molberg et al., 2001*).

CD4+ cells are involved in the pathophysiology of MS (*Chitnis*, 2007). Regulatory T cells (Treg) from peripheral blood of animal models have demonstrated capacity to suppress various types of immune responses, including autoimmune attack against the CNS by activated effector T cells (Teff). Treg have a central role in protecting an individual from autoimmunity. MS and other autoimmune and inflammatory diseases may have an impaired Treg function and an imbalance in Teff-Treg homeostasis (*Buckner, 2010; Fritzsching et al., 2011; Vélez de Mendizábal et al., 2011*).

The anti-tTGs are auto-antibodies against enzymes, while the AGA (anti-gliadin antibody) is an antibody to a food component. The single most sensitive and specific serologic marker of CD is the IgA anti-tTG isotype 2 (over 90%). The presence of the AGA has been historically considered to be an important hallmark of CD, although lower figures for its sensitivity and specificity in comparison to IgA anti-tTG-2 have led to many people abandoning it as a marker for diagnosis (*Tofledal et al., 2010*). Furthermore, AGA may be present in other inflammatory diseases and also appear in many healthy people (*Uibo et al., 2010*).

The new test for anti-gliadin antibodies that uses deamidated gliadin peptides (DGP) instead of whole gliadin protein mixtures is more specific for detection of CD than is classic AGA (*Dahle et al., 2010*). IgG anti-DGP is now considered to have as much sensitivity and specificity as IgA anti-tTG-2 antibody test for detection of CD (*Vermersch et al., 2010; Volta & de Giorgio, 2010*).

The term 'non-celiac gluten sensitivity' has been used to describe the presence of positive AGA in patients without intestinal involvement, but with associated extra-intestinal manifestations (*Troncone & Jabri, 2011*). An immune-mediated pathogenesis, initiated by gluten, is considered in patients affected by neurologic disorders, with positive AGA and immunologic abnormalities of the CNS and PNS, especially if some have a favorable response to GFD with lower AGA titers. (*Fernández et al., 2005*).

Anti-tTG-6 antibody is the best serologic marker for assessing neurological GS, whereas antibody to tTG-3 is the best marker for dermatitis herpetiformis, but these assays are not yet available for routine clinical practice (*Stamnaes et al., 2010*).

The relationship between CD and MS in the same patient is a controversial issue in the medical literature. In two case series with a sample of more than 300 MS patients from Italy, all patients lacked specific antibodies related to CD. In these studies, however, positive antibodies were only detected in one individual of the control group. This individual appeared to be affected by CD (*Nicoletti et al., 2008; Salvatore et al., 2004*).

GS was studied in a sample of 161 MS patients from Iran, testing serum IgG and IgA AGA, and compared with a healthy control group. Neither IgG nor IgA AGA showed significant differences between MS patients and controls. Anti-tTG antibodies and histopathologic studies were negative in selected patients with positive IgG or IgA AGA results (*Borhani Haghighi et al., 2007*)

On the basis supposition that vitamin D deficiency caused by malabsortion may increase the risk of MS and high serum concentrations of 25-hydroxycholecalciferol having a protective effect against MS, a Swedish study investigated the possible relationship between CD and MS in a register of patients with diagnosis of CD between 1964–2003. The study found no increased risk of MS in patients with CD. However, the authors excluded 12 patients who had previously been diagnosed as having MS and also 4 patients in whom MS was detected in the first year of the follow-up (*Ludvigsson et al., 2007*). It is also possible that the mildest cases of MS were not diagnosed, particularly in the period preceding the introduction of MRI.

By contrast, a study from Norway in 38 MS patients found significantly higher titers of IgA and IgG AGA in the MS group in comparison to the control group ($p < 0.001$) (*Reichelt & Jensen, 2004*).

A study from Israel that sought to determine the prevalence of AGA and anti-tTG antibodies in MS patients analyzed the serum of a series of 98 MS patients compared with 140 controls. The authors found a significant increase in the titers of IgG-AGA and tTG-2 in the MS patients. Seven patients (7.1%) had a positive IgG-AGA, whereas only 2 controls (1.4%) had positive titers (p=0.03) and 4 patients (4.1%) had positive IgG anti-tTG-2 while all the controls tested were negative (p=0.02). However, IgA-AGA and tTG-2 were not significantly higher in the MS group in comparison to the control group (*Ben-Ami Shor et al., 2009*).

Our group analyzed, in a prospective and observational study, the prevalence of serologic, genetic and histologic CD markers, in a series of 72 RRMS patients from Asturias (Spain) and in their 126 first-degree relatives, compared to 123 healthy controls (*Rodrigo et al., 2011*).

Of the 72 RRMS patients, 60 (83%) were women and, among them, 32 had children. The female-male ratio was 5:1. The age of the patients ranged from 24 to 58 years. The mean duration of MS was 11 years. At the beginning of the study, the mean annual relapse rate was 1.1 and the median Expanded Disability Status Scale (EDSS) was 2 (range, 0-5). Forty-four patients (67 %) had been treated with immunomodulatory agents.

IgA anti-tTG-2 antibodies were positive (values > 2 U/ml) in 7 RRMS patients (10%) compared to 3 healthy controls (2.4%) (p=0.04). No differences were found in the frequency of HLA-DQ2 marker of genetic susceptibility for CD between the MS (29%) and control (26%) groups (p>0.5).

An upper GI endoscopy with multiple duodenal biopsies was performed on all patients included in the study. Duodenal biopsies were studied by two expert pathologists and classified according to the histologic classification for CD screening, described by Marsh in 1992 and modified seven years later by the European Pathologists Consensus Conference (*Oberhüber et al., 1999*).

The small bowel biopsies showed mild or moderate villous atrophy (types 3 A/B of Marsh) in 8 MS patients (11.1%), who were simultaneously diagnosed with CD. Of these, 7 patients showed slightly increased serologic levels of anti-tTG-2; 6 mild gastrointestinal symptoms and 1 moderate weight loss. We also found a high proportion of CD among first-degree relatives of the RRMS patients (18.6%).

All the 8 CD patients were put on a GFD, which was followed with good adherence. All of them improved considerably with respect to their gastrointestinal and neurological symptoms during the 3 years of follow-up.

5. Possible therapeutic implications

At present, MS therapy is not associated with a particular diet (*Riccio et al., 2011*). Historically the GFD has occasionally been used in MS patients and there have been anecdotal reports indicating both positive effects after its implementation (*Hafner, 1976*) as well as no benefit (*Hewson, 1984*).

In our case report, the patient has followed a strict GDF as single treatment for the last seven years and she has been in good health, without suffering any further relapses or new digestive symptoms to date. Thus, GFD appeared to 'kill two birds with one stone'.

The development of autoimmunity against multiple targets might be a secondary effect of shared genetic risk factors that predispose individuals to several autoimmune diseases (*Visser et al., 2009; Gutiérrez-Achuri et al., 2011*). In the case of patients with these two autoimmune diseases (CD and MS), we hypothesized whether addressing one of them might result in an improvement in the other. In our experience, GFD has been the most important treatment for CD, but it could potentially be useful for both diseases. The main difficulty for these patients is to follow a strict GFD for the rest of their lives.

MS and NMO patients could be good candidates for a clinical trial with a GFD, if they have had positive anti-tTG-2 IgA or anti-DGP IgG antibody tests and confirmatory villous atrophy in the duodenal biopsies. The prevalence of CD among RRMS patients in our study is higher (11.1%) than in previous studies (*Ben-Ami Shor et al., 2009; Nicoletti et al., 2008; Salvatore et al., 2004*). Therefore, we consider that in clinical practice, it would be prudent to perform testing for the early detection of CD in MS patients.

Continued exposure to gliadin for several years, starting in infancy, may not only be the main cause of activation of CD but also an additional factor that in some patients triggers other autoimmune diseases. Recent genoma-wide association studies (GWAS) in immune-mediated and autoimmune diseases have identified more than a hundred regions of the genoma with susceptibility loci to one of these common diseases. In addition, there is evidence that loci predisposing to one disease can have effects that increase the risk of the patients developing a second disease, although the risk allele for one disease may not be the same as for the other (*Cotsapas et al., 2011*).

Continued studies of these individuals with multiple immune/autoimmune disorders are necessary to help identify shared genetic susceptibility and to apply appropriate treatment strategies for patients (*Baranzini, 2009*).

6. References

Baranzini SE. (2009). The genetics of autoinmune diseases: a networked perspective. *Curr Opin Immunol* 21: 596-605

Ben-Ami Shor D, Barzilai O, Ram M, Izhaky D, Porat-Katz BS, Chapman J, Blank M, Anaya JM, & Shoenfeld Y. (2009). Gluten sensitivity in Multiple Sclerosis. Experimental myth or clinical truth? *Ann N Y Acad Sci* 1173: 343-9

Bergamaschi R, Jarius S, Robotti M, Pichiecchio B, Wildemann B, & Meola G. (2009). Two cases of benign neuromyelitis optica in patients with celiac disease. *J Neurol* 256: 2097-9

Bomprezzi R, Postevka E, Campagnolo D, &Vollmer TL. (2011). A review of cases of neuromyelitis optica. *Neurologist* 17: 98-104

Borhani Haghighi A, Ansari N, Mokhtari M, Geramizadeh B, & Lankarani KB. (2007). Multiple sclerosis and gluten sensitivity. *Clin Neurol Neurosurg* 109: 651-3

Buckner JH. (2010). Mechanisms of impaired regulation by CD4+, CD5+, FOXP3+ regulatory T cells in human autoimmune diseases. *Nat Rev Immunol* 10: 849-59

Catassi C, Kryszak D, Bhatti B, Sturgeon C, Helzlsouer K, Clipp SL, Gelfond D, Puppa E, Sferruzza A, & Fasano A. (2010). Natural history of celiac disease autoimmunity in a USA cohort followed since 1974. *Ann Med* 42: 530-8

Chitnis T. (2007). The role of CD4 T cells in pathogenesis of multiple sclerosis. *Int Rev Neurobiol* 79: 43-72

Compston A, & Coles A. (2008). Multiple sclerosis. *Lancet* 372: 1.502-17

Cotxapas C, Voight BF, Rossin E, Lage K, Neale BM, et al. (2011). Pervasive sharing of genetic effects in autoimmune disease. *PLoS Genet* 7 (8): e1002254

Cox MB, Cairns MJ, Gandhi KS, Carroll AP, Moscovis S, Stewart GJ, Broadley S, Scott RJ, Booth DR, Lechner-Scott J, & ANZgene MS genetics Consortium. (2010). MicroRNAs miR-17 and miR-20a inhibit T cell activation genes and are un-expressed in multiple sclerosis whole blood. *PLoS One* 5 (8): e12132

Dahle C, Hagman A, Ignatova S, & Ström M. (2010). Antibodies against deamidated gliadin peptides identify adult coeliac disease patients negative for antibodies against endomysium and tissue transglutaminase. *Aliment Pharmacol Ther* 32:254-60

De Seze J, Lebrun C, Stojkovic T, Ferriby D, Chatel M, & Vermersch P. (2003). Is Devic's Neuromyelitis optica a separate disease? A comparative study with multiple sclerosis. *Mult Scler* 9: 521-5

Di Sabatino A, & Corazza GR. (2009). Coeliac disease. *Lancet* 373: 1480-93

Dørum S, Arntzen MØ, Qiao SW, Holm A, Koehler CJ, Thiede B, et al. (2010).The preferred substrates for transglutaminase 2 in a complex wheat gluten digest are peptide fragments harboring celiac disease T-cell epitopes. *PLoS One* 5: (11): e14056

Fernández E, Riestra S, Rodrigo L, Blanco C, López-Vázquez A, Fuentes D, Moreno M, & López-Larrea C. (2005). Comparison of six human anti-transglutaminase ELISA-tests in the diagnosis of celiac disease in the Saharawi population. *World J Gastroenterol* 11: 3762-6

Ferro MT, Franciotta D, Riccardi T, D'Adda E, Mainardi E, & Montanelli A. (2008). A case of multiple sclerosis with atypical onset associated with autoimmune hepatitis and silent celiac disease. *Neurol Sci* 29: 29-31

Ford RPK. (2009). The gluten syndrome: A neurological disease. *Med Hypotheses* 73: 438-40

Freeman HJ, Chopra A, Clandinin MT, & Thomson AB. (2011). Recent advances in celiac disease. *World J Gastroenterol* 17: 2259-72

Frisullo G, Nociti V, Iorio R, Patanella AK, Caggiula M, Marti A, Sancricca C, Angelucci F, Mirabella M, Tonali PA, & Batocchi A. (2009). Regulatory T cells fail to suppress CD4+ T-bet+ T cells in relapsing multiple sclerosis patients. *Immunology* 127: 418-28

Frisullo G, Nociti V, Iorio R, Patanella AK, Marti A, Cammarota G, Mirabella M, Tonali PA, & Batocchi AP. (2008). Increased expression of T-bet in circulating B cells from a patient with multiple sclerosis and celiac disease. *Hum Immunol* 69: 837-9

Fritzsching B, Haas J, König F, Kunz P, Fritzsching E, Pöschl J, Ktammer PH, Brück W, Suri-Payer E, & Wildemann B. (2011). Intracerebral human regulatory T cells: analysis of CD4+ CD25+ FOXP3+ T cells in brain lesions and cerebrospinal fluid of multiple sclerosis patients. *PLoS One* 6 (3): e17988

Fromont A, Binquet C, Sauleau EA, Fournel I, Bellisario A, Adnet J, Weill A, Vukusic S, Confavreux C, Debouverie M, Clerc L, Bonithon-Kopp C, & Moreau T. (2010). Geographic variations of multiple sclerosis in France. *Brain* 133: 1889-99

Gleicher N, & Barad DH. Gender as risk factor for autoimmune diseases. (2007). *J Autoimmun* 28: 1-6

Graber DJ, Levy M, Kerr D, & Wade WF. (2008). Neuromyelitis optica pathogenesis and aquaporin 4. *J Neuroinflammation* 5: 22

Green P, Alaedini A, Sander HW, Brannagan TH, Latov N, & Chin RL. (2005). Mechanisms underlying celiac disease and its neurologic manifestations. *Cell Mol Life Sci* 62: 791-9

Green P, & Cellier C. (2007). Celiac disease. *N Engl J Med* 357: 1731-43

Gutierrez-Achury J, Coutinho de Almeida R, & Wijmenga C. (2011). Shared genetics in coeliac disease and other immune-mediated disease. *J Intern Med* 269:591-603

Hadjivassiliou M, Sanders DS, Grünewald RA, Woodroofe N, Boscolo S & Aeschlimann D. (2010). Gluten sensitivity: from gut to brain. *Lancet Neurol* 9: 318-30

Hafner FH. (1976). Letter: Gluten-free diet as treatment for multiple sclerosis. *Postgrad Med* 59: 20

Hernández-Lahoz C, Mauri-Capdevila G, Vega-Villar J, & Rodrigo L. (2011). Neurological disorders associated with gluten sensitivity. *Rev Neurol* 53: 287-300

Hernández-Lahoz C, Rodríguez S, Tuñón A, Saiz A, Santamarta E & Rodrigo L. (2009). Sustained clinical remission in a patient with remittent-recurrent multiple sclerosis and coeliac disease on a gluten-free diet for 6 years. *Neurologia* 24: 213-5

Hewson DC. (1984). Is there a role for gluten-free diets in multiple sclerosis? *Hum Nutr Appl Nutr* 38: 417-20

Hu W, & Luccinetti C. (2009). The pathological spectrum of CNS inflammatory demyelinating diseases. *Semin Immunopathol* 31: 439-53

Invernizzi P, Pasini S, Selmi C, Gershwin ME, & Podda M. (2009). Female predominance and X chromosome defects in autoimmune diseases. *J Autoimmun* 33: 12-6

Jacob S, Zarei M, Kenton A, & Allroggen H. (2005). Gluten sensitivity and neuromyelitis optica: two case reports. *J Neurol Neurosurg Psychiatry* 76: 1028–30

Jarius S, Jacob S, Waters P, Jacob A, Littleton E, & Vincent A. (2008). Neuromyelitis optica in patients with gluten sensitivity associated with antibodies to aquaporin-4. *J Neurol Neurosurg Psychiatry* 79: 1084

Keegan M, Pineda AA, McClelland RL, Darby CH, Rodriguez M, & Weinshenker BG. (2002). Plasma exchange for severe attacks of CNS demyelination: predictors of response. *Neurology* 58: 143-6

Lennon VA, Kryzer TJ, Pittock SJ, Verkman AS & Hinson SR. (2005). IgG marker of optic-spinal multiple sclerosis binds to the aquaporin 4 water channel. *J Exp Med* 202: 473-7

Lennon VA, Wingerchuk DM, Kryzer TS, Pittock SJ, Luccinetti CF, Fujihara K, Nakashima I, & Weinshenker BG. (2004). A serum autoantibody marker of Neuromyelitis optica: distinction from multiple sclerosis. *Lancet* 364: 2106-12

Lublin FD, & Reingold SC. (1996). Defining the clinical course of multiple sclerosis: results of an International survey. *Neurology* 46: 907-11

Ludvigsson JF, Olsson T, Ekbom A, Montgomery SM. (2007). A population-based study of coeliac disease, neurodegenerative and neuroinflammatory diseases. *Aliment Pharmacol Ther* 25:1317-27

Matijaca M, Pavelin S, Kaliterna DM, Bojic L, & Matijaca A. (2011). Pathogenic role of acuaporin antibodies in the development of neuromyelitis optica in a woman with celiac disease. *Isr Med Assoc J* 13: 182-4

Marrie RA, & Horwitz RI. (2010). Emerging effects of comorbidities on multiple sclerosis. *Lancet Neurol* 9: 820-8

McNamara PH, Costelloe L, Langan Y, & Redmond J. (2011). Aquaporin-4 seropositivity in a patient with coeliac disease but normal neurological examination and imaging. *J Neurol* 258: 702-3

Meyts I, Jansen K, Renard M, Bossuyt X, Roelens F, Régal L, Lagae L, & Buyse G. (2011). Neuromyelitis optica-IgG (+) optic neuritis associated with celiac disease and dysgammaglobulinemia: a role for tacrolimus? *Eur J Paediatr Neurol* 15: 265-7

Miller D, Barkhof F, Montalban X, Thompson A & Filippi M. (2005). Clinically isolated syndromes suggestive of multiple sclerosis, part I: natural history, pathogenesis, diagnosis, and prognosis. *Lancet Neurol* 4: 281-8

Molberg Ø, McAdam S, Lundin KE, Kristiansen C, Arentz-Hansen H, Kett K & Sollid LM. (2001). T cells from celiac disease lesions recognize gliadin epitopes deamidated in situ by endogenous tissue transglutaminase. *Eur J Immunol* 31: 1317-23

Nicoletti A, Patti F, Lo Fermo S, Sciacca A, Laisa P, Liberto A, Lanzafame S, Contraffatto D, D'Agate C, Russo A, & Zappia M.(2008). Frequency of celiac disease is not increased among multiple sclerosis patients. *Mult Scler* 14:698-700

Oberhüber G, Granditsch G, & Vogelsang H. (1999). The histopathology of coeliac disease: time for a standardized report scheme for pathologists. *Eur J Gastroenterol Hepatol* 11:1185-94

Okuda DT, Mowry EM, Beheshtian A, Waubant E, Barankini SE, Goodin DS, Hauser SL, & Pelletier D. (2009). Incidental MRI anomalies suggestive of multiple sclerosis. The radiologically isolated syndrome. *Neurology* 72: 800-5

Okuda DT, Mowry EM, Cree BA, Crabtree EC, Goodin DS, Waubant E, & Pelletier D. (2011). Asymptomatic spinal cord lesions predict disease progression in radiologically isolated syndrome. *Neurology* 76: 686-92

O'Riordan JI, Gallagher HL, Thompson AJ, Howard RS, Kingsley DP, Thompson EJ, McDonald WI, & Miller WI. (1996). Clinical, CSF, and MRI findings in Devic's neuromyelitis optica. *J Neurol Neurosurg Psychiatry* 60: 382-7

Orton SM, Herrera BM, Yee IM, Valdar W, Ramagopalan SV, Sadovnick AD, & Ebers GC. (2006). Sex ratio of multiple sclerosis in Canada: a longitudinal study. *Lancet Neurology* 5: 932-6

Pengiran Tengah CD, Lock RJ, Unsworth DJ, & Wills AJ. (2004). Multiple sclerosis and occult gluten sensitivity. *Neurology* 62: 2326-7

Phan-Ba R, Lambinet N, Louis E, Delvenne P, Tshibanda L, Boverie J, Moonen G, & Belachew S. (2011). Natalizumab to kill two birds with one stone: a case of celiac disease and multiple sclerosis. *Inflamm Bowel Dis* 17: E62-3

Polman CH, Reingold SC, Banwell B, Clanet M, Cohen JA, Filippi M, Fujihara K, Havrdova E, Hutchinson M, Kappos L, Lublin FD, Montalban X, O'Connor P, Sandberg-Wollheim M, Thompson AJ, Waubant E, Weinshenker B, & Wolinsky JS. (2011). Diagnostic criteria for multiple sclerosis: 2010 revisions to the McDonald criteria. *Ann Neurol* 69: 292-302

Ramagopalan SV, Dobson R, Meier UC, & Giovannoni G. (2010). Multiple sclerosis: risk factors, prodromes, and potential causal pathways. *Lancet Neurol* 9: 727–39

Reichelt KL, & Jensen D. (2004). IgA antibodies against gliadin and gluten in multiple sclerosis. *Acta Neurol Scand* 110: 239-41

Riccio P, Rossano R, & Liuzzi GM. (2011). May diet and dietary supplements improve the wellness of multiple sclerosis patients? A molecular approach. *Autoimmune Dis* 2010: 249842

Rodrigo L, Hernández-Lahoz C, Fuentes D, Alvarez N, López-Vázquez A, & González S. (2011). Prevalence of celiac disease in multiple sclerosis. *BMC Neurol* 11: 31

Roma E, Panayiotou J, Karantana H, Constantinidou C, Siakavellas SI, Krini M, Syriopoulou VP, & Bamias G. (2009). Changing pattern in the clinical presentation of pediatric celiac disease: a 30-year study. *Digestion* 80: 185-91

Rostami Nejad M, Rostami K, Pourhoseingholi MA, Nazemalhosseini Mojarad E, Habibi M, Dabiri H, & Zali MR. (2009). Atypical presentation is dominant and typical for celiac disease. *J Gastrointestin Liver Dis* 18: 285-91

Ruprecht K, Klinker E, Dintelmann T, Rieckmann P & Gold R. (2004). Plasma exchange for severe optic neuritis: treatment of 10 patients. *Neurology* 63: 1081-3

Salvatore S, Finazzi S, Ghezzi A, Tosi A, Barassi A, Luini C, Bettini B, Zibetti A, Nespoli L, & Melzi d'Eril GV. (2004). Multiple sclerosis and celiac disease: is there an increased risk? *Mult Scler* 10: 711-2

Sapone A, Bai JC, Ciacci C, Dolinsek J, Green P, Hadjvassiliou M, Kaukinen K, Rostami K, Sanders DS, Schumann M, Ullrich R, Villalta D, Volta U, Catassi C, & Fasano A. (2012). Spectrum of gluten-related disorders: consensus on new nomenclature and classification. *BMC Medicine* 10:13

Sellner J, Schirmer L, Hemmer B, Mühlau M. (2010). The radiologically isolated syndrome: take action when the unexpected is uncovered? *J Neurol* 257: 1602-11

Stamnaes J, Dorum S, Fleckenstein B, Aeschlimann D, & Sollid LM. (2010). Gluten T cell epitope targeting by TG3 and TG6; implications for dermatitis herpetiformis and gluten ataxia. *Amino Acids* 39:1183-9

Sugai E, Hwang HJ, Vázquez H, Smecuol E, Niveloni S, Mazure R, Mauriño E, Aeschlimann P, Binder W, Aeschlimann D, & Bai JC. (2010). New serology assays can detect gluten sensitivity among enteropathy patients seronegative for anti-tissue transglutaminase. *Clin Chem* 56: 661-5

Swanton JK, Rovira A, Tintoré M, Altmann DR, Barkhof F, Filippi M, Huerga E, Miszkiel KA, Plant GT, Polman C, Rovaris M, Thompson AJ, Montalban X, & Miller DH. (2007). MRI criteria for multiple sclerosis in patients presenting with clinically isolated syndromes: a multicenter retrospective study. *Lancet Neurol* 6: 677-86

Toftedal P, Nielsen C, Madsen JT, Titlestad K, Husby S, & Lillevang ST. (2010). Positive predictive value of serological diagnostic measures in celiac disease. *Clin Chem Lab Med* 48: 685-91

Troncone R, & Jabri B. (2011). Coeliac disease and gluten sensitivity. *J Intern Med* 269 : 582-90

Uibo O, Uibo R, Kleimola V, Jõgi T, & Mäki M. (1993). Serum IgA anti-gliadin antibodies in an adult population sample. High prevalence without celiac disease. *Dig Dis Sci 38:* 2034-7

Vélez de Mendizábal N, Carneiro J, Solé RV, Goñi J, Bragard J, Martinez-Forero I, Martínez-Pasamar S, Sepulcre J, Torrealdea J, Bagnato F, Garcia-Ojalvo J, & Villoslada P. (2011). Modeling the effector - regulatory T cell cross-regulation reveals the intrinsic character of relapses in Multiple Sclerosis. *BMC Syst Biol* 5: 114

Vermeersch P, Geboes K, Mariën G, Hoffman I, Hiele M, & Bossuyt X. (2010). Diagnostic performance of IgG anti-deamidated gliadin peptide antibody assays is comparable to IgA anti-tTG in celiac disease. *Clin Chim Acta* 411: 931-5

Visser J, Rozing J, Sapone A, Lammers K, & Fasano A. (2009). Tight junctions, intestinal permeability and autoimunity : celiac disease and type 1 diabetes paradigms. *Ann N Y Acad Sci* 1165: 195-205

Vivas S, Ruiz de Morales JG, Riestra S, Arias L, Fuentes D, Alvarez N, Calleja S, Hernando M, Herrero B, Casqueiro J, & Rodrigo L. (2009). Duodenal biopsy may be avoided when high transglutaminase antibody titers are present. *World J Gastroenterol 15: 4775-80*

Volta U, & de Giorgio R. (2010). Gluten sensitivity: an emerging issue behind neurological impairment? *Lancet Neurol* 9: 233-5

Wingerchuk DM, Lennon VA, Lucchinetti CF, Pittock SJ, & Weinshenker BG. (2007). The spectrum of neuromyelitis optica. *Lancet Neurol* 6: 805–15

Wingerchuk DM, & Weinshenker BG. (2005). Neuromyelitis optica. *Curr Treat Options Neurol* 7: 173-82

Section 3

Detection of Cereal Toxic Peptides Based on New Laboratory Methods

7

Sensitive Detection of Cereal Fractions that Are Toxic to Coeliac Disease Patients, Using Monoclonal Antibodies to a Main Immunogenic Gluten Peptide

Carolina Sousa, Ana Real, Mª de Lourdes Moreno and Isabel Comino
Department of Microbiology and Parasitology, Faculty of Pharmacy, University of Seville, Seville, Spain

1. Introduction

Coeliac disease (CD) is a common autoimmune disorder that has genetic, environmental, and immunological components. Though under-diagnosed, it is one of the most prevalent chronic gastrointestinal diseases in humans, and exhibits unusually large clinical, histological, immunological, and genetic heterogeneity (Alaedini & Green, 2005; Sollid & Khosla, 2005). The clinical spectrum of CD has been expanded in recent years, with the identification of asymptomatic patients, patients with minimal symptoms (the most difficult to detect), and patients with extra-intestinal symptoms (Sollid & Khosla, 2005). Regardless of symptomatic presentation, the active disease in virtually all CD patients requires dietary exposure to a common environmental antigen, gluten. The ingestion of gluten proteins contained in wheat, barley, and rye, and in some cases oats (Arentz-Hansen et al., 2004; Comino et al., 2011), leads to characteristic inflammation, villous atrophy, and crypt hyperplasia in the CD patient's upper small intestine.

Gluten is a complex mixture of polypeptides. The main immunogenic peptides of gluten belong to a family of closely related proline- and glutamine-rich proteins called prolamines (15% proline and 35% glutamine residues). Gliadin, hordein, secalin, and avenin are the prolamines of wheat, barley, rye, and oats, respectively (Sollid & Khosla, 2005).

CD is triggered by peptides that result from the fragmentation of prolamines, and are not digested by human proteases because the high proline and glutamine content prevents complete proteolysis by gastric and pancreatic enzymes, and long oligopeptides that are toxic to coeliac sprue patients build up in the small intestine (Sollid & Khosla, 2005). *In vitro* and *in vivo* studies in rats and humans have demonstrated that a 33-mer peptide from α-gliadin is not digestible by gastric, pancreatic, and intestinal brush-border membrane endoproteases (Shan et al., 2002). This and similar peptides have been identified as the principal contributors to gluten immunotoxicity.

At present, treatment with a gluten-free diet (GFD) is the only available therapy for CD patients. However, it is not easy to maintain a diet with zero gluten content because gluten contamination of food is commonplace (Collin et al., 2004). Even products specifically targeted at dietary treatment of CD may contain tiny amounts of gluten proteins, either because of the cross-contamination of originally gluten-free cereals during their milling, storage, and manipulation, or because of the presence of wheat starch as a major ingredient. Gluten is a common ingredient in the human diet; after sugar, it is perhaps the second most widespread food substance in Western civilization. Since about 10% of gluten seems to be made up of potentially toxic gliadin peptides (Sollid & Khosla, 2005), the characterization and quantification of the toxic peptides of the gluten in foodstuffs is crucial to avoid coeliac damage and enable monitoring of their enzymatic detoxification.

2. Gluten testing

2.1 Antibodies testing for gluten-free foods

A standardized method of analysis is needed to quantitatively determine the gluten content of food and provide the basis for enforcing regulations regarding use of the term "gluten-free" in food labelling. People with coeliac disease should feel confident that foods labelled "gluten-free" have been assessed for gluten using the same "best available" methodology. According to the *Codex Alimentarius*, only food with a gluten content under 20 ppm can be considered gluten-free. Food containing between 20 ppm and 100 ppm of gluten is considered to be very low in gluten content according to EU regulations, but there is no full agreement among countries about the term "gluten-free food". Unfortunately, there is not a well-defined correlation between the amount of gluten ingested and the severity of clinical symptoms, which makes finding a threshold value difficult. Various antibodies (Ab) have been raised against different gliadin epitopes. The anti ω-gliadin Ab is used in a sandwich format that was approved as an official method by the AOAC (Association of Official Agricultural Chemists; Skerritt & Hill, 1991). However, the content of ω-gliadin in wheat varies significantly, from 6% to 20%, and this method cannot accurately detect and quantify barley prolamines (Thompson & Mendez, 2008). The ω-gliadin (Skerritt) ELISA was developed in 1991 and was considered a first reference assay. Subsequent assays have improved on some of the important limitations of the techniques based on the Skerritt antibody ELISA. Other antibodies were raised against different epitopes of α-gliadin, such as PN3 (residues 31-49) for the toxic 19-mer peptides (Ellis et al., 1998), CDC5 (residues 56-75; Nassef et al., 2008), Abs against T-cell stimulatory peptides present in gluten (Mitea et al., 2008), and R5, which recognized highly repeated peptide sequences present in wheat, barley, and rye grains (Valdés et al., 2003). The sandwich R5 ELISA was endorsed as a type I method by the Codex Committee on Methods of Analysis and Sampling (*Codex Alimentarius Commission. Report of the 27th session of the Codex Committee on methods of analysis and sampling 2006, ALINORM 06/29/23*) for gluten determination. One criticism is that it overestimates barley hordein (Thompson & Méndez, 2008). It is also unable to accurately quantify hydrolyzed gluten.

2.2 Antibodies to toxic gluten peptides

Recent advances in the coeliac field strongly recommend updating the concept of "gluten detection" to "potential relative immunotoxicity of gluten" for the safety of coeliac consumers of food. Two monoclonal antibodies (moAbs), A1 and G12, were raised against the immunodominant peptide 33-mer (LQLQPFPQPQLPYPQPQLPYPQPQLPYP QPQPF, residues 57 to 89; Morón et al., 2008a).

2.2.1 Detection of gliadin immunogenic peptide by anti-33-mer moAbs

The 33-mer peptide from α-2 gliadin is a principal contributor to gluten immunotoxicity (Shan et al., 2002). Thus the production of moAbs against this toxic gluten peptide could be of great importance in both research and diagnosis. We obtained moAbs against the 33-mer peptide (A1 and G12 moAbs) (Morón et al., 2008a). To test the relative sensitivity of each moAb for the 33-mer peptide, we immobilized different concentrations of the C-LYTAG-33-mer polypeptide, and detected with A1 and G12 moAbs in an indirect ELISA. The affinity of each moAb for the antigen was quantified by calculation of the concentration of the antigen giving a 50% reduction of the peak signal in the ELISA (IC50). The sensitivity of the G12 moAb for the toxic 33-mer peptide was about eight times higher than that of A1 (Figure 1A). To test for moAb specificity, we studied the cross-reactivity (CR) values of these moAbs against commercial gliadin, also by indirect ELISA. The G12 moAb presented an IC50 of almost double that obtained with the A1 moAb, suggesting that A1 had broader reactivity with gliadin epitopes than did G12, which is more specific for the 33-mer (Figure 1B).

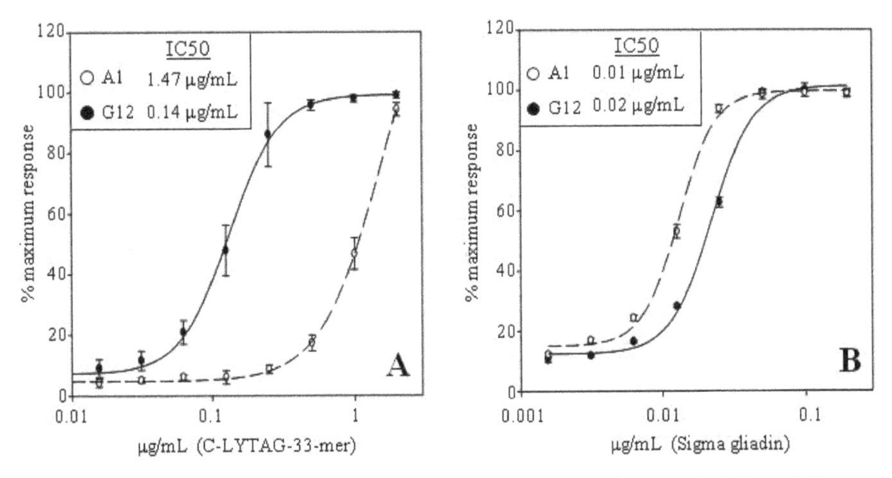

Fig. 1. Standard curve of the detection of C-LYTAG-33-mer polypeptide (A) and Sigma gliadin (B) by indirect ELISA using G12 (black) and A1 (white) moAbs. Each point of the curve represents the mean ±standard deviation of n=4 assays. IC50 values of the moAbs to the two antigens are indicated.

2.2.2 Characterization of A1 and G12 moAb sensitivity for coeliac-toxic cereals

We investigated whether the G12/A1 moAbs were able to detect the presence of gliadin 33-mer-related epitopes in prolamines from various cereals (Morón et al., 2008a; 2008b). To obtain quantitative data on the capacity of these antibodies to detect coeliac-toxic prolamines, we performed an indirect ELISA with samples of wheat, barley, rye, oats, rice, and maize (Figure 2). The assay proved to be highly specific for wheat, rye, and barley, as no signal was observed in samples containing prolamines from rice or maize (Figure 2). The G12 and A1 moAbs detected oats with lower sensitivity, indicating that there are peptides in avenin with sequence similarity to the 33-mer. This is consistent with the identification of proline- and glutamine-rich epitopes in avenins that are toxic in some CD patients (Arentz-Hansen et al., 2004). The lower sensitivity for oat avenins may be due to the lower proportion of oat-flour protein content consisting of prolamines relative to the proportion of gliadins, hordeins, or secalins in their respective grains.

The A1 moAb was clearly more sensitive than the G12 moAb for the detection of the prolamine fractions from wheat, barley, rye, and oats. Although they were targeted at the toxic 33-mer peptide of wheat gliadin, both moAbs were more sensitive for barley than for wheat (Figure 2), with the affinity for barley of the A1 moAb being almost three-fold higher than that of the G12. The A1 was also more sensitive for the prolamines of rye than for those of wheat.

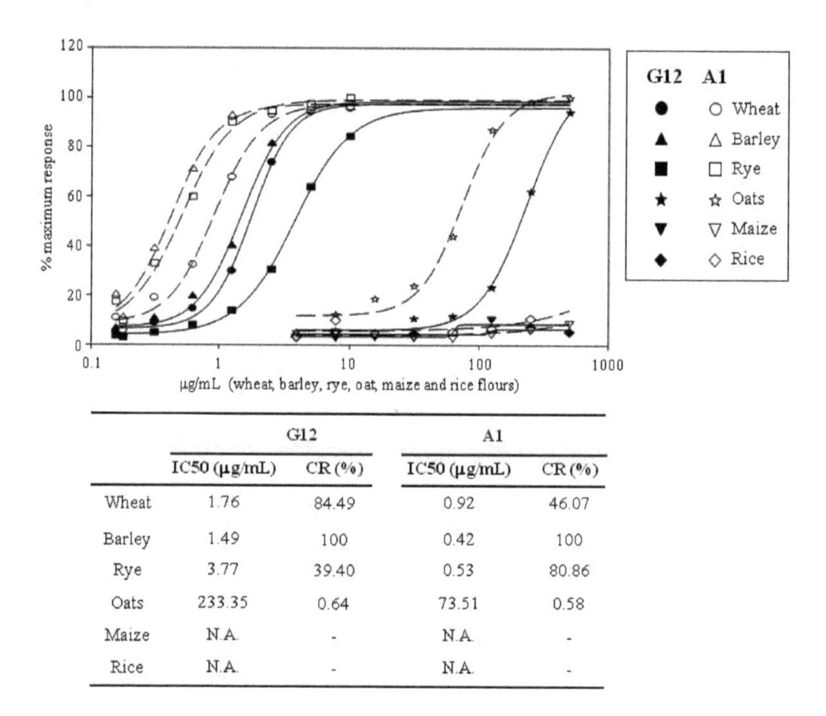

	G12		A1	
	IC50 (µg/mL)	CR (%)	IC50 (µg/mL)	CR (%)
Wheat	1.76	84.49	0.92	46.07
Barley	1.49	100	0.42	100
Rye	3.77	39.40	0.53	80.86
Oats	233.35	0.64	73.51	0.58
Maize	N.A.	-	N.A.	-
Rice	N.A.	-	N.A.	-

Fig. 2. Comparative reactivity of prolamines from wheat, barley, rye, oats, maize, and rice from indirect ELISAs using G12 (black) and A1 (white) moAbs. Each point of the curve shows the mean of n=3 assays. IC50 and CR values of the moAbs to prolamines are indicated. N.A.: Not applicable.

2.2.3 Development of a competitive ELISA assay using the anti-gliadin 33-mer moAbs

The preparation of many foodstuffs involves heating or enzymatic processes that may partially hydrolyze or deamidate gluten. As a result, the quantity of gluten extracted from foodstuffs processed by heat or fermentation may be underestimated by indirect or sandwich ELISA. We therefore developed a competitive ELISA method using the G12 moAb. The result was a highly sensitive competitive assay with a limit of detection of 0.44 ng/mL and a limit of quantification of 3.95 ng/mL. The gliadin concentration giving a 50% reduction in the maximum signal (i.e., IC50) in the standard curve of the competitive ELISA was determined to be 26.92 ng/mL. The repeatability and reproducibility of the method were calculated from various standard curves performed on the same ELISA plate (intra-assay) and on different ELISA plates (inter-assay), respectively. For the standards situated between 25 ng gliadin/mL and 1.56 ng gliadin/mL, the intra-assay was 1.38–3.75%, and the inter-assay was 1.65–10.30% for the same standards. To determine whether the competitive assay was able to detect small fragments originated by gliadin digestion, we analyzed a sample of gliadin that had been digested with trypsin and pepsin. We observed that the developed assay could detect the peptides coming from the degradation of gliadin by these enzymes. We also analyzed a sample of hydrolyzed baby cereals in which the gliadin had been partially hydrolyzed during processing. These cereals contain a mixture of wheat, barley, rye, oat, and rice flours. The ethanolic extract obtained from the foodstuff was analyzed using the competitive ELISA. The partially hydrolyzed prolamines present in the sample were able to compete, and the quantitative assay could be performed.

We developed a similar assay using the A1 moAb. The repeatability and reproducibility of the method were calculated from various standard curves performed on the same ELISA plate (intra-assay), and on different ELISA plates (inter-assay). The intra-assay coefficient of variation of the standards situated between 100 ng/mL of gliadin and 1.56 ng/mL of gliadin was found to be between 1.37% and 5.21%, while the inter-assay coefficient of variation was between 3.16% and 11.78% for the same standards.

2.2.4 Analysis of the epitope recognition of G12 and A1 moAbs

To determine the epitope recognized by the G12 and A1 moAbs within the 33-mer peptide, fusions of the C-LYTAG coding sequence of the pALEXb plasmid (Biomedal S.L., Seville, Spain) were constructed with coding sequences of hepta- and octapeptides comprising the complete sequence of the 33-mer peptide (Figure 3A). The resulting plasmids were introduced by transformation into the REG1 strain of *Escherichia coli,* allowing for overexpression of the encoded fusion proteins upon induction (Biomedal S.L., Seville, Spain). The overexpressed bacterial extracts were analyzed by indirect ELISA using the anti-33-mer A1 and G12 moAbs. Similarly, the anti-C-LYTAG 6B5L1 moAb (Biomedal, S.L., Seville, Spain) was used to establish that the designed protein was expressed intact in all cases. A reference signal in the bacterial extract containing the C-LYTAG-33-mer fusion protein was observed for all the moAbs assayed (A1, G12, and 6B5L1) (Figure 3B). Saturating signals were obtained in the indirect ELISA analysis using the anti-C-LYTAG 6B5L1 moAb for all the analyzed fusion proteins, indicating that all fusion proteins were overexpressed (Figure 3B).

With regard to the determination of the sequence of recognition of the anti-33-mer moAbs (G12 and A1), a positive signal was detected only in the bacterial extracts containing the fusion peptides Pro63-Tyr69 (PQPQLPY) and Gln64-Pro70 (QPQLPYP) for the G12 moAb and in the bacterial extracts containing the fusion peptide Gln66-Pro72 (QLPYPQP) for the A1 moAb (Figure 3B). These results thus indicate that the region of recognition within the

33-mer peptide for the G12 moAb is QPQLPY (common to the fusion proteins Pro63-Tyr69 and Gln64-Pro70) and that for the A1 moAb is QLPYPQP.

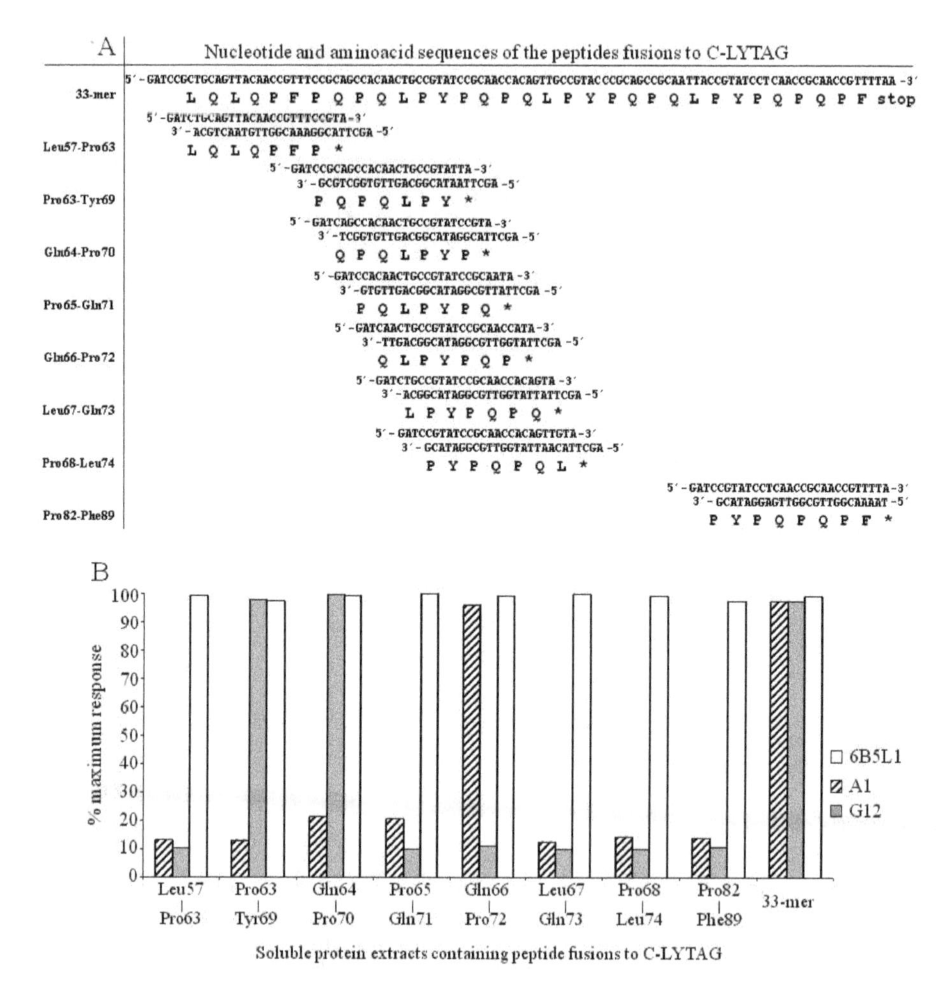

Fig. 3. Analysis of anti-33-mer moAb recognition regions in recombinant 33-mer peptide fragments expressed in *E. coli*. A. Nucleotide sequences and the deduced amino acid sequences of the encoded peptide fusions to C-LYTAG. B. Detection of C-LYTAG-peptide fusions by an indirect ELISA with the use of G12, A1, and 6B5L1 moAbs.

2.2.5 Study of the relative affinity of the G12 moAb for different peptide variants derived from the regions of recognition

The recognition sequence of the G12 moAb (QPQLPY) is repeated three times within the gliadin 33-mer peptide. To determine the relative affinity of G12 for this epitope, and for similar sequences present elsewhere in toxic prolamines, we constructed hexapeptide variants of the G12 epitope, two of which were designed based on their presence in the prolamines of barley and rye (Figure 4A and 4C). The affinity of the G12 moAb for different hexapeptide variants was determined in a competitive assay in which immobilized gliadin was challenged with QPQLPY-derivative peptides as soluble competitors (Figure 4A). The G12 moAb had high affinity for the peptide QPQLPF, reduced only four-fold relative to the previously identified epitope recognized by this moAb in the 33-mer, QPQLPY (Figure 4B). While the conservative replacement of tyrosine (QPQLPY) with phenylalanine (QPQLPF) did not drastically reduce the affinity of the G12 moAb, substitution with leucine (QPQLPL) reduced the affinity a thousand-fold, indicating the importance of this last position in determining affinity. A dramatic reduction in affinity was also observed for the peptide QPQQPY, with the affinity of the anti-33-mer G12 moAb decreasing as follows: QPQLPY>QPQLPF>>QPQLPL>QPQQPY.

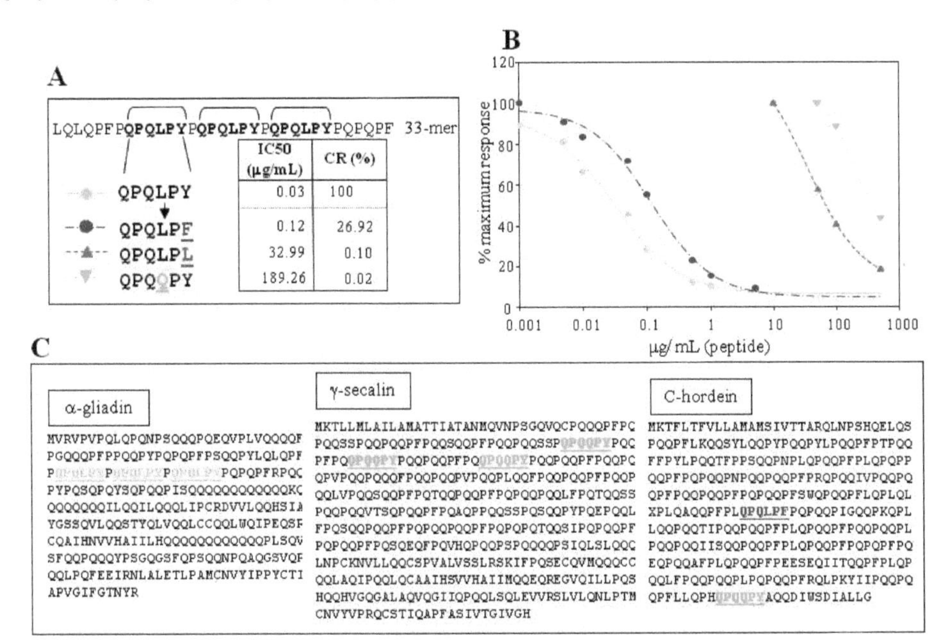

Fig. 4. Relative affinity of the G12 moAb for different peptide variants derived from its recognition region (QPQLPY). A. Amino acid sequences of the peptides. The G12 recognition sequence in the 33-mer peptide is in bold face. IC50 and CR values of the G12 moAb to peptides are indicated. B. Competition assay measuring the affinity of the G12 moAb for the peptides. Two separate assays were performed with the antibody, each with three repetitions. C. Localization of the peptides in the α-gliadin (accession number: JQ1047), c-secalin (accession number: ABO32294.1), and C-hordein (accession number: AAA92333.1) sequences. The same colour code for labelling the peptides has been used in A, B, and C.

2.2.6 Determination of the peptide sequence preferences for A1 moAb binding

We also studied the relative affinity of the A1 moAb for its recognition sequence (QLPYPQP) and for related peptide variants by a competitive assay (Figure 5A). The peptides assayed for A1 were more numerous than those for G12 due to the longer heptapeptide recognition sequence contained in the 33-mer and to the suspected broader specificity of A1 for other prolamine sequences based on indirect ELISA assays (Figure 2). Figure 5 shows the affinity of the A1 moAb for the different peptides assayed; the IC50 was used to compare the affinity of A1 for each peptide.

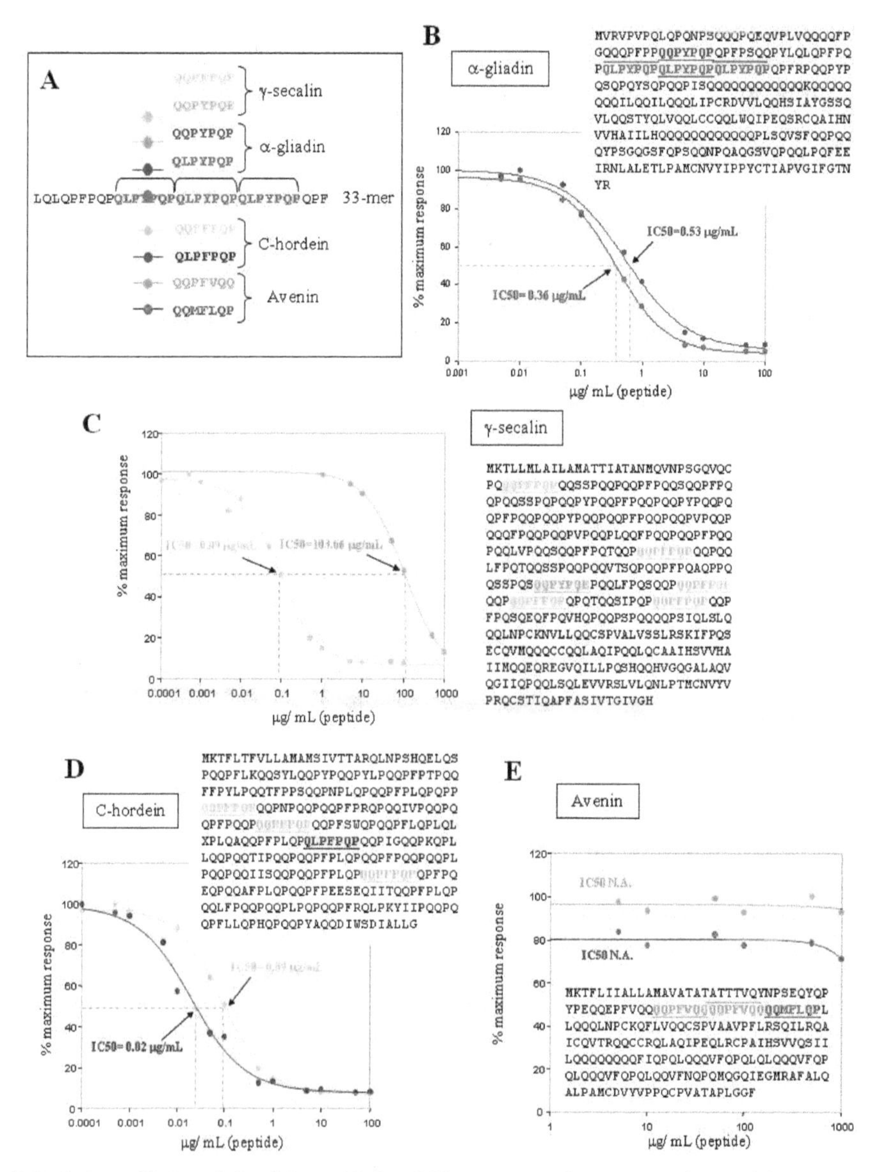

Fig. 5. Relative affinity of the A1 moAb for different peptide variants derived from its recognition region (QLPYPQP). A. Amino acid sequences of the peptides. The A1

recognition sequence in the 33-mer peptide is in red. B, C, D, and E. Competition assay for detection of the affinity of the A1 moAb for the peptides and their localization in α-gliadin (B; accession number: JQ1047), c-secalin (C; accession number: ABO32294.1), C-hordein (D; accession number: AAA92333.1), and avenin (E; accession number: AAA32716.1). Two separate assays were performed with the moAb, each with three repetitions. IC50 values of the A1 moAb to peptides are indicated. N.A.: Not applicable. The colour code for labelling the peptides is the same as that used in A.

Notably, two peptides present in secalin and hordein (QQPFPQP and QLPFPQP, Figures 5C and 5D, respectively) showed higher affinity for the A1 moAb than did the 33-mer-derived recognition sequence peptide (QLPYPQP). This suggests that the fourth residue in the recognition sequence is substantially important to A1 recognition, whereas the second position is not. Consistent with this, gliadin peptides QLPYPQP and QQPYPQP showed comparable affinity for the moAb (Figure 5B). The affinity of the anti-33-mer A1 moAb for epitopes present in coeliac-toxic cereals decreased as follows: QLPFPQP>QQPFPQP>QLPYPQP>QQPYPQP>>QQPYPQE.

The affinity for the sequence included in the wheat gliadin 33-mer was not as high as for QQPFPQP, which is one of the most abundant sequences in secalin and hordein, similarly to the 33-mer epitope in gliadin. This may explain why, despite its lower affinity for the 33-mer peptide relative to the G12 moAb, the A1 moAb had a higher sensitivity for the whole range of toxic cereals tested in this study. The A1 moAb may therefore be useful as a sensitive detection tool for identifying coeliac-toxic peptides in complex foodstuffs.

Preliminary attempts to find an avenin epitope gave no positive results (Figure 5E). The prolamines in oats represent much less of the total seed proteins than those in the other cereals. Furthermore, the amount of proline residues contained in avenins (10%) is about two-thirds that in the prolamines of wheat (gliadins and glutenins), barley (hordeins), and rye (secalins). In any case, we tested certain previously proposed potential avenin epitopes located in the avenin regions with the highest content of proline residues, regions also rich in glutamine, but could not obtain any reactivity to the A1 moAb.

To study the relative importance of glutamine and proline residues in epitope selection by the A1 moAb, single substitutions or deletions were made to these amino acids in the recognition sequence (QLPYPQP). We performed the analysis with the A1 moAb rather than with the G12 moAb because A1 has higher sensitivity for prolamines from toxic cereals. When the first glutamine of the A1 recognition sequence was eliminated (LPYPQP), the affinity for A1 decreased significantly, consistent with the results from epitope scanning with the C-LYTAG fusions (Figure 3). Substitutions of each proline residue in the recognition sequence with a serine residue decreased A1 affinity markedly. This effect was greatest when the substitution was made in the second proline position (QLPYSQP), resulting in a CR that was practically zero.

These results indicate that the initial glutamine residue and all three prolines of the epitope QLPYPQP were important for their recognition by A1, suggesting that this moAb could serve as a tool for monitoring enzymatic degradation of toxic peptides by potentially therapeutic glutamine- and proline-specific proteases.

2.2.7 Use of the A1 moAb to monitor gluten detoxification by candidate glutenases

Oral administration of glutamine- and proline-specific proteases (i.e., glutenases) is a potential therapeutic alternative (or adjunct) to a gluten-free diet (Stepniak & Koning, 2006; Cerf-Bensussan et al., 2007). However, validation of the efficacy of these enzymes at detoxifying gluten *in vitro* must precede clinical testing, and such validation currently relies on low-throughput, technically challenging cell-culture-based assays (Siegel et al., 2006; Gass et al., 2007; Stepniak & Koning, 2006) or on polyclonal anti-gliadin-antibody-based ELISA assays that are only grossly quantitative (Gass et al., 2007). A competitive ELISA using an anti-33-mer moAb would enable high-throughput, highly quantitative testing of gluten detoxification by candidate therapeutic glutenases.

We digested commercial whole-wheat bread under mock gastric conditions for 60 min with pepsin supplemented either with EP-B2 at varied concentrations (Figure 6A), or with a fixed EP-B2 concentration plus varied concentrations of SC PEP (Figure 6B). Dilution series of the quenched digests were prepared in parallel with a calibration dilution series of chemically synthesized 33-mer peptide, and these were tested against fixed 33-mer in an indirect competitive ELISA using A1 moAb. Treatment of whole-wheat bread with EP-B2 reduced the concentration of the 33-mer and close analogues by up to 10-fold in a dose-dependent manner (Figure 6A). This is consistent with the observation that EP-B2 cleaves the 33-mer after Gln66, Gln73, and Gln80 (Bethune et al., 2006), cleavages expected to extirpate the affinity of A1 for the resultant fragments.

The combination of EP-B2 + SC PEP further reduced antigen concentrations by at least an additional 10-fold to levels undetectable by our methods (Figure 6B). This is again consistent with previously published results, in which EP-B2 substantially detoxified similar bread digests, but the synergistic combination of EP-B2 with SC PEP was required to dramatically reduce the intestinal T-cell reactivity of these digests (Gass et al., 2007). The intensity of the signal obtained with the A1 moAb in our assay was therefore proportional to the potential damage caused to a CD patient by a commercial gluten source (Morón et al., 2008b).

2.2.8 Analysis of the recognition of anti-33-mer moAbs for deamidated and innate gluten peptides

CD is closely associated with genes that code for human leukocyte antigens DQ2 and DQ8. These have been shown to bind with high affinity to gliadin-derived peptides in which specific glutamine residues in key positions have been converted to glutamic acid by transglutaminase-2-mediated deamidation (Alaedini & Green, 2005; Sollid & Khosla, 2005). A moAb capable of discriminating between native and deamidated gluten peptides would be a valuable research tool for monitoring the fate of digested prolamine peptides. To test the relative sensitivity of each moAb for the deamidated 33-mer peptide, a peptide (QPQLPYPQP) was designed that represented a region of recognition common to the two moAbs, together with the same peptide deamidated (QPELPYPQP).

The affinities of the A1 and G12 moAbs for these peptides were determined by a competitive assay in which immobilized gliadin was challenged with peptides as competitors. The affinity of the G12 moAb for the deamidated peptide was about forty times higher than that of the A1 moAb. However, both moAbs recognized the non-deamidated peptide with >100-fold greater affinity than they did the deamidated peptide. In

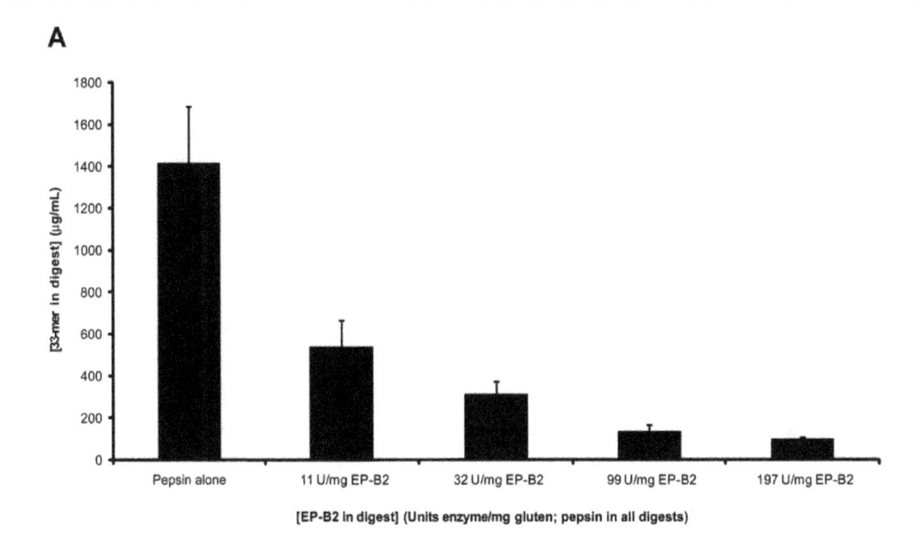

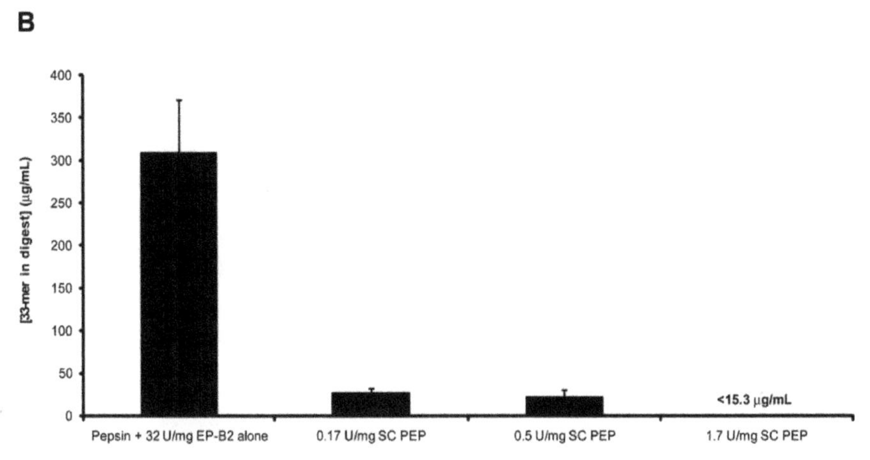

Fig. 6. Indirect competitive ELISA using A1 moAb to test whole-wheat bread digests for 33-mer content. A. Concentration of 33-mer (mg/mL) in whole-wheat bread digests containing 0.6 mg/mL pepsin supplemented with specified concentrations of recombinant proEP-B2 (U/mg gluten). B. Concentration of 33-mer (mg/mL) in whole-wheat bread digests containing 0.6 mg/mL pepsin and 32 U/mg EP-B2 supplemented with specified concentrations of recombinant SC PEP (U/mg gluten). The concentration of 33-mer in each digest was determined by comparison with a synthetic 33-mer standard curve. Two separate assays were performed with the antibody, each with three repetitions.

combination with a previously characterized, commercially available moAb that has 20-fold greater affinity for the deamidated form of an overlapping gluten peptide than for its non-deamidated counterpart, G12 and A1 moAbs may be useful for future studies on transglutaminase-2-mediated gluten peptide deamidation.

The innate immune response to gluten plays a key role in the development of CD (Fehniger & Caligiuri, 2001; Bernardo et al., 2007). This response is mediated by interleukin 15 (a typical cytokine of the innate immune system) and elicited by the toxic peptide p31-49 (19-mer), derived from alpha-gliadin. To test whether the anti-33-mer A1 and G12 moAbs recognized peptide p31-49, competitive ELISAs with each moAb were performed. The A1 moAb was able to detect p31-49 (IC50 3.18 mg/mL). The G12 moAb showed no affinity for the 19-mer peptide.

These results were consistent with our previous identification of the QQPYPQP peptide, included in p31-49, as a permissive epitope for the A1 moAb. Therefore, this moAb shows an interesting range of peptide recognition that includes gliadin peptides involved in both the adaptive and the innate immunological responses in CD.

3. The oats controversy: selection of oat varieties with no toxicity in coeliac disease

There is an ongoing debate concerning the presence or absence of gluten in oats. Traditionally, treatment with a GFD has excluded not only wheat, barley, and rye, but also oats. Oats differ from other cereals in their prolamine content. The percentage of proline and glutamine (amino acids abundant in toxic regions) in avenin is lower than in other toxic cereals (Figure 8).

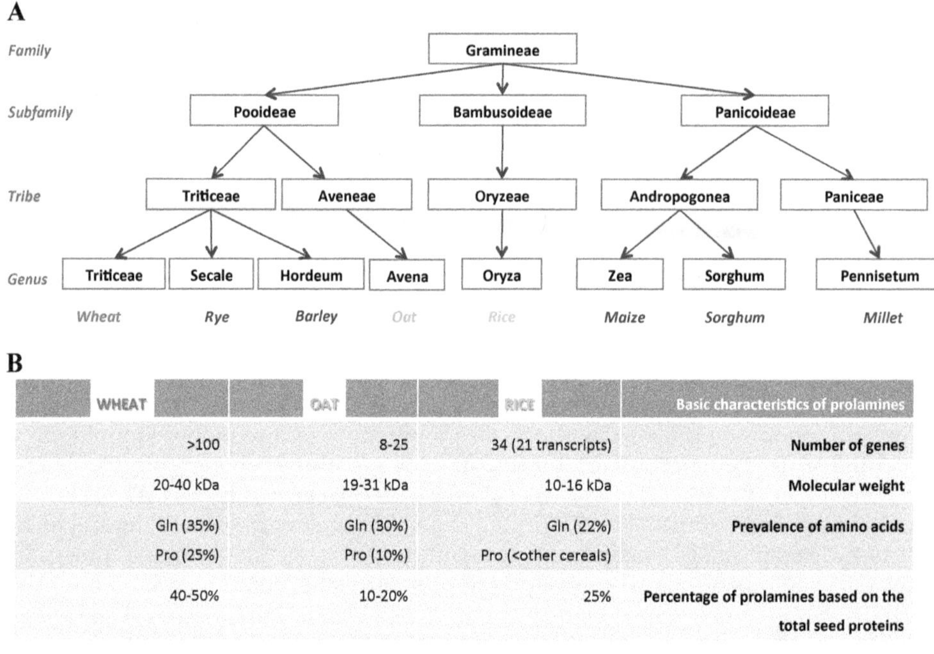

WHEAT	OAT	RICE	Basic characteristics of prolamines
>100	8-25	34 (21 transcripts)	Number of genes
20-40 kDa	19-31 kDa	10-16 kDa	Molecular weight
Gln (35%) Pro (25%)	Gln (30%) Pro (10%)	Gln (22%) Pro (<other cereals)	Prevalence of amino acids
40-50%	10-20%	25%	Percentage of prolamines based on the total seed proteins

Fig. 8. Taxonomy and basic characteristics of the prolamines of oats in relation with other cereals. A. Taxonomy of oats in relation with other cereals. B. Basic characteristics of the prolamines of wheat, oats, and rice.

However, there is still some debate about the safety of oats (Pulido et al., 2009). Several *in vivo* and *in vitro* studies have indicated that the majority of coeliac subjects can tolerate moderate amounts of pure oats. Some countries permit the use of oats in "gluten-free" products, e.g. Gluten-Free Oats®. According to the Codex Standard for food for special dietary use for persons intolerant to gluten, CODEX STAN118-1979 (revised 2008, http://www.codexalimentarius.net/web/more_info.jsp?id_sta=291), oats can be tolerated by most, but not all, people who are gluten-intolerant. Therefore, the permitting of oats that are not contaminated with wheat, rye, or barley in foods covered by this standard may be determined at the national level. Moreover, according to the Commission Regulation (EC) No 41/2009 (http://eur-lex.europa.eu/LexUriServ/LexUriServ.do?uri=OJ:L:2009:016:0003:0005:EN:PDF) concerning the composition and labelling of foodstuffs suitable for people intolerant to gluten, a major concern is the contamination of oats with wheat, rye, or barley that can occur during grain harvesting, transport, storage, and processing. Therefore, the risk of gluten contamination in products containing oats should be taken into consideration with regard to labelling of those products. Certain cross-reactivity with gliadin-specific antibody has been attributed to wheat contamination in oat-based food (Pulido et al., 2009).

However, other authors shown clear evidence that avenins have the ability to induce the activation of mucosal T-cells, causing gut inflammation and villous atrophy (Pulido et al., 2009). Arentz-Hansen et al. (2004) described the intestinal deterioration suffered by some CD patients following the consumption of oats while on GFD. Avenin can trigger an immunological response in these patients similar to the response produced by the gluten of wheat, rye, or barley. The monitoring of 19 adult coeliac patients who consumed 50 g/day of oats over twelve weeks showed that one of the subjects was sensitive to oats. Therefore, it is crucial to clarify either qualitatively or quantitatively the potential immunotoxicity of oats to coeliac patients (Arentz-Hansen et al., 2004; Pulido et al., 2009).

In a previous work, we obtained two moAbs, G12 and A1, against the 33-mer peptide (Morón et al., 2008a). Our results suggested that the reactivity of these moAbs was correlated with the potential immunotoxicity of those dietary grains from which the proteins were extracted (Morón et al., 2008b; Ehren et al., 2009). These antibodies are able to recognize with great sensitivity peptides (besides the 33-mer peptide) immunotoxic for coeliac patients. The sensitivity and epitope preferences of these antibodies were found to be useful for detecting gluten-relevant peptides to infer the potential toxicity of food for coeliac patients. The G12 moAb showed cross-reactivity that served to detect a certain amount of oat avenins, although with lower sensitivity than the hordein, gliadin, and secalin (Morón et al., 2008a) The oats controversy appears to be a unique case for exploring this issue, because cases of intermediate immunotoxicity could be expected and the correlation of potential toxicity and analytical signal could be assessed.

3.1 Relative affinity of the G12 moAb for different varieties of oats

Different oat varieties monitored for their purity and by their distinct protein pattern (Figure 9), were used to examine differences in G12 moAb recognition by ELISA and Western blot.

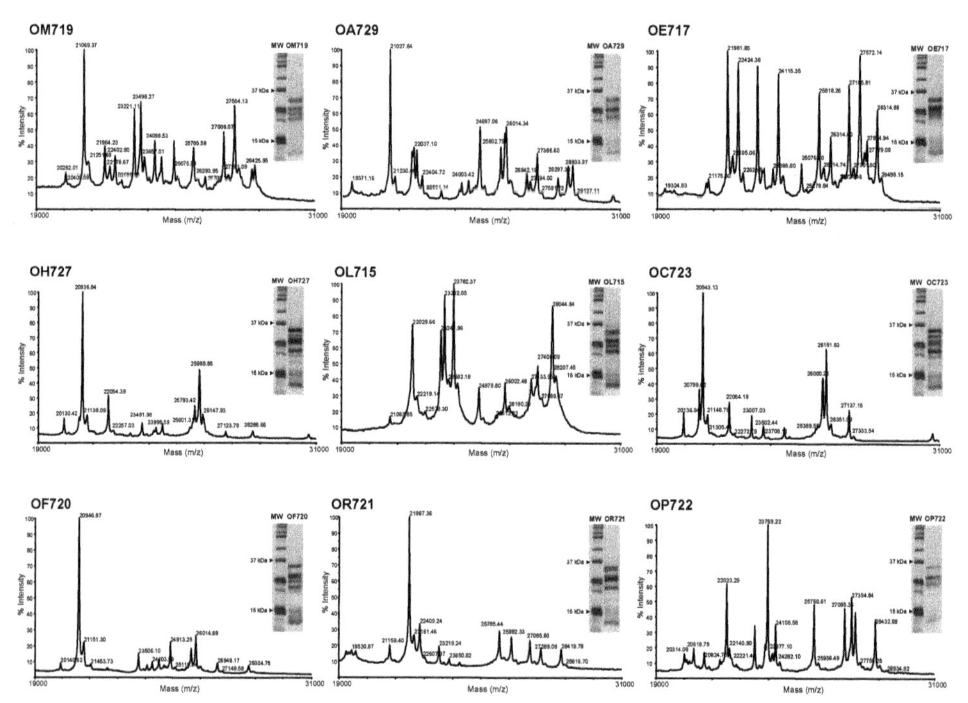

Fig. 9. Comparison of avenin fractions extracted from oat varieties studied. Avenin spectra were determined by matrix-assisted laser desorption/ionization time-of-flight mass spectrometry of the 9 oat varieties. Analysis of proteins extracted from the oat varieties by SDS-PAGE. MW: Protein molecular weight marker.

To determine whether the G12 moAb had distinct reactivity to the different oat varieties, the affinity of the G12 moAb was determined by competitive ELISA. The G12 moAb showed different affinity for the oat varieties tested (Figure 10A). Therefore, three groups of oat varieties could be clearly distinguished depending on their recognition by the G12 moAb: a group of high affinity towards the antibody (OM719, OA729 and OE717), a group of intermediate recognition (OH727, OL715, and OC723), and another group comprising oats that were not recognized by the G12 moAb (OF720, OR721, and OP722). The alternative anti-33-mer A1 moAb provided equivalent results (data not shown).

In order to quantify the affinity of the oat varieties for the G12 moAb, the IC50 and the CR were determined for each variety (Figure 10B). The IC50 is defined as the concentration that produces a reduction of 50% in the peak signal in the ELISA. The CR was determined as (IC50 of the oat variety that presents the greatest affinity for the antibody/IC50 of each variety assayed) x 100. Varieties OE717 and OA729 respectively showed a CR of around 60% and 75% with respect to the most sensitive variety (OM719). Varieties OH727, OL715, and OC723, with a CR of 25%, 24%, and 12%, respectively, were recognized by the G12 moAb, but with a lower sensitivity. The avenins of OF720, OR721, and OP722 were not recognized by the G12 moAb, as in the case of the negative control (rice).

In order to confirm the ELISA results with another immunological technique and to identify protein patterns with cross-reactivity to the anti-33-mer antibody, immunoblotting electrophoresis analyses were performed. The results (Figure 10C) showed that the G12 moAb had affinity for the varieties OM719, OA729, OE717, OH727, OL715, and OC723. However, the antibody did not react with varieties OF720, OP722, and OR721. The variability in reactivity demonstrated by Western blot thus correlated with the previously presented ELISA results. These results suggested the presence of different prolamine subunits in the oat varieties, differing in both their amino acid composition and length.

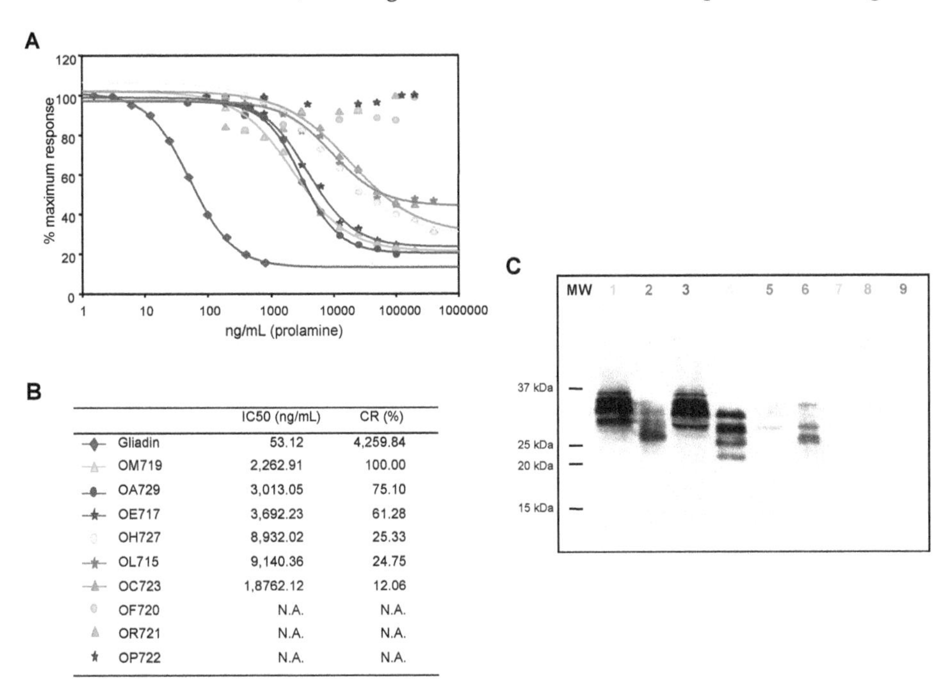

	IC50 (ng/mL)	CR (%)
Gliadin	53.12	4,259.84
OM719	2,262.91	100.00
OA729	3,013.05	75.10
OE717	3,692.23	61.28
OH727	8,932.02	25.33
OL715	9,140.36	24.75
OC723	1,8762.12	12.06
OF720	N.A.	N.A.
OR721	N.A.	N.A.
OP722	N.A.	N.A.

Fig. 10. Relative affinity of the G12 anti-33-mer moAb for different oat varieties and gliadin. A. Competitive ELISA using the G12-HRP anti-33-mer antibody to determine the relative affinity of this antibody against the different varieties of oats. Three assays were performed, with three replicates of each. Gliadin was used as positive control. B. IC50 and CR of the different oat varieties. N.A.: Not applicable. C. Western blot analysis of toxic fractions from different prolamines extracted from the grains of oats. Membranes were stained with G12 antibody. The colour code for labelling the varieties is the same as that used in A and B.

3.2 Determining the concentration of immunoreactive peptides in oats

To evaluate the relative amount of immunotoxic epitopes present in the prolamines of different oat varieties, one variety was chosen from each of the three groups previously identified for their affinity towards the G12 moAb. Thus, OM719 represented the group with greatest affinity towards the G12 moAb, OH727 those of intermediate reactivity, and OF720 those not recognized by this antibody.

The presence of immunoreactive peptides was determined by the G12 moAb competitive ELISA, using the 33-mer peptide as the standard curve. The presence of 33-mer and close analogues in the most reactive oat variety, OM719, was of the order of 1,340 ng/mg of avenin (Figure 11). In OH727, the levels of 33-mer were some 4-fold lower than in OM719. However, in the case of OF720, the concentration of 33-mer was reduced more than 1,300-fold with respect to OM719, reaching levels undetectable by this method.

This result was consistent with earlier results obtained using IC50 and CR, and by Western blot, and at the same time indicated the enormous difference between some varieties and others regarding the presence of sequences that are immunoreactive for coeliac patients.

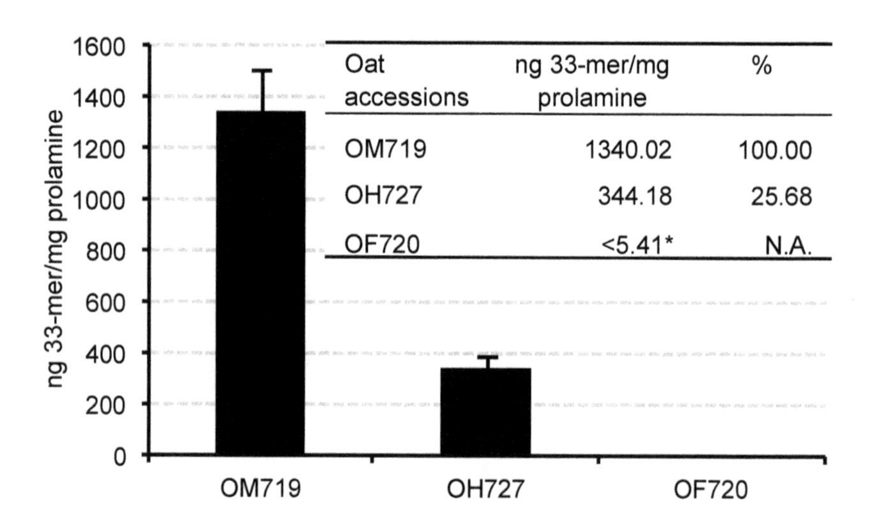

Oat accessions	ng 33-mer/mg prolamine	%
OM719	1340.02	100.00
OH727	344.18	25.68
OF720	<5.41*	N.A.

Fig. 11. Detection of concentration of 33-mer peptide in different oat varieties. The concentration of 33-mer was determined by competitive ELISA using the G12 monoclonal antibody. Different dilutions were tested independently for each oat variety, each with three repetitions.

3.3 Correlation between G12 moAb reactivity and immunogenicity of different oat varieties

To determine whether the variations in the reactivity of the anti-33-mer G12 in the different oat varieties were correlated with the greater or lesser immunogenicity of the cereal, we directly challenged the cereal extracts with appropriate cells obtained from coeliac patients. The clinical and immunological characteristics of coeliac patients are presented in Table 1.

Immunogenicity was determined by T-cell proliferation and IFN-γ production. Three cultivars of oats were selected -one variety was chosen from each previously identified group *(OM719, OH727 and OF720)*. We tested whether there was a correlation between their potential immunotoxicity for coeliac patients and their reactivity with the G12 moAb.

The avenin of the oat varieties, gliadin, and oryzein were subjected to peptic, trypsic, and chymotrypsin sequential digestion and treated with tTG. Cell proliferation and IFN-γ release in culture medium were measured as indices of lymphocyte activation.

Patient	Sex	Age (years)	Atrophy grade MARSH	AAEM	AATG	HLA DQB1	HLA DRB1
Coeliac 1	Male	6	III b	+	252	0201-0202	3-7
Coeliac 2	Female	3	III a	+	20	0201-0202	3-7
Coeliac 3	Male	13	III b	-	2	0202-0301	7-11
Coeliac 4	Female	5	III b	+	102	0201-0604	3-11
Coeliac 5	Female	9	III b	+	139	0201-0202	3-7
Coeliac 6	Female	2	III b	+	15	0302-0301	4-4
Coeliac 7	Female	4	III b	+	28	0201-0501	1-3
Coeliac 8	Female	7	II	+	111	0201-0202	3-7
Coeliac 9	Male	10	III b	+	165	0202-0301	7-11
Coeliac 10	Male	5	III b	+	118	0201-0202	3-7

Table 1. Clinical data of coeliac patients. AAEM: anti-endomysial antibody. AATG: anti-transglutaminase antibody expressed U/mL.

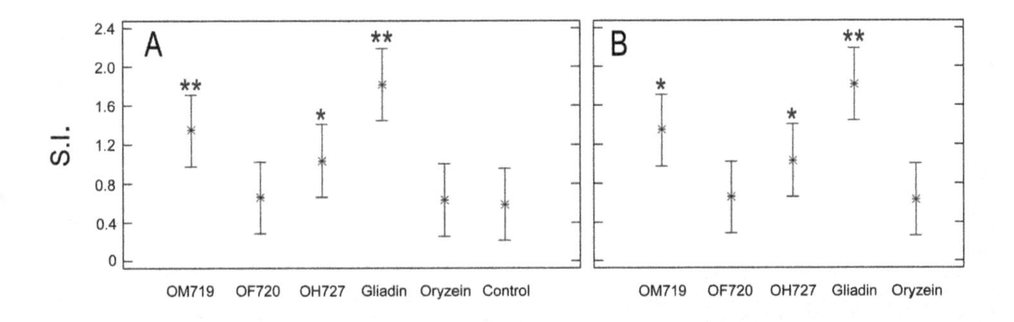

Fig. 12. Proliferative responses of T-cells to deamidated peptides of prolamine from three different oat varieties. PBMCs were exposed to tTG-treated prolamine-digest stimulation for 48 h. Gliadin and oryzein were used as positive and negative control, respectively. The experiments were performed in duplicate, and the mean S.I. value ± SDM is shown. A. The S.I. values of T-cells exposed to prolamine digests were statistically significant with respect to the control (healthy patient) and B. with respect to oryzein. *$p<0.05$, **$p<0.005$.

We found a significant increase of T-cell proliferation in cultures incubated with OM719 and gliadin (S.I.=1.3 ± 0.7 and 1.8 ± 0.9, respectively), and with OH727 (S.I.=1.02 ± 0.5). This clearly showed that gliadin and OM719 displayed the highest activity, and were potentially the most immunogenic (Figure 12). The incubation with OF720 increased cell proliferation (S.I.=0.65 ± 0.4) similarly to that with oryzein (S.I.=0.62 ± 0.3). We included the values presented in healthy patients (control) as reference values to compare the effect of peptides in coeliac patients, under the same conditions of cell culture. Release of IFN-γ in the culture medium after the exposure of coeliac peripheral T-lymphocytes to deamidated avenin peptides was assessed (Figure 13). According to this assay, gliadin and prolamines from OM719 were very immunogenic, with the highest values of IFN-γ release (9.4 ± 0.76 pg/mL and 7.9 ± 0.57 pg/mL, respectively), while the exposure to OH727 induced a lower mean value of IFN-γ (4.8 ± 0.95 pg/mL). Finally, OF720 and oryzein were the least immunogenic (3.4 ± 1.09 pg/mL and 2.3 ± 0.89 pg/mL, respectively).

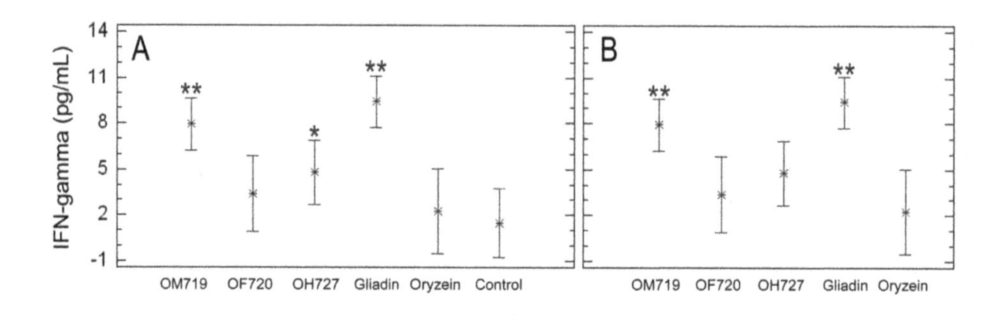

Fig. 13 IFN-γ production by T-cells with prolamine digests from three different oat varieties. T-lymphocytes were stimulated with digested prolamines after treatment with tTG. IFN-γ production was evaluated by ELISA after 48 h of incubation. Results are shown as means of duplicate wells and expressed as pg/mL. Gliadin and oryzein were used as positive and negative control, respectively. A. Significant with respect to healthy control and B. with respect to oryzein. *$p<0.05$, **$p<0.005$.

4. Conclusion

Immunotoxic gluten peptides that are recalcitrant to degradation by digestive enzymes appear to trigger CD. A 33-mer peptide from α-2 gliadin has been identified as a principal contributor to gluten immunotoxicity. A gluten-free diet is currently the only therapy for CD patients; therefore, the characterization and quantification of the toxic portion of gluten in foodstuffs is crucial to avoid coeliac damage. Our work was to develop tools for immunological assays to measure cereal fractions that are immunotoxic to CD patients. Two monoclonal antibodies, G12 and A1 (anti-33-mer antibodies), were developed against a highly immunotoxic gliadin 33-mer peptide.

Compared with other ELISAs, those based on these antibodies showed a broader specificity for prolamines that are toxic to CD patients, along with a higher degree of sensitivity, accuracy, and reproducibility. Furthermore, these antibodies have shown no cross-reactivity with any known food ingredient including soybean, as observed in the Codex standard R5 ELISA.

Gliadin and other immunotoxic prolamines are sometimes hydrolyzed in food and drinks, which may result in the underestimation of the net amount of toxic fractions by other less-specific antibodies that are not targeted at strictly immunotoxic peptides. The anti-33-mer antibodies have shown their practical efficacy as analytical tools in quantifying food toxicity for CD patients. These antibodies were assessed, and shown to be very suitable to provide a routine assay to determine gluten content, since their sensitivity and specificity were superior to previously described gluten immunoassays. Furthermore, the reactivity of these moAbs was correlated with the potential immunotoxicity of those dietary grains from which the proteins were extracted. T-cell reactivity analysis and enzymatic detoxification of the proteins showed that the signal of these antibodies was correlated with the sample's potential toxicity for coeliac patients.

We show, using the anti-33-mer antibodies raised against the toxic fragment, that oat immunogenicity for coeliac disease patients varies according to the variety of cultivar. We showed that the intensity of the signal obtained with the antibody was proportional to the potential damage caused to CD patients. We have proved that the reactivity of these antibodies with different varieties of oats was correlated with the immunotoxicity of those dietary grains from which the proteins were extracted, thereby providing a rational explanation of why some oats trigger immunological response, and a solution of how to avoid the presence of such varieties in gluten-free diets. The possibility of assessing the potential immunotoxicity to coeliac patients with a simple assay is an attractive idea with obvious applications in food analysis. Our study gives new insights about the dilemma of oats in coeliac disease, and suggests practical methods to select varieties of oats that are tolerable for coeliac patients, and at the same time, offers the possibility of measuring potential immunotoxicity by a simple immunological method, regardless of the cereal's origin. The experimental design to resolve those issues served to shed light on an ongoing controversy regarding the contradictory conclusions from clinical studies to establish the tolerance of coeliac patients to oats. Our work should also be taken into consideration by food safety regulations - in particular, the labelling of gluten-free products that may contain oats. Therefore, this work may potentially have a social impact besides its relevance in basic and clinical research of coeliac disease.

This work suggests considering whether the most practical way to measure food safety for coeliac patients is to quantify the amount of the immunoreactive prolamine epitopes, rather than the amount of any gluten in a given sample. The two antibodies have been used to develop different analytical techniques, including ELISA (competitive and sandwich) and immunochromatographic strips for routine assays (Glutentox®, Biomedal S.L., Seville, Spain). The A1- and G12-based immunoassays appear to be a promising approach to detect, with a direct relationship, any sample's net toxicity for coeliac patients.

5. Acknowledgment

Carolina Sousa gratefully acknowledges funds from the Asociación de Celíacos de Madrid (ACM, Madrid, Spain), the Ministerio de Ciencia e Innovación, and the Instituto Andaluz de Biotecnología (IAB).

6. References

Alaedini, A. & Green, P.H.R. (2005). Narrative review: celiac disease: understanding a complex autoimmune disorder. Annasl of Internal Medicine, Vol.142, No.4, (February 2005), pp.289–299, ISSN 0003-4819.

Arentz-Hansen, H., Fleckenstein, B., Molberg, Ø., Scott, H., Koning, F., Jung, G., Roepstorff, P., Lundin, K.E. & Sollid, L.M. (2004). The molecular basis for oat intolerance in patients with celiac disease. PLoS Medicine, Vol.1, No.1, (October 2004), pp.84–92, ISSN 1549-1277.

Bernardo, D., Garrote, J.A., Fernández-Salazar, L., Riestra, S. & Arranz, E. (2007). Is gliadin really safe for non-celiac individuals? Production of interleukin 15 in biopsy culture from non-celiac individuals challenged with gliadin peptides. Gut, Vol.56, No.6, (June 2007), pp.889-890, ISSN 1468-3288.

Bethune, M.T., Strop, P., Tang, Y., Sollid, L.M. & Khosla, C. (2006). Heterologous expression, purification, refolding, and structural-functional, characterization of EP-B2, a self-activating barley cysteine endoprotease. Chemistry & Biology, Vol.13, No.6, (June 2006), pp.637–647, ISSN 1074-5521.

Bethune, M.T. & Khosla, C. (2008). Parallels between pathogens and gluten peptides in celiac sprue. PLoS Pathogens, Vol.4, No.2, (February 2008), pp.e34, ISSN 1553-7366.

Cerf-Bensussan, N., Matysiak-Budnik, T., Cellier, C. & Heyman, M. (2007). Oral proteases: a new approach to managing coeliac disease. Gut, Vol.56, No.2, (February 2007), pp.157-160, ISSN 1468-3288.

Collin, P., Thorell, L., Kaukien, K. & Mäki, M. (2004). Alimentary Pharmacology & Therapeutics, Vol.19, No.12, (June 2004), pp.1277–1283, ISSN 1365-2036.

Comino, I., Real, A., de Lorenzo, L., Cornell, H., López-Casado, M.A., Barro, F., Lorite, P., Torres, M.I., Cebolla, A. & Sousa, C. (2011). Diversity in oat potential immunogenicity: basis for the selection of oat varieties with no toxicity in coeliac disease. Gut, Vol.60, No.7, (February 2011), pp.915-922, ISSN 1468-3288.

Ehren, J., Morón, B., Martin, E., Bethune, M.T., Gray, G.M. & Khosla, C. (2009). A food-grade enzyme preparation with modest gluten detoxification properties. PLoS One, Vol.4, No.7, (July 2009), pp.e6313, ISSN 1932-6203.

Ellis, H.J., Rosen-Bronson, S., O'Reilly, N. & Ciclitira, P.J. (1998). Measurement of gluten using a monoclonal antibody to a coeliac toxic peptide of A-gliadin. Gut, Vol.43, No.2, (August 1998), pp.190-195, ISSN 1468-3288.

Fehniger, T.A. & Caligiuri, M.A. (2001) Interleukin 15: biology and relevance to human disease. Blood, Vol.97, No.1, (January 2001), pp.14-32, ISSN 1528-0020.

Gass, J., Bethune, M.T., Siegel, M., Spencer, A. & Khosla, C. (2007). Combination enzyme therapy for gastric digestion of dietary gluten in celiac sprue patients. Gastroenterology, Vol.133, No.2, (August 2007), pp.472-480, ISSN 0016-5085.

Khosla, C., Gray, G.M. & Sollid, L.M. (2005). Putative efficacy and dosage of prolyl endopeptidase for digesting and detoxifying gliadin peptides. Gastroenterology, Vol.129, No.4, (October 2005), pp.1362–1363, ISSN 0016-5085.

Mitea, C., Havenaar, R., Drijfhout, J.W., Edens, L., Dekking, L. & Koning, F. (2008). Efficient degradation of gluten by a prolyl endoprotease in a gastrointestinal model: implications for coeliac disease. Gut, Vol.57, No.1, (January 2008), pp.25-32, ISSN 1468-3288.

Morón, B., Cebolla, A., Manyani, H., Alvarez-Maqueda, M., Megías, M., Thomas, M. del C., López, M.C. & Sousa, C. (2008a). Sensitive detection of cereal fractions that are toxic to celiac disease patients by using monoclonal antibodies to a main immunogenic wheat peptide. The American Journal of Clinical Nutrition, Vol.87, No:2, (February 2008), pp.405-414, ISSN 1938-3207.

Morón, B., Bethune, M.T., Comino, I., Manyani, H., Ferragud, M., López, M.C., Cebolla, A., Khosla, C. & Sousa, C. (2008b). Toward the assessment of food toxicity for celiac patients: characterization of monoclonal antibodies to a main immunogenic gluten peptide. PloS One, Vol.3, No.5, (May 2008), pp.e2294, ISSN 1932-6203.

Nassef, H.M., Bermudo, Redondo, M.C., Ciclitira, P.J., Ellis, H.J., Fragoso, A. & O'Sullivan, C.K. (2008). Electrochemical immunosensor for detection of celiac disease toxic gliadin in foodstuff. Analytical Chemistry, Vol.80, No.23, (December 2008), pp.9265-9271, ISSN 0003-2700.

Pulido, O., Gillespie, Z., Zarkadas, M., Dubois, S., Vavasour, E., Rashid, M., Switzer, C. & Goderfroy, S.B. (2009). Introduction of oats in the diet of individuals with celiac disease: A systematic review, In: Advances in Food and Nutrition Research, Steve L. Taylor, pp.235-285, ISBN 978-0-12-374440-1, USA.

Shan, L., Molberg, Ø., Parrot, I., Hausch, F., Filiz, F., Gray, G.M., Sollid, L.M. & Khosla, C. (2002) Structural basis for gluten intolerance in celiac sprue. Science, Vol.297, No.5590, (September 2002), pp. 2275–2279, ISSN 1095-9203.

Siegel, M., Bethune, M.T., Gass, J., Ehren, J., Xia, J., Johannsen, A., Stuge, T.B., Gray, G.M., Lee, P.P. & Khosla C. (2006). Rational design of combination enzyme therapy for celiac sprue. Chemistry & Biology, Vol.13, No.6, (June 2006), pp.649–658, ISSN 1074-5521.

Skerritt, J.H. & Hill, A.S. (1991). Enzyme immunoassay for determination of gluten in foods: collaborative study. Journal -Association of Official Analytical Chemists. Vol.74, No.2, (March-April 1991), pp.257-264, ISSN 1060-3271.

Sollid, L.M. & Khosla, C. (2005). Future therapeutic options for celiac disease. Nature Clinical Practice. Gastroenterology & Hepatology, Vol.2, No.3, (March 2005), pp.140–147, ISSN 1743-4386.

Stepniak, D. & Koning, F. (2006). Celiac disease-sandwiched between innate and adaptive immunity. Human Immunology, Vol.67, No.6, (June 2006), pp.460-468, ISSN 0198-8859.

Thompson, T. & Mendéz, E. (2008). Commercial assays to assess gluten content of gluten-free foods: why they are not created equal. Journal of the American Dietetic Association, Vol.108, No.10, (October 2008), pp.1682-1687, ISSN 0002-8223.

Valdés, I., García, E., Llorente, M. & Méndez E. (2003). Innovative approach to low-level gluten determination in foods using a novel sandwich enzyme-linked immunosorbent assay protocol. European Journal Gastroenterology & Hepatology, Vol.15, No.5, (May 2003), pp.465–474, ISSN 1473-5687.

Section 4

Advanced Therapies in Celiac Disease

8

Enzyme Therapy for Coeliac Disease: Is it Ready for Prime Time?

Hugh J. Cornell[1] and Teodor Stelmasiak[2]
[1]RMIT University, Melbourne,
[2]Glutagen Pty Ltd, Maribyrnong,
Australia

1. Introduction

Coeliac disease (CD) is a form of gluten intolerance in which the small bowel is damaged by proteins present in wheat, rye, barley and some varieties of oats (Mäki & Collin, 1997). . These proteins cause severe damage to the duodenum and jejunum (villous atrophy) and can produce a variety of symptoms such as abdominal pain and cramping, bloating diarrhoea, nausea and lethargy.

The discovery of the disease by Dicke led to treatment by means of a gluten-free diet, which needs to be maintained for the rest of life (Dicke et al, 1953). If left untreated, severe malabsorption causes the loss of vital nutrients, resulting in conditions such as osteoporosis. In addition, anaemia and long-term immune and autoimmune mechanisms can induce lymphomas (van Heel & West, 2006) .

Diagnosis thus needs to be effected early in life and screening tests are available that are based on antibodies to tissue transglutaminase. If positive, biopsies are necessary to confirm the diagnosis of CD (Sollid, 2002).

In people of European descent about one in 100 people suffer from CD, but the disease is considerably under-diagnosed. This is partly because, over the last two decades, the symptoms have changed and become more covert (van Heel & West, 2006). Hence, it is vital that the correct diagnosis be made, taking advantage of serology and endoscopic biopsy, and if positive, a gluten free diet commenced. In addition, we recommend that enzyme supplementation be utilized in order to hasten repair to tissue and help to begin a greatly improved lifestyle (Cornell & Stelmasiak, 2007).

The background to our work on enzyme therapy began with studies of etiology of CD and were essentially of a biochemical nature. Although treatment with a gluten-free diet had been hailed as a major breakthrough in patient management, the disease was still poorly understood and further studies were considered absolutely necessary. Like other studies of CD, they were based on showing that the proteins in the gluten fraction of wheat were the causative agents (Anderson et al, 1952). Later, Frazer et al, (1959) showed that a peptic-tryptic digest of gluten was still toxic to patients with CD and obtained an indication that this toxicity was abolished by further treatment of the digest with an extract of hog mucosa, suggesting an enzyme deficiency was the cause of CD. Bronstein et al (1966) showed the peptic-tryptic-pancreatinic digests of the lower molecular weight group of proteins, called gliadin, were toxic in vivo. The following experiments were conducted to investigate the toxic factors present.

Fractionation of such a gliadin digest by ion exchange showed that it contained a fraction (Fraction 9) that was incompletely digested by small intestinal mucosa from children with coeliac disease in remission (Cornell & Townley, 1973). Undigested residues showed up after electrophoresis of the mucosal digests.

Small intestinal mucosa from children with active coeliac disease was cultured in the presence of each fraction of the gliadin digest. Electron microscopy was used to observe the changes to the tissue. Fraction 9 was again seen as being different from the other fractions in that it prevented recovery of the tissue and thus was shown to be highly toxic (Townley et al.,1973).

Feeding tests using the xylose tolerance method in children showed that Fraction 9 was the only fraction to cause a reduction in urinary xylose excretion, thus confirming its toxicity *in vivo* (Cornell&Townley, 1974).

Collaboration with Anderson and Rolles (Cornell & Rolles, 1978) showed that there was a partial enzyme deficiency in a number of the first degree relatives of the coeliac probands, and helped explain the wide-range of symptoms observed in coeliac disease.

These studies confirmed that residues of undigested peptides were higher from coeliac patients in remission than from controls.

Further work was then focused on the structures of the peptides present in Fraction 9 and the types of mechanisms that might operate in CD. Further collaboration in regard to other assays of toxicity was of the utmost importance as was the introduction of tests on synthetic peptides.

2. The structures of the toxic peptides

A considerable amount of research has been necessary to define the toxic peptides present in such a complex mixture as a gliadin digest. The basis for these experiments was finding that the toxicity of gliadin, in the form of a low molecular weight digest (approximately 1500 Daltons average) was concentrated in Fraction 9 (Cornell & Townley, 1973). Hence it was decided to further fractionate Fraction 9 and perform amino acid analysis on the sub-fractions. Alongside these analytical experiments, it was, of course necessary to evaluate the *in vitro* toxicity of the various sub-fractions. This was achieved by the use of a screening assay based on the observation that rat liver lysosomes were disrupted by a peptic-tryptic digest of gluten (Dolly & Fottrell, 1969). Using an assay based on lysosome disruption it was confirmed that Fraction 9 was the most toxic of the ion-exchange fractions obtained and this herewith gave confidence in the value of the assay as a screening test for toxicity (Cornell & Townley, 1973b).

The justification for the use of the rat liver lysosome assay mainly came from the work of Riecken et al.(1966), who showed that human lysosomes lost their integrity in patients with active coeliac disease, but this integrity was regained on a gluten-free diet. The value of prednisolone in promoting recovery of mucosa in coeliac disease is known to be due to stabilization of lysosomal membranes (Weissman, 1966).

Fraction 9 was not only shown to be the most active fraction, but peptides remaining after digestion of Fraction 9 with remission coeliac mucosa still had an appreciable effect of lysosomal membranes, whereas those remaining after digestion of Fraction 9 with normal intestinal mucosa had only little effect (Cornell & Townley,1973b).

The mucosal digestion experiments were repeated with an extract of porcine intestinal mucosa in comparison with remission coeliac mucosa and normal mucosa. Protection of the lysosomes was high with the porcine and normal human mucosal extracts but was low with remission coeliac mucosal extract (Cornell& Stelmasiak, 2004).

These experiments showed the value of lysosomes in our understanding of an enzyme deficiency in coeliac disease. Most importantly, they have opened the way for enzyme therapy, which began with tests on animal intestinal extracts. Lysosomal assays thus form the basis of our assays for detoxification of gliadin.

The rat liver lysosome assay was employed in two different ways:

- The first way was to evaluate the toxicity of fractions of a gliadin digest and the synthetic peptides corresponding to the A-gliadin structure. Confirmation of the *in-vitro* toxicity of the latter in a chick assay (Mothes et al., 1985) could then be undertaken. For this purpose, the toxicity of each of the fractions was calculated from

$$T\,(\%) = \frac{Z - A}{Z} \times 100$$

where T = toxicity

Z = absorbance at 410nm after dilution with buffer and

A = absorbance at 410nm after incubation at 37°C for 1.5 hours and then dilution with buffer.

Toxicity is thus a percentage reduction in absorbance caused by disruption of the lysosomes and has been shown to be highest in the case of Fraction 9, compared to all the other fractions of the gliadin digest (Cornell & Townley, 1973b).

- The second way in which the assay was used was to evaluate the percentage protection offered by various animal and human mucosal extracts, plant extracts and commercial enzymes. Pre-incubation of the gliadin digest with enzyme solution, followed by incubation with lysosomes and dilution with buffer was necessary. Absorbance at 410nm of this mixture (E) was then used to calculate P (%) as follows:

$$P\,(\%) = \frac{E - A}{Z - A} \times 100$$

P can also be calculated from

$$P\,(\%) = \frac{T - T_E}{T} \times 100$$

where T_E = Toxicity after pre-incubation with enzyme.

Mucosal digestion was carried out by homogenizing tissue in PBS (30mg/mL) followed by filtration. The assay normally used 0.20ml of the filtrate per tube, 0.10ml of gliadin digest (50mg/mL) and 0.10ml of a rat liver lysosome suspension. This latter suspension was of such concentration that 0.10ml when diluted with PBS gave an absorbance reading of 0.9-1.0 at 410mm (Cornell & Townley, 1973b).

The starting point for all subsequent studies was to determine the composition of the toxic peptides present in Fraction 9. This was achieved by HPLC of Fraction 9 on ODS Hypersil followed by amino acid analysis of the sub-fractions (Cornell et al.1992). The most active fractions, as determined by the lysosomal screening assay, were then subjected to amino acid sequencing. This led to the identification and amino acid sequence of two peptides - one corresponding to residues 5-20 of A-gliadin from wheat (Fraction 13) and the other (Fraction 20) corresponding to residues 75-86 of A-gliadin, the A-gliadin sequence having been determined by Kasarda et al.(1994).

Sub-fraction 13 was shown to contain two peptides of similar amino acid composition and indicating about 16 residues in each. Both were close in composition to the peptide 5-20 of A-gliadin, which contains the PSQQ and QQQP motifs, seen to be important to toxicity by De Ritis et al. (1988).

Sub-fraction 20-1 (rechromatographed Sub-fraction 20) was shown to be identical to residues 75-86 of A-gliadin and specific amino acid deletions were useful in showing that toxicity in the chick assay was lost below the size of the octapeptide 77-84 (Cornell & Mothes,1993). Peptide 75-84 still retained toxicity. Peptides within the sequence 75-86 appear to be immunogenic peptides, as shown by their ability to cause the release of gamma-interferon from red blood cells of patients with CD (Cornell et al., 1994).

Sealy-Voyksner et al (2010) have identified several peptides in gluten digests that are relevant to the immunological response in patients with CD. Some of these correspond to segments of α - and ß-gliadins, and were close matches to those in previous studies on A-gliadin (Mc Lachlan et al.2002). Importantly, one of these peptides contained the PQQPYP motif found in the active peptide 75-86 of A-gliadin (Cornell & Mothes, 1993).

The work of De Ritis et al (1988), was an important finding as it enabled McLachlan et al (2002) to use a proteomics approach to investigate common sequences in wheat, rye and barley - the most toxic cereals to patients with CD - and compare them with oats (having questionable toxicity in CD) and maize and rice (non-toxic cereals). They found that QQQP was present in a number of sequences in wheat, but QQQPS was also found in the non-toxic cereals, maize and rice. This led to the conclusion that the flanking amino acids were also important and extended motifs needed to be examined. When this was done it turned out that an extended motif common to wheat, rye and barley was QQQPFP. A shorter motif, QQQPF was also present in oats and may be present in the cultivars of this cereal which have been shown to have activity in some 'in-vitro' assays (Silano et al., 2006).

Regarding the PSQQ motif, proposed by De Ritis et al. (1988) the relevant extended motifs were FPSQQ, PSQQP, PFPSQQ and FPSQQP, but these were associated only with wheat and barley, not rye.

The proteomics approach opened the way for looking at other motifs which may be associated with CD toxicity. Mention has already been made of HPLC of Fraction 9 and amino acid analysis of the fractions. These experiments showed that there were two sub-fractions which were toxic to rat liver lysosomes and that amino acid analysis and amino acid sequence determinations pointed to structures corresponding to residues 5-20 and 75-86 of A-gliadin. The latter peptide proved to be the most abundant one of sequence RPQQPYPQPQPQ. It was thought that the key sequence in this peptide could be a four amino acid motif like QQPY, since the proteomic studies indicated that wheat, rye and barley all contained the extended motifs PQQPY and QQPYP which are both present in peptide 75-86(McLachlan et.al.,2002). Other searches had shown that peptide 31-49 of A-gliadin (LGQQQPFPPQQPYPQPQPF) was toxic "in vivo" to patients with CD (Sturgess et al.1994). It can be seen that the extended (5 amino acid) sequences are also both present in this peptide. Fetal chick assays were also carried out on a series of peptides related to peptide 75-86(Cornell & Mothes, 1993). These assays showed that all peptides in this region had appreciable toxicity except peptide 76-86 with an N-terminal proline residue.

Regarding peptide 5-20 (VPQLQPQNPSQQQPQE), it is seen that not only the PSQQ motif, but the QQQP motif, is also present. The extended motifs PSQQQ, NPSQQQ and PSQQQ are found only in wheat. Again, it was found that searches for the four amino acid motif QPYP, resulted in matches for wheat, rye, barley, oats and the non-toxic rice indicating the need for using an extended motif.

The significance of this work only became apparent when the mucosal digestion studies of synthetic peptides and fetal chick assays were carried out. The use of the latter assay in connection with synthetic peptides prepared with selective amino acid deletions, showed that peptide 11-19 was the most active peptide within the sequence of 5-20. It was considerably more active than peptide 8-19, reported by Kocna et al. (1991), who used the same assay. The octapeptide 12-19, which contains motifs PSQQ and QQQP in overlapping sequence, was still toxic in the assay. This reinforced the view that sequences of eight-amino acids are large enough to retain toxicity, whereas the hexapeptide 13-18 is not (Cornell & Mothes, 1993).

Peptide 11-19 gave higher amounts of residues after digestion with remission coeliac mucosa than were obtained with normal mucosa. Moreover, these residues still retained the serine residue, presumably associated the PSQQ motif, because the amino acid composition of the residues matched the octapeptide sequence 12-19, QNPSQQQPQ (Cornell & Rivett, 1995). It is interesting that peptide 206-217, has been shown to be toxic *in vivo* (Mantzaris & Jewell, 1991). Its sequence of LGQGSFRPSQQN contains the PSQQ motif, which may be a problem with digestion by coeliac mucosa.

Mucosal digestion and amino acid analysis of residues from peptide 75-86 were also very informative (Cornell, 1998). Again, like peptide 11-19, digestion with remission coeliac mucosa was not complete and residues corresponding to octapeptides were obtained. These residues seemed to correspond to peptide 77-84 (QQPYPQPQ) which was shown to be toxic in the fetal chick assay. Such residues also contain the QQPYP extended motif, suggesting that an enzyme deficiency in remission coeliac mucosa is the reason why these undigested residues remain and also why the extended motifs present in residues 12-19, QNPSQQQPQ (from peptide 11-19) and 77-84, QQPYPQPQ (from peptide 75-86) both contain the extended amino acid sequences corresponding to the three most toxic cereal proteins.

With regard to the activity of other peptides of A-gliadin, Vader et al.,(2002) have shown that gluten-specific T-cell responses in HLA-DQ2 positive adult coeliac patients are directed at multiple peptides of gliadin and glutenin. An interesting example is peptide 56-68 of A-gliadin (LQLQPFPQPQPY). By the criterion of activation of coeliac intestinalCD4+ T-clones (Halstensen et al., 1993), it is the dominant epitope, yet it is not able to cause damage *in vitro*. Another two examples are the A-gliadin peptides 31-43 and 31-49. The former peptide does not activate coeliac intestinal CD4+ T-clones (McAdam & Sollid, 2000). Peptide 31-49 (LGQQQPFPPQQPYPQPQPF) which is toxic in vivo (Sturgess et al., 1994) has the De Ritis motif QQQP and the tyrosine motifs QQPY and QPYP, both of which are associated with coeliac-toxic cereals (McLachlan et al., 2002). However, peptide 31-43 has only the QQQP and QQPY but not QPYP, so the latter may have great importance in toxicity. Like peptide 31-49, the 33-mer peptide of alpha-2 gliadin (Shan et al.,2002) also has the PYPQ motif.

Toxic action seen on fetal rat jejunum, but not on mature jejunum, is consistent with development of protective enzymes or immune mechanisms. Experiments *in vitro* production of interferon indicated that the serine-containing peptides, like peptide 11-19 of A-gliadin, were weakly immunogenic (but potent in their cytotoxicity) compared with the tyrosine-containing peptides like peptide 75-86 of A-gliadin (Cornell & Wills-Johnson, 2001). Other workers (McAdam & Sollid, 2000; Shan et al., 2002) have reported immunogenic peptides containing tyrosine. Peptides 57-73 of A-gliadin and 57-89 of α-2 gliadin do not have PSQQ or QQQP motifs, but the latter has the QPYP motif common to all three coeliac toxic cereals (McLachlan et al., 2002).

Secondary structural differences in the peptides 11-19 and 75-86 have been suggested by molecular modelling. This work indicates that peptide 11-19 favours an α-helical structure, whereas peptide 75-86 has high β-turn content Similarly, peptides in an avenin from oats, which also appear to be highly immunoreactive, have been shown to have a high β-turn content using circular dichroism(Alfonso et al.,1998).

3. Etiology of coeliac disease

Studies of possible enzyme deficiency have been rewarding, in that, using different techniques, all the results have pointed to two particular peptides from A-gliadin that seem to have different modes of action in regard to their toxicity, yet both are incompletely digested by remission coeliac mucosa (Cornell & Rivett,1995; Cornell,1998).

An enzyme deficiency has been indicated not only from studies of native gliadin but also from studies using synthetic peptides. At this point it would be of benefit to readers to list the findings which support an enzyme deficiency.

a. One fraction of a gliadin digest (Fraction 9) was incompletely digested by small intestinal mucosa from patients with CD in remission. This fraction was completely digested by small intestinal mucosa from normal individuals as were all the other fractions of the digest by mucosa from normal and those with CD (Cornell & Townley, 1973).
b. Cultures of small intestinal mucosa from patients with active CD improved after 24 hours in media containing fractions other than Fraction 9 or in the absence of gliadin. This was in complete contrast to tissue from patients in the presence of Fraction 9. Tissue from normal individuals was not damaged, except to a small extent with

Fraction 9. Electron microscopy was thus able to differentiate the damage caused by the presence of toxic gliadin peptides in the culture medium (Townley et al., 1973).

c. Using the tanned red blood cell technique, it was shown that antibodies against the fractions from ion exchange of the gliadin digest were highest against Fraction 9, suggesting that in patients with active CD, undigested peptides from Fraction 9 had mounted a significant immune response, compared with other fractions, which had presumably been better digested (Cornell,1974).
d. The xylose tolerance test showed that in children with CD in remission, some damage to the small intestine was indicated by reductions in levels of xylose excretion in their urine after ingestion of Fraction 9. No significant changes in urinary xylose were seen with the other fractions when combined (Cornell & Townley, 1973).
e. Fraction 9 displayed high activity in a fetal chick assay and was shown to contain two active peptides, one corresponding to residues 5-20 and the other to residues 75-86 of A-gliadin (Cornell et al., 1992). When these peptides were subjected to specific deletions of amino acids it was found that the most active peptide was the nonapeptide 11-19 while the dodecapeptide 75-86 was seen to be close to the maximum activity in this group of peptides (Cornell & Mothes,1993,1995).
f. Coeliac mucosal digestion of each of these peptides showed that undigested residues of octapeptides were obtained in greater amounts than those obtained from digestion with mucosa from normal individuals (Cornell & Rivett, 1995; Cornell, 1998).
g. Importantly, these undigested octapeptides were found to contain sequences of amino acids found by ourselves and others to be associated with toxicity (De Ritis et al.1988; McLachlan et al., 2002).

The connection between the most active fraction and undigested peptide residues being found in the same fraction indicates that the reason for this toxicity is due to insufficient activity of an enzyme in patients with CD. This proposal was first put forward by Frazer et al. (1959) on the basis that patients on a gluten-free diet relapsed after being fed a peptic-tryptic digest of gluten, but this did not happen when the gluten digest was subjected to further digestion with a hog intestinal extract.

It must be said that apart from our work and that of our collaborators, little else has been contributed to support an enzyme deficiency in CD. Perhaps some commonality is seen in the work on a 33-mer peptide of α-2gliadin, which was observed to be difficult to digest (Shan et al., 2002).These undigested peptides have significant immunogenicity which are thought to be responsible for toxicity, but so far, no toxicity data have been presented. Current work in this area is directed towards an understanding of the type of enzyme which appears to be missing or defective in CD. One way of gaining this information is by examining the structures of peptides which remain after coeliac mucosal digestion. The other way is to examine the types of peptides that are the most effective for digesting the gliadin down to small fragments which are no longer toxic in the assay employed. These approaches will be discussed in Sections 5 and 6 of the chapter.

4. A unified theory of CD

Quite often, CD is referred to an autoimmune disease, meaning that the body, by mistake, produces antibodies that damage its own tissues (Maki, 1996). Although antibodies are produced in patients with CD to tissue transglutaminase (tTG), which potentiates the action of dietary gluten, the source of the problem is a group of proteins which are foreign to the body and if these are not broken down to amino acids and small peptides, an immunological response will be mounted and tissue will be damaged. If the proteins are broken down to amino acids and small peptides, the tissue will remain in a normal and healthy state (Cornell & Stelmasiak, 2007).

These harmful proteins are present in wheat, barley and rye and to a much smaller extent in oats. The wheat gluten contains two major groups of proteins, referred to as glutenins and gliadins. The latter group contains proteins of lower molecular weight (≈ 30,000 Daltons) and are regarded as being the more harmful to those with CD. Most work has been done on these gliadins, not only because of their higher toxicity, but also because they are simple chain proteins and can be readily extracted from gluten or flour by 70% v/v ethanol (Mothes et al., 1999). They are referred to as prolamins. Prolamins from rye are called secalins, those from barley as hordeins and those from oats as avenins.

Some humans are born with a genetic predisposition to CD which may become obvious after exposure to dietary gluten, as when an infant is introduced to solid foods. The HLA typing with the genes referred to as DQ2 and DQ8 and genetic testing is useful for excluding a diagnosis of CD. However, only about 3% of people with either or both these genes will develop CD. The prevalence of HLA-DQ2 alone is about 25% in the North European population yet only about 1% has CD, suggesting that additional genes are involved in CD (Kagnoff, 2007). Mäki and Collin (1997) reported that more specific factors, probably non-HLA genes are involved. Both genetic and environmental factors appear to play a role in development of CD.

The older theory of an enzyme deficiency in CD must be given serious consideration because it is hard to imagine what type of substance in a hog intestine extract, other than an enzyme, can result in detoxification of a gluten digest. (Frazer et al., 1959). Moreover, the work summarised in Section 3 by the writers carries some weight insofar as certain toxic peptides in A-gliadin seem not to be completely digested by mucosa from children with CD in remission. Strengthening this even more is the finding of motifs of amino acids from two peptides which appear in the residues from mucosal digestion of children with CD in remission that we and others have shown to be associated with the toxicity of gliadin

The concept of an enzyme deficiency is more plausible than the proposal that proline-rich epitopes are exceptionally resistant to enzymatic processing (Hausch et al., 2002). '*In vitro*' mucosal digestion with small intestinal homogenates from normal individuals show consistently lower amounts of peptide residues from toxic peptides compared to residues from coeliac mucosal digestion. However if the amounts of peptides used are excessive, compared with mucosal dry matter, one would expect more residual peptides from the normals. For those interested in the historical overview of the assays and toxicity studies, the reader is referred to an older review (Cornell, 1996).

Coupled with an enzyme deficiency is the need to recognise the plethora of immunological reactions that appear to be responsible for the pathology of CD. We fully affirm the importance of immunological reactions in the pathogenesis of CD as proposed by Falchuk and Strober (1974). However, Biagi et al. (1999) dispute that the pathology is the result of abnormal presentation of gliadin. We contend that these pathogenetic mechanisms are the result of partially digested gliadin (or other toxic cereal peptides) that accumulate in the small intestine as the result of an enzyme deficiency. The immune response might be magnified by prior cytotoxic action. Experiments with two types of toxic peptides we have described tend to verify this view.

Several hypotheses have been proposed to account for the susceptibility of certain individuals to CD. Two major hypotheses have been referred to as the Enzymopathic (enzyme deficiency) Hypothesis (Frazer et al., 1959) and the Immunological Hypothesis (Falchuk & Strober, 1974). A third hypothesis is based on a defect in the permeability of the intestinal mucosa (Bjarnason & Peters, 1983).

The evidence for damage to tissue as a result of immunological mechanisms is overwhelming but the argument that it represents an aberrant reaction because of abnormal presentation of gliadin is less convincing (Biagi et al., 1999). The modern view is that HLA class II molecules in antigen-presenting cells expose processed peptides to immunocompetent T-cells thereby triggering pathogenesis (Sollid, 2002).T-lymphocytes respond by releasing cytokines which cause inflammation and damage of enterocytes and other cells in the small intestine.

Vader et al (2002) studied gluten specific T-cell responses in HLA-DQ2 positive adult patients with CD and showed that they were directed at multiple peptides derived from gliadin and glutenin. There is a broad spectrum of sensitivity to gluten in patients with CD and this can be explained partly by multiple levels of immune regulation (Schuppan & Hahn, 2002) and partly by enzymatic processes governing the extent of digestion of gliadin peptides (Cornell & Rolles, 1978).

Regarding the hypothesis of permeability defect in the intestine mucosa ("Leaky Gut" syndrome), the general argument is that there is increased permeability of the epithelium. One group claims that this is caused by a myosin variant and leads to increased antigen presentation(Monsuur et al.,2005) whilst another group claims that sustained release of zonulin occurs, concomitant with an increase in permeability (Drago et al.2006). The zonulin release was less in normals, suggesting better digestion of gliadin occurred.

The writers have proposed a "Unified Hypothesis of CD" (Cornell & Stelmasiak, 2007) to account for the specific causative effects of gluten, which cannot be explained simply by saying that gliadin peptides are difficult to digest. Certainly, there has been some evidence to suggest that individuals other than those with CD have problems caused by gluten-containing food (Jones et al., 1982). The fact of the matter is that the majority of people do not encounter this problem, except for some first degree relatives, who have been shown to have partial deficiency in regard to their ability to digest gluten completely (Cornell & Rolles, 1978). The etiology of CD has many similarities to that of dermatitis herpetiformis, except that the manifestation of this condition is the formation of a rash and itchiness (Fry, 1992). Both are quite different in etiology to wheat allergy.

It raises the important point that some gliadin peptides may not inflict damage to cells until they are modified in some way. Mölberg et al. (1998) have shown that tissue transglutaminase appears to modulate the reactivity of gliadin-specific T-cells. This effect is mediated by a specific deamidation of gliadin peptides which binds them strongly to DQ2 molecules and allows recognition by certain T-cells. It is an important example of enzymatic modification of antigens that results in activation of pathological processes.

Returning to the basic etiology of CD, the writers maintain that there are multiple peptides in a peptic-tryptic-pancreatinic digest of gliadin that require a specific enzyme for complete digestion to harmless peptides. This enzyme is deficient or defective in individuals with CD. The enzyme attacks peptides that contain certain sequences of amino acids that are present in the three coeliac-toxic cereals, wheat, rye and barley. Without this enzyme patients with CD are unable to digest the gliadin peptides and damage to the small intestine mucosa ensues (Cornell & Stelmasiak, 2007).

Two different types of active peptides have been discerned and the use of synthetic peptides of A-gliadin have made it possible to say that a group of serine-containing peptides such as 11-19 of A-gliadin have displayed potent cytotoxicity, while those such as tyrosine-containing peptide 75-86, have potent immunogenicity (Cornell&Wills-Johnson,2001).It is because of the fact that both these peptides are not digested by coeliac mucosa down to small harmless peptides, but instead resist digestion past the octapeptide stage, that we invoke the concept of damage both by cytotoxic and immunologic mechanisms (Cornell & Stelmasiak,2007). The latter are suggested from their ability to produce interferon-γ from red blood cells from patients with CD (Cornell et al.,1994) This is not so for the serine-containing group of toxic peptides. Hence the writers have proposed a hypothesis which combines the two main theories, henceforth referred to as the Unified Hypothesis (Cornell & Stelmasiak, 2007). The etiology and pathogenesis of CD are closely linked in complex events and this term seems to be a satisfactory way of explaining all of those events according to present day knowledge.

Other workers have pointed out the difficulty of digesting certain proline-rich peptides which can involve immunological reactions leading to intestinal damage. Hausch et al. (2002) comment on immunodominant epitopes that are considered difficult to digest because of the low activity of enzymes capable of N-terminal and C-terminal attack on proline residues (DPPIV and pancreatic endoproteases respectively). These epitopes are probably more important from the point of view of their particular key amino acid sequences, particularly ones that contain tyrosine, rather than their high proline content. The bioactivity of wheat and problems with the digestion of some of its components in CD have been pointed out (Cornell & Hoveling, 1998). The 33-mer peptide of α-2 gliadin (Shan et al., 2002) is also difficult to digest and again, the repeating sequences containing proline, tyrosine and glutamine are probably of importance to its immunogenicity. From a clinical point of view, they also provide the rationale for the application of enzyme therapy. Sollid offers an explanation that proline has a dominant role in the specificity of tissue transglutaminase and could facilitate binding to the above 33-mer fragment (Sollid, 2002).

5. The basis of enzyme therapy

The elucidation of structures in gliadin that are resistant to digestion by remission coeliac mucosa has provided a promising basis for treatment, providing the amount of gluten ingested is not excessive. The way in which this could be evaluated was offered by the use of the rat liver lysosome assay, based on the principle that the lysosomes are disrupted by toxic gliadin peptides. If the gliadin is detoxified by an enzyme capable of digesting the peptides responsible for damage to the lysosomes, that enzyme could form the basis of suitable therapy for patients with CD.

It was kept in mind that, to be effective therapy, the product would have to be able to counteract 50mg of gluten/day (Catassi et al.2007). Hence there would be no way of achieving high degrees of protection unless the patients remained on a nominal gluten-free diet in order to achieve a degree of protection and used enzyme therapy as an adjunct treatment, i.e., as a safeguard.

Another use of the rat-liver lysosome assay, which throws direct light on the enzyme deficiency in CD, is the way it was used to show that there was residual activity in Fraction 9 after incubation of small intestinal mucosa from children with CD in remission. In five experiments, the mean reduction in absorbance was 45% for coeliac mucosa and 23% for normal mucosa. Controls without Fraction 9 registered 18%, close to the normal mucosa. Thus, there appears to be incomplete digestion of Fraction 9 in those with CD compared with normals ($p<0.001$) (Cornell & Townley, 1973b).

This conclusion had also been indicated by toxicity studies with fetal rat mucosa (Cornell et al., 1988) and gave confidence in the use of lysosomes as a screening test. Similarly, good correlations between the lysosome screening test and results of fetal chick assay were obtained (Cornell & Mothes, 1995).As an animal model for studies of CD small intestinal tissue from fetal animals has been very useful, presumably because these animals do not have fully developed protective enzyme systems. This, of course, is completely in agreement with the idea of defective digestion being a key component of tissue damage by gliadin peptides.

The authors embarked on a program to study adult animal intestine with a view to determining if complete digestion of toxic gliadin peptides could be achieved and thereby used as a means of providing the missing or defective enzymes in patients with CD. In these studies of animal intestinal mucosa, the authors showed that no significant toxic peptide residues remained after digestion of the gliadin digest with the normal human, pig, cow and sheep intestinal mucosa, whereas toxic residues were obtained after incubation with remission coeliac mucosa. Highest degrees of protection (85-90%) against gliadin were offered in the lysosomal assay by the pig and cow extracts, followed by human and sheep (70-76%). By contrast, remission coeliac mucosa offered only 15% protection, not very different from the controls without mucosa (Cornell & Stelmasiak, 2004).

These results led to our first experiments with animal mucosa in which we decided to investigate the use of pig mucosal extracts for enzyme therapy in CD. It was of great importance to note that digestion by the intestinal mucosa of these animals was comparable to that by normal human mucosa and far more complete than that seen in patients with CD in remission. These animals have been ingesting various forms of gluten for millions of years longer than have humans and have evolved efficient digestive systems. Some humans are well behind in this aspect and conjecture on this matter is strengthened by a further group of individuals who have varying degrees of gluten intolerance (Van Heel & West, 2006).

Pig intestinal mucosa was chosen for a series of investigations designed to show that the active principle in this mucosa was an enzyme. It was therefore necessary to begin with large quantities of pig mucosa and refine it to the extent of producing enough active enzyme to be characterized and possibly identified.

The evaluation of products from all stages of the purification were monitored by the rat liver lysosome assay (refer Section 2) using a 2 hour at 37°C period of incubation of the fraction of pig mucosa with the gliadin digest before testing residual toxicity against the lysosomes. When the enzyme was effective, the residual toxicity was low; hence high values of protection (P) were obtained.

The first stage of refinement involved the use of an ion-exchange resin. Ion exchange resins were considered favourably because their bead form allows high flow rates and they can be readily regenerated using sodium hydroxide. Pilot scale experiments using filtered extract from 4kg pig intestinal mucosa yielded a product enriched in gliadin detoxifying enzymes from the use of the weakly basic Amberlite anion exchange resin, IRA95.

The active principle in the pig intestinal mucosa was found to be bound by the ion-exchange column at pH 7.5 and could be eluted by phosphate buffer of pH 5.0 containing 0.3mol/L sodium chloride. The eluate was desalted by membrane filtration and freeze dried. A refined enzyme extract was obtained as a fawn-coloured powder in yields of 3-4% on freeze-dried mucosa extract.

Further fractionation using laboratory-sized columns of the weakly acidic (carboxymethyl) ion exchanger CM Sephadex C50, were used to prepare more enriched fractions. In this case, the most enriched fraction was obtained by raising the pH of the phosphate eluting buffer (0.05 mol/L) and applying a linear salt (sodium chloride) gradient to 0.3 mol/L. The most active fraction (Fraction 4) eluted at pH 6.2 and 0.20 mol/L sodium chloride.

The specific activity of each of the most active fractions was calculated from the results of the rat liver lysosome assay. Results of these evaluations are shown in Table 1. Note that specific activity is calculated from protection (%) offered per mg sample.

Sample	Specific Activity (P/mg)
Crude enzyme extract	12
Fraction from Amberlite IRA 95	17
Fraction 4 from CM Sephadex C-50	34

Table 1. Specific activity of pig extract and crude fractions thereof

Other enzyme levels determined on Fraction 4 were protease levels by the benzoylarginine ethyl ester (BAEE) method, which is a good measure of total protease levels (Arnon,1970) Refer Table 2.

PEP levels in Fraction 4 were carried out using Z-gly-pro-p-nitroanilide (Kocna et al., 1980). Crude pig extract showed levels of 6.4×10^{-4} U/mg and this was increased to 2.1×10^{-3} U/mg after ion exchange on Amberlite IRA 96. Pure PEP (Seikagu, Japan) has a specific activity of 20 U/mg so the above levels showed that PEP was not an important contributor to activity, as measured by the lysosome assay.

An important finding was that prolidase activity, measured by the ability of the enzymes present to hydrolyse Ac-Pro-Gly was 0.025 U/mg in the crude extract while Fraction 4 was 0.06 U/mg (Cornell et al., 2010).

Neither the crude extract nor the material absorbed on IRA 95 contained any significant amounts of enzyme activity measured according to the BAPNA (benzoylarginine p-nitroanilide assay) (Gravett et al., 1991). This assay was used extensively in studies of activity in papaya oleo-resin (see Section 6).

Fraction No	Yield (%)	Elution Conditions	RLL assay (P%)*	BAEE assay U/mg	PEP assay U/mg
1	17.7	unabsorbed	45	0.10	4.3×10^{-4}
2	5.2	change of pH	51	0.45	5.6×10^{-5}
3	7.3	change of pH	45	0.31	8.0×10^{-5}
4	7.4	0.10-0.20 mol/L NaCl	90	0.10	5.8×10^{-5}
5	2.7	0.25 mol/L NaCl	35	0.42	1.0×10^{-5}
6	9.2	0.25-0.50 mol/L NaCl	18	0.78	1.8×10^{-5}
Starting Extract	-	-	68	0.36	6.4×10^{-4}

*4mg fraction/assay tube

Table 2. The results of activity and enzyme assays on fractions obtained by chromatography of the refined pig intestinal extract on CM Sephadex C-50 Column (3.2 × 20 cm).

Fraction 4 was digested with trypsin and submitted for mass spectrometric fragmentation analysis but the only known protein found was pig albumin which has a molecular weight of 68KDa, similar to that of the active enzyme produced during processing, even though temperatures were held at 5°C. Without processing, the active enzyme in fresh pig extract is in the range of 120-170kDa obtained using Sephacryl S300, but Fraction 4 appears to have a very broad peak of activity between 50 and 80 kDa, which explains the contamination with pig albumin. No matches were obtained between the analysed sequences of the enzyme and the library of known pig enzymes. Specific activities of the higher (80 kDa) and lower (50 kDa) fractions on Sephacryl S-300 were 90 and 36 respectively, higher than the result (17) for the starting material.

Fraction 4 was further purified using size exclusion HPLC on Bio Sep SEC-S2000 in 0.05 mol/L phosphate buffer, pH 6.8. The column allowed applications of up to 3mg of sample. Highest activity was obtained in fractions that corresponded to molecular weight in the range 60-100 kDa. By absorbance at 214mm, 6 peaks were obtained, with the highest lysosomal activity in the range corresponding to peaks 2 and 3. Some autolysis of the enzymes may have occurred during processing. These results are in agreement with the size exclusion experiments using Sephacryl S-300 (refer Table 2).

Estimates of specific activity on the fractions of highest lysosomal activity are in the range 180-220. This has allowed partial sequencing of active enzymes but the samples were not pure enough to show significant homology between the active enzyme and known enzymes present in the pig.

Fractionation of pig small intestine extract has been useful for characterising the active enzyme, according to monitoring with the rat liver lysosome assay. Among these can be listed:

a. Optimal pH of 8.4
b. Strongly inhibited by phenylmethyl sulfonyl fluoride (PMSF)
c. Unstable to heating at 85°C
d. Unstable to acid (pH 2)
e. Molecular weight may be greater than 100 kDa before autolysis

The identity of the enzyme in pig is likely to be similar to that of the missing enzyme in humans. It seems to fit the general description of a prolidase and appears to attack coeliac-active peptides on the N-terminal side of proline residues and is a necessity for digesting key motifs associated with toxicity that contain proline. Hence the enzyme is likely to be an imino-oligopeptidase, a proline specific enzyme not implicated in detoxification of gliadin up to this time.

In conclusion, an enzyme capable of detoxifying gliadin was found in pig intestinal mucosa and appears to be a prolidase. It can be partially separated from prolyl endopeptidase (PEP) which has less activity than the prolidase in the rat liver lysosome assay, considered to be relevant to measurement of protection against gliadin toxicity.

Enrichment of the prolidase can be achieved by elution of higher salt concentration in phosphate buffers on weakly acidic cation exchanges or by reason of its higher molecular weight. The prolidase has a higher pH optimum (8.4) compared with PEP (7.5).

Because of the ability of the prolidase to attack the N-terminal side of proline residues, it is ideal for disrupting toxic residues common to wheat, rye and barley such as QQQP, QQPYP and PQQPY. By this means, toxicity of peptides derived from these three cereals is able to be curtailed and small amounts of the cereals will be able to be tolerated. PEP attacks these sequences on the C-terminal side of proline residues, which may not be as effective in reducing toxicity. Even with sequences such as 11-19 of A-gliadin (QNPSQQQPP), that appear to be only present in wheat, it was observed(Cornell&Rivett,1995) that the N-P bond remained intact, which would not be the case after attack by a prolidase.

6. Strategies for treatment of CD

Since the publication of the first clinical trial of enzyme therapy, other groups have also contributed to knowledge in this area. Shan et al. (2002) have shown that a 33-mer T-cell stimulatory peptide, which appears to cause difficulties in digestion by normal digestive enzymes, can be degraded by prolyl oligopeptidase from *Flavobacterium meningosepticum*. Others have shown that this enzyme has only limited efficiency in the detoxification of gliadin peptides in CD (Matysiak-Budnik et al., 2005). Furthermore this enzyme is not deficient in remission coeliac mucosa, as one would expect if it were a key factor (Donlon & Stevens, 2004).

Other types of enzymes which have been investigated for use in enzyme therapy are those from *Aspergillus niger*. Stepniak et al. (2006) have identified a prolyl endopeptidase (AN-PEP) from *A.niger* which was able to degrade T-cell stimulatory peptides *in vitro* under conditions like those in the gastrointestinal tract. Its action was considerably faster than the prolyl endopeptidase from *Flavobacterium meningosepticum*.

Enzyme therapy is based on the premise that the digestive deficiency in CD can be corrected by the oral administration of special enzymes formulated in enterically coated tablets so that the contents can be protected from the action of the gastric juices, allowing the required enzymes to pass through to the small intestine where they can complete the digestion of gluten peptides down to harmless small peptides and amino acids. It may not be necessary in some cases to enterically coat the tablet, as some enzymes such as the one from *A.niger* is stable at pH 2 and is completely resistant to digestion with pepsin. However, its pH optimum is 4-5, which is well below that of the contents of the small intestine.

A totally different approach has been taken by Anderson et al. (2000). Since their discovery of a transglutaminase-modified peptide as the dominant A-gliadin T-cell epitope, these workers have pioneered the way for antigen-specific immunotherapy in CD. Using fresh peripheral blood lymphocytes from subjects undergoing challenge from gluten, interferon-γ release was elicited by a 17-amino acid peptide corresponding to residues 57-73 of A-gliadin. This peptide has the structure QLQPFPQPELPYPQPQS, with E at residue 65, being the result of deamidation of the corresponding glutamine residue.

It is interesting to note that tyrosine is present in this peptide as part of the PYPQ motif that could be important in relation to difficulty of proteolytic digestion. However, it will be important to consider sequences in the other coeliac-toxic cereals rye and barley, which feature PQQPY as being common in all three cereals implicated in CD (McLachlan et al., 2002).

If a suitable vaccine is able to be made, some liberties with respect to ingestion of gluten are expected to be allowed. However, the use of a safeguard based on enzyme therapy will probably still be necessary as the enzyme recommended is able to detoxify peptides that produce an immune response and also those that have cytotoxic action(Cornell et al.,2010) .

Plant enzymes were considered a better option than animal enzymes, despite the fact that the enzyme most likely to be missing or defective in CD is bound to be closely related to one from a higher animal. The reason for not continuing with our plans to market an animal-based product were due to the prevalence of animal diseases, such as bovine spongiform encephelopathy (BSE or "mad cow disease") and porcine adenoviruses. In addition, religious restraints put on products from these two animals in particular would be a barrier to their marketing. Other people may have dietary concerns. It was therefore decided to look at plant sources and among these were papaya latex, bromelain, chymotrypsin, fungal proteases and *Aspergillus oryzae*. These materials were compared against pure papain and prolyl endopeptidase.

It was found that papaya latex concentrate with a protection (P%) of 93 was far the most active preparation. Crystalline papain, the major papaya enzyme, gave a P value of only 7. Prolyl endopeptidase (P=35) gave results comparable to highly purified prolyl endopeptidase from *Chryseobacterium meningosepticum*, but in terms of specific activity, it was much lower than pure caricain, which gave a result of 9,412 (see later in this section).

The evaluation of these sources of enzymes for purpose of making an enzyme supplement to digest gliadin efficiently, was carried out using the rat liver lysosome assay (refer Section 2). Up until this stage, the assay was used for evaluation of the toxicity of gliadin peptides and for testing the residual toxicity (activity) after small intestinal mucosal digestion. By incubating the toxic gliadin digest with a sample of each enzyme, a comparison of the effectiveness of these enzymes could be made. A two hour period of incubation of the enzyme with the gliadin digest at 37°C was given before testing the residual activity of the gliadin against the lysosomes. Calculations of specific activity were also able to be made by dividing the protection (P %) by the mass of enzyme-containing product.

The enzyme caricain (papaya protease omega) is a cysteine protease (Dubey et al., 2007) found in the latex of Carica papaya. Caricain is one of the several proteases present which degrade proteins. They are endopeptidases of broad and narrow specificity, with the major ones being papain, chymopapain, glycyl endopeptidase and caricain. They are synthesised by the plant as inactive forms (zymogens) that are converted into the active forms within a short time after the latex is removed from the plant (Azarkan et al., 2003).

The optimum pH of caricain is 6.8 and its isoelectric point is 10.5. As expected, it is eluted from cation exchangers such as SM Sephadex only at high concentrations (>0.7 mol/L) of sodium chloride. It is classified internationally as E.C.3.4.22.30 and its function is that of an endopeptidase. The structure consists of a proenzyme of 106 amino acids and an active enzyme of 242 amino acids (Groves et al., 1996). Recent experiments with purified carciain indicated that the reaction which controls detoxification of a wheat gliadin digest at pH 7.5 and 37°C is a 1st Order reaction with rate constant 1.7×10^{-4} sec^{-1} (Cornell & Stelmasiak, 2011). The enzyme was able to offer about 80% protection to rat liver lysosomes when used at a concentration of 1.7% on substrate after 2 hours incubation at 37°C, representing a specific activity of 9,412. These experiments were valuable in demonstrating that caricain is a very effective enzyme in detoxifying gliadin and promises to be a prime starting point for enzyme therapy. Papaya enzymes are deemed to be extremely safe (Australian Government Report, 2008) if extracted from the fruit of Carica papaya.

A further development in the use of papaya was the concept of synergism between two active enzymes. This was evident with combinations of the pig intestinal extract and the papaya latex. Table 3 shows that this combination showed a significant improvement over what would be expected from the mean protection (P %) of two separate batches of pig intestinal extract and papaya latex. The experiment was repeated with bromelain but, in this case, there was nothing to be gained in protection although the combination gave higher protection than expected from the mean. There has been a report of combination enzyme therapy using prolylendopeptidase and an enzyme from germinating barley(Siegel et al.,2006) and this is worthy of further study with plant enzymes.

Enzyme 1	P (%)	Enzyme 2	P (%)	Combination P(%)
Pig intestinal extract	61	Papaya latex	71	92
Pig intestinal extract	48	Papaya latex	54	68
Bromelain	21	Papaya latex	62	61

Note: Each enzyme evaluated at 6mg/mL in mixture of two and also at 12mg/mL separately. Results are the means of two determinations.

Table 3. Results of some combinations of crude enzymes to test for synergistic activity. The protection index (P%) from the rat liver lysosome assay was used as the indicator.

7. Preliminary clinical studies

Clinical studies to confirm the value of enzyme therapy were of prime importance as only *in vitro* testing had been carried out up to the stage of using animal intestinal extracts. All the *in vitro* experiments had indicated that pig intestinal extracts completed the digestion of a toxic gliadin digest. The first trial was conducted to verify that these extracts could complete digestion *in vitro*. A large scale batch of pig intestinal extract was prepared for a clinical trial at The Royal Melbourne Hospital. This trial was carried out to test the efficacy of such an extract in countering the effects of a mild gluten challenge in patients with CD. Participants were 21 biopsy-proven adults with CD who were on a gluten-free diet. The design of the trial was of double-blind crossover type using the extract in enterically coated capsules and a placebo in the same type of capsules. Six patients were also biopsied and histological changes compared for treatment and placebo (Cornell et al., 2005).

In those patients who developed symptoms (8 of the 21) these symptoms were ameliorated with the enzyme ($p<0.02$), suggesting that the therapy was beneficial. Further evidence was provided by the histological studies which showed that 5 of the 6 patients chosen at random showed small bowel abnormalities at the start of the trial, but that further damage as a result of the gluten challenge was reduced in 3 of these patients. Antibodies to tTG and gliadin (Dahele et al., 2001) were roughly correlated with severity of histological damage at the start of the trial but no significant reduction in titres was obtained during the course of the trial. This clinical trial was successful in demonstrating that the enzyme deficiency in coeliac disease could be partly corrected by the use of enzymes in a tablet administered orally at the start of a meal. As the tablets were enterically coated, it allowed the enzyme to pass through the stomach unaffected by the hydrochloric acid and pepsin present and to pass into the small intestine where it rapidly disintegates to release the enzymes for complete digestion of any small amount of gluten that may be ingested. In this way it acts as a safeguard and allows more latitude in selection of food. It will thus take the worry out of eating at restaurants, homes of friends and other places where there is a question about the gluten content of the food. It could represent the most important breakthrough in patient management since the introduction of the gluten-free diet over 50 years ago.

A further clinical trial is being conducted to evaluate histological changes in the small intestine of coeliac patients brought about by enzyme therapy using plant enzymes. The aim of this trial is to determine whether the active enzyme in papaya is able to repair damage small intestinal mucosa caused by small amounts of gluten in the diet. It will involve 20 biopsy-proven participants with CD who have been on a gluten-free diet for at least 12 months. Participants will undergo biopsy at the beginning and end of the test period (3 months) while taking either enterically coated tablets of a papaya oleo-resin extract or a placebo. Thus it is a double-blind design but without crossover and has a longer treatment period than the first trial, but without defined gluten challenge. As for the first trial, blood tTG levels are being monitored; participants with higher than normal levels have been favoured for this trial. Changes in small bowel histology during the course of treatment are the major indicators of whether the enzyme is effective, with confirmation from the examination of changes in the participants on placebo.

A combination of a gluten-free diet and enzyme therapy should ensure that traces of gluten in the diet are eliminated, thus providing a sound basis for maintaining the small intestine in sound condition. Otherwise, traces of gluten can bring about alterations in architecture of the small intestine, particularly in the region of the duodenum, and this is seen in a significant number of patients on a normal gluten-free diet without the benefit of enzyme therapy. In the light of experience, the use of such an enzyme safeguard is justified because it is well known that contamination alone makes the gluten content of coeliac diets doubtful. Added to that are the problems of inadequate labelling and the lack of knowledge of the disease by some food suppliers.

We are confident that enzyme supplementation will detoxify gluten in not only wheat, but also in rye, barley and oats. It will be a safer alternative than drugs and will be ready long before any other techniques can be implemented such as changing gluten into a non-toxic form or commercial production of a safe vaccine against gluten. We are convinced that our work with enzyme supplements is critical for the better management of coeliac disease and will reduce the incidence of ongoing intestinal dysfunction.

All of our work on digestion of gliadin is in complete agreement with the experiments of earlier workers, who found that the combined amino acids, present as building blocks in gluten, are not injurious to patients with gluten-sensitive enteropathy. It is extremely important to note that virtual complete digestion of gluten guarantees that there will be no adverse reaction to that mixture of amino acids and small peptides, in contrast to the disease state, where incompletely digested larger peptides are capable of causing damage by various mechanisms. The use of enzyme therapy is a significant step towards ensuring that these incompletely digested gluten peptides are at an absolute minimum concentration in the small bowel.

We are aware of other approaches to the problem of gluten ingestion but in the case of long-term solutions, there is still the likelihood of enzyme therapy being required as it targets all the toxic peptides, not just the immunoactive ones. Enzyme therapy will still be needed as a safeguard.

Early diagnosis of CD and enzyme therapy will safeguard against damage and consequences of long-term ingestion of gluten (osteoporosis, malabsorption of vital nutrients and lymphomas) and should reduce concerns about children and adults being uncertain of the gluten content of food, particularly that prepared outside the home.

Enzyme therapy provides a form of natural product therapy based on sound scientific principles for treatment of a number of conditions relating to gluten intolerance. It has further advantages of easy administration and its low cost could compensate for the extra costs of gluten-free foods, particularly if greater emphasis was placed on fruit, vegetables, meat and fish rather than gluten-free cakes and pastry. Gluten-free bread, cereals and pasta will need to be the main special foods purchased.

Enzyme therapy is now becoming well documented, although there is still a degree of scepticism, brought about by a strong leaning to the "immunological" theory of coeliac disease, rather than the older "enzyme deficiency" theory. Market trials are showing the value of a tablet containing the active enzyme, in that symptoms are markedly reduced. A significant percentage of coeliacs on a gluten-free diet are still experiencing symptoms of a mild to moderate nature and are thus risking further damage to their small intestine. Others with relatively few symptoms are certain to have some abnormalities in that region of the gut.

At present, we are considering commercialization of tablets manufactured to contain 300mg of crude papaya enzyme (15mg pure caricain) one of which is able to detoxify about 1.5g gluten, about 5 dry cracker biscuits, or one third of a slice of bread.

8. Applications of enzyme therapy

Enzymes are such versatile materials that their application to therapy should be widespread. Before enzyme therapy was considered for CD, enzymes were on the market for pancreatic insufficiency. Lipases, amylases and proteases are commonly present, in capsule or tablet form, that are useful for individuals with this condition. Pepsin, bromelain and papain are often used in conjunction with such enzymes to provide products that are useful as digestive supplements. For lactose deficiency, tablets containing the enzyme (β-D-galactosidase) can be used or drops that can be added to milk or infant formulae. Apart from the present application of enzyme therapy to CD, there are other conditions where gluten is considered to be harmful and where a gluten-free diet is recommended. One such condition is dermatitis herpetiformis, in which the small intestine often shows only patchy damage, but the disease manifests itself as an itchy rash (Fry, 1992). A gluten-free diet is essential in order to prevent the troublesome rash but also to guard against damage to the small intestine. So far, we have been only able to test enzyme therapy with caricain in one individual and the results are promising insofar as the effects of a wheat-based cereal and bread were almost eliminated by the use of one tablet at the beginning of each breakfast meal. A small controlled clinical trial is now being planned.

Gluten may be a dietary factor in certain neurological disorders, e.g. schizophrenia. Dr Curtis Dohan was a pioneer of work on the harmful effects of gluten in schizophrenia. One study involved 110 patients, half of whom were on a diet free from cereal grains and milk. Those on the special diet showed improvement in their condition and were discharged almost twice as quickly (Dohan&Grasberger, 1973).A subsequent trial showed that schizophrenics maintained on a cereal grain-free and milk-free diet regressed during a period of a "blind" gluten challenge (Singh&Kay, 1976) .The cause of these ill-effects appear to center around gluten peptides that act as opioids. (Fukudome & Yoshikawa, 1992).

As schizophrenia is a very serious neurological illness, the use of enzyme therapy in conjunction with a gluten-free diet could be a useful form of patient management. If enzyme therapy and a gluten-free diet were used in conjunction with the medication it could turn out that the amounts of neuroleptic drugs used at present could be reduced, which would almost certainly mean less serious side effects.

Autism is another neurological condition which is often accompanied by gastrointestinal symptoms. Since the first report from Asperger (1961), who noted that many children with CD showed psychiatric conditions, there has been a strong focus on autism and its associated difficulties in intellectual and social development of the young. Because gluten contains many opioid sequences, these have again been thought to be a direct cause. In this condition and others with a neurological basis a gluten-free diet is helpful suggesting a role for enzyme supplementation.

Irritable bowel syndrome (Biesiekierski et al., 2011) is a condition in which abdominal pain, flatulence and bloating are commonly observed. It is commonly believed that wheat and/or gluten is responsible for many individuals with this condition and this has been largely responsible for the proliferation of many gluten-free foods. Better public education on CD has perhaps given the lead in this direction. However, those suffering from irritable bowel syndrome appear to outnumber those with CD.

Further work in this area will be undertaken to determine if enzyme therapy will be helpful. It may be successful in some individuals and not in others as there appear to be a number of dietary triggers in irritable bowel syndrome (Shepherd et al., 2008). Ulcerative colitis and Crohn's disease are examples of conditions where a gluten-free diet has been of some help, suggesting that enzyme therapy could be a useful adjunct treatment.

Another application of enzyme therapy could be in management of patients with silent CD. This condition is where the individual has villous atrophy yet displays no symptoms. Examples were provided by Matysiak-Budnik et al (2007) who studied individuals diagnosed with CD in childhood but who were asymptomatic as adults on a normal diet. The majority (48/61) showed different degrees of villous atrophy (silent CD) while 13 had no detectable atrophy (latent CD). Latent patients did not differ significantly from the 7 control patients on a gluten-free diet, but did have CD-specific serum antibodies. However, this was not free of risk as 2 latent patients relapsed clinically and histologically on follow-up. The use of enzyme supplementation would be recommended in cases of silent CD as otherwise risks of malignancy are raised, among other conditions. There is a wide range of symptoms and enteropathy caused by gluten (Picarelli et al., 1996).

Finally, mention should be made of the status of first degree relatives of patients with CD. The finding that 82.3% do not have CD (Biagi et al., 2008) is in keeping with general experience. However, it is likely that many of these individuals will have some intolerance, in keeping with their partial enzyme deficiency (Cornell & Rolles, 1978) and therefore could be in the need of enzyme supplementation whilst on a normal or low gluten diet.

9. Conclusions

- Whether you agree with an enzyme deficiency in CD or simply believe that gliadin and certain other cereal proteins are difficult to digest down to non-toxic small peptides, enzyme therapy is an obvious answer to this problem. In our opinion it is the most useful advance in patient management since the gluten-free diet and deserves funding for further research. It could turn out to be a way of reversing damage to the small intestine caused by small amounts of gluten over extended periods of time.
- A significant proportion of patients with CD show minimal symptoms despite challenge with gluten and are in need of enzyme supplementation as a means of protecting them from intestinal damage. This applies particularly to those patients, who are regarded as having silent CD and therefore in need of early diagnosis and treatment. Otherwise, the consequences can be very serious (Maki&Collin, 1997). Measurement of antibodies to tissue transglutaminase (tTG) is presently the most reliable diagnostic test with follow-up by biopsy (Van Heel & West, 2006). Modern practice makes use of deamidated gliadin peptide assays.
- The use of extracts of pig intestinal mucosa confirmed that they were helpful in reducing the severity of symptoms induced in patients with CD (Cornell et al, 2006). This was taken to mean that such extracts were able to supply an enzyme or enzymes that were deficient in these patients. The enzymes in pig mucosa that make up for this deficiency are likely to be prolidases or oligoiminopeptidases capable of hydrolysing N-terminal peptide bonds associated with proline residues. Such residues are contained within motifs of amino acids that are associated with toxicity and are left intact after

digestion with remission coeliac mucosa. Examples of these motifs are PQQPY, QQPYP found in wheat, rye and barley (Mc Lachlan et al.2002).

- The uses of enzymes from Carica papaya, especially caricain, seem to be effective *in vitro* tests. A highly purified caricain preparation has performed extremely well in these tests and has led to the setting up of a clinical trial to test the value of caricain in enzyme therapy (Cornell & Stelmasiak, 2011).
- Enzyme therapy is expected to act as a safeguard and relieve those who suffer from CD from the worry of maintaining a strict gluten-free diet. Products of high potency should allow some latitude with oats, a very nutritious cereal, which is not part of a gluten-free diet in several countries. The immunotoxicity of oats has been shown to depend on the particular cultivar (Silano et al., 2002). Furthermore, it has been shown that there are three levels of antigenicity according to their reactivity to antibodies against the 33-mer peptide of an alpha-gliadin. High, medium and absent reactivity were observed, correlating with measured activation of T-lymphocytes from patients with CD and hence potential immunotoxicity. (Comino et al., 2011). Oat intolerance may be responsible for villous atrophy seen in patients who are eating oats but otherwise are adhering to a strict gluten-free diet (Arentz-Hansen et al., 2004).
- Although it is generally recognised that the function of HLA molecules is to present small peptides to T-cells, there is not a strong argument that HLA DQ2/DQ8 are primary causes of CD since a large proportion 25-30% of the Caucasian population also have this typing and do not have CD (Sollid, 2002). Instead, it is more reasonable to say HLA DQ2/DQ8 are predisposing factors and that the etiology is another genetic defect that manifests as an enzyme deficiency. Specific deamidation of a glutamine residue results in enhanced binding to those molecules and is important in the ensuing immunological reactions, but this probably only happens with peptides that have resisted digestion.
- CD has a wide spectrum of clinical presentation and mucosal damage. Furthermore it is spread widely throughout the world with it now being recognised in parts of the Orient (Jiang et al., 2009). It could now be regarded as a systemic disease because of its effect on the various organs of the body. Another aspect of the deleterious effect of gluten is the likely, but not always proven, effect in other disorders such as schizophrenia, autism, irritable bowel syndrome and other situations where individuals do not tolerate gluten (the so-called non-coeliac gluten intolerance).
- At the molecular level, there has been much progress in our understanding of those parts of the gliadin molecule that are the cause of further reactions that damage the small intestinal mucosa. Two regions of the A-gliadin molecule that remain undigested by remission coeliac mucosa are peptides from residues 12-19 and 77-84 and the problems seem to center around motifs associated with toxicity such as PSQQ, QQQP and QQPY. It should be noted that QQPYP and PQQPY are present in all three coeliac-toxic cereals - wheat, rye and barley (McLachlan et al., 2002).
- There appears to be a great need for enzyme therapy as a form of management in CD. It will reduce the worry connected with the necessity of keeping to a strict gluten-free diet, particularly when the food has been prepared outside the home or where contamination by wheat, rye or barley products is a possibility. By the use of a natural enzyme from the papaya plant, this should be able to be accomplished safely. However, clinical trials will be the arbiter of this project.

- The availability of new, highly sensitive and specific serological tests has led to the realization that CD is the most common food intolerance in the world (Accomando & Cataldo, 2004). We have always been aware of the need to understand the mechanisms that operate in this disease and resulting from these studies was the investigation of animal and plant enzymes as a form of therapy (Cornell & Stelmasiak, 2009). Coupled with this advance is the need for diagnosis of CD at an early age, making enzyme therapy an important lifetime management program. We think enzyme therapy is ready for "prime time".

10. References

Accomando, S. & Cataldo, F. (2004). The global village of coeliac disease. *Dig. Liver Dis.* Vol. 36. pp.492-498.

Alfonso, P., Soto, C., Albar, J.P., Camafeita, E., Escobar, H., Suárez, L., Rico, M., Bruix, M., & Méndez, E. (1998). Beta structure motif recognition by anti-gliadin antibodies in coeliac disease. *FEBS letters*. Vol. 427. pp. 36-40.

Anderson, C.M., Fraser A.C., French J.M., Gerrard J.W., Sammons, H.G. & Smellie, J.M. (1952). Coeliac disease: gastrointestinal studies and the effect of dietary wheat flour. *Lancet.* Vol.1. pp. 836-842.

Anderson, R. P., Degano, P., Godkin, A.J., Jewell, D.P. & Hill, A.V. (2000) *In vivo* antigen challenge in coeliac disease identifies a single transglutaminase-modified peptide as the dominant A-gliadin T-cell epitope. *Nature Med.* Vol. 6. pp. 337-342.

Arentz-Hansen, H., Fleckenstein, B., Molberg, Ø., Scott, H., Koning, F., Jung, G., Roepstorff, P., Lundin, K., & Sollid, L. M. (2004). The molecular basis for oat intolerance in coeliac disease patients. *PLoS Med.* Vol.1. pp. 84-92.

Arnon, R. (1970). The cysteine proteases: papain. *Methods Enzymol.* Vol. 19. pp. 226-244.

Australian Government Report. (2008). The biology of Carica Papaya L. *Dept. of Health Report.* Version 2. pp. 25-26.

Azarkan, M., El Moussaoui, A., Van Wuytswinkel, D., Dehon, G. & Looze, Y. (2003) Fractionation and purification of the enzymes stored in the latex of *Carica papaya. J Chromatog.B* Vol. 790. pp. 229-238.

Biagi, F., Campanella, J., Bianchi, P.I., Zanellati, G., Capriglione, I., Klersy, C. & Catassi, C., Fabiani, E., Iacono, G., D'Agate, C., Francavilla, R., Biagi, F., Volta, V., Accomando, S., Picarelli,A., De Vitis, I., Pianelli, G., Gesuita, R., Carle, F., Mandolesi, A., Bearzi, I. & Fasano, A. (2007). A prospective, double-blind, placebo-controlled trial to establish a safe gluten threshold for patients with coeliac disease. *Am J Clin Nutr.* Vol. 85. pp.160-166.

Biagi, F., Zimmer, K.P., Thomas, P.D., Ellis, H.J. & Ciclitira, P. (1999). Is gliadin misrepresented to the immune system in coeliac disease? A hypothesis. *Q J Med.* Vol.92. pp. 119-122.

Biesiekierski, J.R., Newnham, E.D., Irving, P.M., Barrett, J.S., Haines, M., Doecke, J.D., Shepherd, S.J., Muir, J.G. & Gibson, P.R. (2011). Gluten causes gastrointestinal symptoms in subjects without coeliac disease: a double-blind randomized placebo-controlled trial. *Am J Gastroenterol.* Vol. 106. pp. 508-514.

Bjarnason, I. & Peters, T.J. (1983). A persistent defect in small intestinal permeability in coeliac disease demonstrated by a 51-Cr-labelled EDTA absorption test. *Lancet.* Vol. 1. pp. 323-325.

Bronstein, H.D., Haeffner, L.J., & Kowlessar, O.D. (1966). Enzymatic digestion of gliadin: The effect of the resultant peptides in adult coeliac disease. *Clin Chim Acta.* Vol.14. pp.141-155.

Burgin-Wolff, A., I. Dahlbom, F. Hadziselimovic, & C. J. Petersson. (2002). Antibodies against human tissue transglutaminase and endomysium in diagnosing and monitoring coeliac disease. *Scand J Gastroenterol.* Vol. 37. pp. 685-691.

Comino, I., Real, A., de Lorenzo L, Cornell H, López-Casado MÁ, Barro F, Lorite P, Torres MI, Cebolla A, Sousa C. (2011). Diversity in oat potential immunogenicity: basis for the selection of oat varieties with no toxicity in coeliac disease. *Gut.* Vol. 60. pp. 915-922.

Corazza, G.R. (2008 The incidence of coeliac disease in adult first degree relatives. *Dig Liver Dis.* Vol.40. pp. 97-100.

Cornell, H.J. (1974). Circulating antibodies to wheat gliadin fractions in coeliac disease. *Arch Dis Child.* Vol. 49. pp. 454-458.

Cornell, H.J. (1996). Coeliac disease: A review of the causative agents and their possible mechanisms of action. *Amino Acids,* Vol. 10. pp. 1-19.

Cornell, H.J. (1998). Partial *in vitro* digestion of active gliadin-related peptides in coeliac disease. *J Protein Chem.* Vol. 17. pp. 739-744.

Cornell, H. J., Auricchio, R. S., Ritis, G. De, Vincenzi, M. De, Maiuri, L., Raia, V. & Silano, V. (1988) Intestinal mucosa of coeliacs in remission is unable to abolish toxicity of gliadin peptides on *in vitro* developing fetal rat intestine and cultured atrophic coeliac mucosa. *Pediatric Research.* Vol. 24, pp. 233- 237.

Cornell, H.J., Doherty, W. & Stelmasiak T. (2010). Papaya enzymes capable of detoxification of gliadin. *Amino Acids.* Vol.38. pp. 165-175.

Cornell, H. J. & Hoveling, A. W. (1998). In: *Wheat chemistry and utilization.* pp.350-360. Technomic Publishing Company, Inc. Lancaster, PA, U.S.A., ISBN 1-56676-348-7.

Cornell, H.J., Macrae, F.A., Melny, J. Pizzey, C., Cook, F., Mason, S., Bhathal, P.& Stelmasiak, T. (2005). Enzyme therapy for management of coeliac disease. *Scand. J. Gastroent.* Vol.40.pp. 1304-1312.

Cornell, H.J., Mothes, T. (1993) The activity of wheat gliadin peptides in *in vitro* assays for coeliac disease. *Biochim Biophys Acta* ; Vol. 1181. pp. 169-173.

Cornell, H.J. , Mothes, T. (1995) Further studies of the *in vitro* activity of synthetic gliadin peptides in coeliac disease. *Biochim Biophys Acta.* Vol.1270. pp. 168-172.

Cornell, H.J., & Rivett, D.E. (1995). *In vitro* mucosal digestion of synthetic gliadin-derived peptides in coeliac disease. *J Protein Chem.* Vol. 14. pp. 335-339.

Cornell, H.J. & Rolles, C.J. (1978). Further evidence of a primary mucosal defect in coeliac disease. *Gut.* Vol.19. pp. 253-259.

Cornell, H.J. & Stelmasiak, T. (2004) Enzyme supplementation in coeliac disease.*Proceedings of the 11th International Symposium on Coeliac Disease.* Belfast, Northern Ireland. p.196.

Cornell, H.J. & Stelmasiak T. (2007). A unified hypothesis of coeliac disease with implications for management of patients. *Amino Acids.* Vol. 33, pp.43-49.

Cornell, H.J. & Stelmasiak, T. (2009). Strategies for improved outcomes for those with coeliac disease. In: *Coeliac Disease: Etiology, Diagnosis and Treatment.* M.A. Edwards, (Ed).pp. 207-211. ISBN: 978-1-61209-873-9., Nova Science Publishers Inc., N.Y.

Cornell, H.J. & Stelmasiak, T. (2011) Caricain a basis for enzyme therapy for coeliac disease. *Sth Afr J Sci.* Vol.9/10. pp.107-111.

Cornell, H.J. & Townley, R.R.W. (1973a). Investigating possible intestinal peptidase deficiency in coeliac disease. *Clin Chim Acta.* Vol.43. pp.113-125.

Cornell, H.J. & Townley, R.R.W. (1973b). The effect of gliadin peptides on rat-liver lysosomes in relation to the pathogenesis of coeliac disease. *Clin ChimActa.* Vol.49. pp.181-188.

Cornell, H.J. & Townley, R.R. (1974). The toxicity of certain cereal proteins in coeliac disease. *Gut.* Vol.15. pp. 862-869.

Cornell, H.J., Skerritt, J.H., Puy, R. & Javadpour, M. (1994). Studies of *in vitro* γ - interferon production in coeliac disease as a response to gliadin peptides. *Biochim Biophys Acta*; Vol.1226. pp.126-130.

Cornell, H.J., Wieser, H. & Belitz, H.D. (1992). Characterisation of the gliadin-derived peptides which are biologically active in coeliac disease. *Clin Chim Acta.* Vol. 213. pp. 37-50.

Cornell, H.J. & Wills-Johnson, G. (2001). Structure-activity relationships in coeliac-toxic gliadin peptides. *Amino Acids.* Vol. 21. pp. 243–253.

Dahele, A.V., Aldhous, M.C., Humphreys, K., & Ghosh, S. (2001). Serum IgA tissue transglutaminase antibodies in coeliac disease and other gastrointestinal diseases. *Q J Med.* Vol.94. pp. 195-205.

De Ritis, G., Auricchio, S., Jones, H.W.,Lew, E.J.L., Bernardin, J.E. & Kasarda, D. (1988). *In vitro* (organ culture) studies of the toxicity of specific A-gliadin peptides in coeliac disease. *Gastroenterology.* Vol. 94, pp. 41-49.

Dicke, W.K., Wejiers, H.A., and van de Kamer, J.H. (1953). Coeliac disease. II. The presence in wheat of a factor having a deleterious effect in cases of coeliac disease. *Acta Paediatrica,* Vol. 42, pp. 34-42.

Dohan, F.C. & Grasberger, J.C. (1973). Relapsed schizophrenics: earlier discharge from the hospital after cereal-free, milk-free diet. *Am J Psychiatry* Vol.130. pp. 685-688.

Dolly, J.O. & Fottrell, P.F. (1969). Effect of different peptide fractions from wheat gliadin on rat liver lysosomes. *Irish J Med Sc.* Vol. 2. p. 47.

Donlon, J., & Stevens, F.M. (2004). No lack of prolyl oligopeptidase (POP) in the coeliac mucosa. *Proceedings of the 11th International Symposium on Coeliac Disease.* Belfast, Northern Ireland. p.19.

Drago, S., El Asmar, R., Di Pierro, M.,Clemente, G. M., Tripathi, A., Sapone, A., Thakar, M., Iacono, G., Carroccio, A., D'Agate, C., Not, T., Zampini, L., Catassi, C. & Fasano A. (2006). Gliadin, zonulin and gut permeability: Effects on coeliac and non-coeliac intestinal mucosa and intestinal cell lines. *Scand J Gastroenterol..* Vol.41. pp. 408-419.

Dubey, V.K., Pande, M., Singh, B.K., & Jagannadham, M.V. (2007). Papain-like proteases: applications of their inhibitors. *Afr J Biotechnol.* Vol. 6. pp. 1077-1086.

Fry, L. (1992). Dermatitis herpetiformis. In: *Coeliac disease* , M. Marsh, (Ed.), Oxford, UK, Blackwell Scientific Pub.

Falchuk, Z.M. & Strober, W. (1974). Gluten sensitive enteropathy: synthesis of anti-gliadin antibody *in vitro*. *Gut.* Vol. 15. pp. 947-952.

Frazer, A.C., Fletcher, R.F., Ross, C.A.C., Shaw, B., Sammons, H.G. & Schneider, R. (1959). Gluten-induced enteropathy: The effect of partially digested gluten. *Lancet.* Vol. 274. pp. 252-255.

Fukudome, S.I., & Yoshikawa , M. (1992). Opioid peptides derived from wheat gluten: Their isolation and characterization. *FEBS letters.* Vol.296. pp.107-111.

Gravett, P.S.,Viljoen,C. & Osthvizen, M. (1991). A steady-state kinetic analysis of the reaction between arginine esterase E-I from *Bitis Gabonica* venom and synthetic arginine substrates and the influence of pH, temperature and solvent deuterium isotope. *In. J Biochem.* Vol. 23. pp. 1085-1099.

Groves, M. R., Taylor, M. A., Scott, M., Cummings, N. J., Pickersgill, R. W. & Jenkins, J. A. (*1996*). The prosequence of procaricain forms an α-helical domain that prevents access to the substrate-binding cleft. *Structure.* Vol.4.pp. 1193-1203.

Halstensen, *T.S.*, Scott, H., Fausa, O. & Brandtzaeg, P., (1993). Gluten stimulation of coeliac mucosa *in vitro* induces activation (CD25) of lamina propria CD4+ T cells and macrophages but no crypt cells hyperplasia. *Scand J Immunol.* Vol. 38. pp. 581–590.

Hausch, .F, Shan, L., Santiago, N.A., Gray, G.M. & Khosla, C: Intestinal digestive resistance of immunodominant gliadin peptides. *Am J Physiol Gastrointest Liver Physiol.* (2002). Vol. 283. pp. G996-G1003.

Lucarelli, S., Frediani, T., Zingoni, A.M., Ferruzzi, F., Giardini, O., Quintieri, .F, Barbato, M., D'Eufemia, P. & Cardi, E. (1995). Food allergy and infantile autism. *Panminerva Med.* Vol.37. pp.137-141.

Jiang, L.L., Zhang, B.L. & Liu, Y.S. (2009). Is adult coeliac disease really uncommon in Chinese? *J Zhejiang Univ Sci. B.* Vol. 10. pp. 168-171.

Jones VA, McLaughlan P, Shorthouse M, Workman E, Hunter JO. (1982) Food intolerance: a major factor in the pathogenesis of irritable bowel syndrome. *Lancet.* Vol.2. pp.1115-1117.

Kagnoff *M. (*2007*)* Coeliac disease: pathogenesis of a model immunogenetic disease. *J Clin Invest.* Vol.117. pp.41-49.

Kasarda, D.D., Okita, T.D., Bernardin, J.E., Baecker, P.A., Nimmo, C.C., Lew, E.J.L., Dietler, M.D. & Greene, F.C. (1984). Nucleic acid (cDNA) and amino acid sequences of ÿ-type gliadins from wheat (*Triticum aestivum*). *Proc Natl Acad Sci USA.* Vol. 81. pp. 4712-4716.

Kocna, P., Fric, P.,Slabý, J.& Kasafírek, E. (1980). Endopeptidase of the brush border membrane of rat enterocyte: separation from aminopeptidase and partial characterization. *Hoppe-Seyler Z Physiol Chem.* Vol. 361. pp.1401–1412.

Kocna, P., Mothes, T., Krchnak, V. & Fric. *P. (*1991*)* Relationship between gliadin peptide structure and their effect on the foetal chick duodenum. *Z. Lebensm. Unters. Forsch.* Vol. 192. pp. 116-119.

Riecken, A.O., Stewart, J.S., Booth, C.C. & Pearse, A.G.E. (1966). A histochemical study of the role of lysosomal enzymes in idiopathic steatorrhoea before and during a gluten-free diet. *Gut.* Vol.7. pp.317-332.

Mäki, M. (1996). Coeliac disease and autoimmunity due to unmasking cryptic epitopes. *Lancet.* Vol.348. pp.1046-1047.

Mäki, M. & Collin, P. (1997). Coeliac disease. *Lancet,* Vol. 349, pp.1755-1759.

Matysiak-Budnik, T., Candalh, C., Cellier, C., Dugave, C., Namane, A., Vidal-Martinez, T., Cerf-Bensussan, N. & Heyman, M. (2005). Limited efficiency of prolyl-endopeptidase in the detoxification of gliadin peptides in coeliac disease. *Gastroenterology.* Vol.129. pp.786-796.

Matysiak-Budnik, T., Malamut, G., de Serre, N.P., Grosdidier, E., Seguier, S., Brousse, N., Caillat-Zucman, S., Cerf-Bensussan, N., Schmitz, J. & Cellier, C. (2007). Long-term follow-up of 61 coeliac patients diagnosed in childhood: evolution toward latency is possible on a normal diet. *Gut.* Vol.56. pp. 1379-1386.

Mantzaris, G.J., & Jewell, D.P. (1991*). In-vivo* toxicity of a synthetic dodecapeptide from A-gliadin in patients with coeliac disease. *Scand J Gastroenterol.* Vol. 26. pp. 392–398.

McAdam, S.N. *&* Sollid LM. *(*2000). Getting to grips with gluten. *Gut.* Vol. 47. pp. 743-745.

McLachlan, A., Cullis, P.G., Cornell, H.J. (2002) The use of extended motifs for focussing on toxic peptides in coeliac disease. *J Biochem Mol Biol Biophys.* Vol. 6. pp. 319-324.

Molberg, O., Mcadam, S.N., Korner, R., Quarsten, H., Kristiansen, C., Madsen, L., Fugger, L., Scott, H., Noren, O., Roepstorff, P., Lundin, K.E., Sjostrom, H. & Sollid, L.M. (1998). Tissue transglutaminase selectively modifies gliadin peptides that are recognized by gut-derived T cells in coeliac disease. *Nat Med* . Vol.4. pp.713-717.

Monsuur, A.J., de Bakker, P.I.W., Alizadeh, B.Z., Zhernakova, A., Bevova, M.R., Strengman, E., Franke, L., van't Slot, R., van Belzen, M.J., Lavrijsen, I.C.M. et al. (2005). *Nature Genetics.* Vol.37. p.1341-1344.

Mothes, T., Osman, A.A., Seilmeier, W. & Wieser, H. (1999). The activity of single gliadin components in a foetal chick intestine assay for coeliac disease. *Eur Food Res Technol.* Vol. 210. pp. 93-96.

Mothes, T., Muhle, W., Muller, F. & Herkens, W.T.J.M. (1985). Influence of gliadin on fetal chick intestine in tissue culture. *Biol Neonate.* Vol.48. pp.59- Shan, L., Molberg, Ø., Parrot, I., Hausch, F., Filiz, F., Gray, G.M., Sollid, L.M. & Khosla, C. (2002.) Structural basis for gluten intolerance in coeliac sprue. *Science.* Vol. 297. pp. 2275-2279.

Sealy-Voyksner, J. A., Khosla, C., Voyksner, R. D. & Jorgensen, J. W. (2010). Novel aspects of quantitation of immunologenic wheat gluten peptides by liquid chromatography-mass spectrometry/mass spectrometry. *J.Chromatogr A.* Vol.25, pp. 4167-4183.

Siegel, M., Bethune, M. T., Gass, J., Ehren, J., Xia, J., Johannsen, A., Stuge, T. B., Gray, G. M., Lee, P. P. & Khosla, C. (2006). Rational design of combination enzyme therapy for coeliac sprue. *Chem Biol.* Vol. 13, pp. 637-647.

Silano, M., Di Benedetto, R., Maialetti, F., De Vincenzi, A., Calcaterra, R., Cornell, H.J. & De Vincenzi, M. (2007). Avenins from different cultivars of oats elicit response by coeliac peripheral lymphocytes. *Scand J Gastroenterol.*Vol. 42. pp.1302-1305.

Singh, M.M. & Kay, S.R. (1976). Wheat gluten as a pathogenic factor in schizophrenia. *Science.* Vol. 191. pp. 401-402.

Shepherd, S,J., Parker, F.C., Muir, J.G. & Gibson, P.R. (2008) Dietary triggers of abdominal symptoms in patients with irritable bowel syndrome: randomized placebo-controlled evidence. *Clin Gastroenterol Hepatol.* Vol. 6. pp. 765-771.

Shan, L.,Molberg, Ø., Parrot, I., Hausch, F., Filiz, F., Gray, G.M., Sollid, L.M. & Khosla, C. (2002). Structural basis for gluten intolerance in coeliac sprue. Science. Vol. 297. pp. 2275-2279.

Shuppan,D., Junker, Y. & Barisani, D. (2009). Coeliac disease: from pathogenesis to novel therapies. *Gastroenterology.* Vol. 137. pp. 1912-1933.

Shuppan, D. & Hahn, E.G. (2002). Gluten and the gut - lessons for immune regulation. *Science.* Vol.297. pp. 2218-2220.

Sollid, L.M. (2002). Coeliac disease: Dissecting a complex inflammatory disorder. *Nature Reviews Immunology.* Vol.2, pp. 647- 655.

Stepniak, D., Spaenij-Dekking, L., Mitea, C., Moester, M., de Ru, A., Baak-Pablo, R., van Veelen, P., Edens, L. & Koning F. (2006). Highly efficient gluten degradation with a newly identified prolyl endoprotease: implications for coeliac disease. *Am J Physiol Gastrointest Liver Physiol* . Vol. 291. pp. G621–G629.

Storch, W. (1978). About the differentiation of antibodies against the connective tissue. *Acta Histochem.* Vol.62. pp. 57-67.

Sturgess, R., Day, P., Ellis, H.J., Lundin, K.E., Gjertsen, H.A., Kontakou, M. & Ciclitira, P.J. (1994). Wheat peptide challenge in coeliac disease. *Lancet.* Vol. 343.pp. 758-761.

Townley, R.R.W., Bhathal, P.S., Cornell, H.J. & Mitchell, J.D. (1973). Toxicity of wheat gliadin fractions in coeliac disease. *Lancet.* Vol.1. pp.1363-1364.

Vader, W., Kooy, Y., van Veelen, P., de Ru, A., Harris, D., Benckhuijsen, W.,Pena, S., Mearin, L., Drijfhout, J.W. & Koning, F. (2002). The gluten response in children with coeliac disease is directed toward multiple gliadin and glutenin peptides. *Gastroenterology.* Vol. 122. pp. 1729-1737.

Van Heel, D.A. & West J. (2006). Recent advances in coeliac disease. *Gut,* Vol.55, pp. 1037-1046.

Weissmann, G. (1964). Lysosomes, autoimmune phenomena, and diseases of connective tissue. *Lancet.* Vol. 284, pp. 1373 – 1375.

Section 5

Follow-up of Patients with Celiac Disease

9

Principles and Strategies for Monitoring Individuals with Celiac Disease

Mohsin Rashid
Dalhousie University
Canada

1. Introduction

Gluten-free diet is an effective therapy for celiac disease. There are few diseases in medicine where a nutritional intervention alone can produce such rapid, gratifying results. One may therefore question the need for following these patients long-term. In the past, a rather simplistic approach was taken towards treatment and follow-up of patients with celiac disease. "Go home, don't eat anything with gluten and you'll be fine", patients were told. But as more individuals were diagnosed with celiac disease and our understanding of this disorder improved, several important issues emerged. Firstly, it was recognized that gluten-free diet is complex, costly and socially restrictive, and that cross contamination of the diet with gluten was very common. For a gluten-free diet to be fully effective, adherence to the diet must be strict and life-long, thereby adding further challenges. Gluten-free diet should be viewed as a "prescribed therapy" rather than a mere change in life style. Furthermore, celiac disease is not simply a malabsorptive gastrointestinal disorder. It is a multisystem, auto-immune disease that carries a significant health burden and risk of complications (Freeman et al. 2011). These factors necessitate ongoing, careful monitoring of patients with celiac disease. The following six key elements of management of celiac disease include long-term follow-up (NIH, 2004):

Consultation with a skilled dietitian
Education about the disease
Lifelong adherence to a gluten-free diet
Identification and treatment of nutritional deficiencies
Access to an advocacy group
Continuous long-term follow-up by a multidisciplinary team

This chapter highlights the important issues in long-term follow-up of patients with celiac disease and offers guidelines for practicing physicians and allied health professionals involved in their management. Issues around the diagnosis of celiac disease and details of the gluten-free diet will not be covered. Because this is a rapidly evolving field, recommendations for follow-up may get modified over time.

2. Importance of follow-up

Because most patients with celiac disease recover symptomatically with therapy they may not perceive the need for follow-up. This view may be shared by some of their health care providers. Hence, not all patients with celiac disease receive regular follow-up care. In a study of 126 adults with celiac disease in United Kingdom, only 62% were receiving formal follow-up care (Bebb et al., 2006). Of these, 92% were being followed at a hospital clinic and 8% by their general practitioner.

Follow-up is essential not only to assess symptomatic recovery and to monitor complications but also to assist the patient in adhering to the diet (Pietzak, 2005). Follow-up care is the key to dietary compliance. There is good objective evidence that proactive follow-up measures can reinforce adherence to the gluten-free diet, both in children and adults (Bardella et al. 1994, Hogberg et al. 2003, Ljugman & Myrdal, 1993, Lamontagne et al, 2001). Follow-up visits also provide an opportunity to give patients updated information on new developments in the field.

3. Who should provide follow-up?

Gastroenterologists are often the ones who establish or confirm the diagnosis of celiac disease. But who should provide their long term follow-up care... the patient's family physician, internist/paediatrician or the gastroenterologist? A survey of Canadian gastroenterologists revealed that 76% routinely provided long-term follow-up care to patients with celiac disease (Silvester & Rashid, 2010). Significantly more paediatric gastroenterologists provided long-term follow-up, as compared with adult gastroenterologists. Also, the elements of follow-up varied, including the frequency of laboratory testing and of repeat duodenal biopsies. The most commonly cited reason (86%) for not providing long-term follow-up was that the patient`s primary care physician was providing this care. Other reasons included, a) not having an organized system to recall patients; b) lack of time and c) the belief that follow-up was not required once the patient was on a gluten-free diet. In some cases, the patients themselves did not want follow-up.

Who eventually provides long-term care to patients with celiac disease may depend on the availability of resources, both personnel and funding, the severity of the patient's illness and the complexity of the disease course. It is probably prudent that all patients be followed by their gastroenterologists for at least the first year after diagnosis. Thereafter, the family physician or internist can follow the patient and request gastroenterologist's input as needed. All children with celiac disease should be followed by either their pediatricians or gastroenterologist.

There is less controversy about the role of the dietitian in follow-up of these patients. Treatment of celiac disease is primarily nutritional and the dietitian's role is therefore of paramount importance. In one survey, the preferred method of follow-up by most patients was to see a dietitian with a doctor being available (Bebb et al. 2006).

Nutritional adequacy of a gluten-free diet is also a concern because it may be deficient in certain vitamins, iron, calcium and fiber (Kupper, 2005). These micronutrient deficiencies require monitoring which is best provided by a dietitian. However, a gluten-free diet is complex and not all dietitians are well-versed in this area. Therefore, ongoing nutritional counseling should be provided by a dietitian skilled in the use of a gluten-free diet (Case, 2005).

4. What constitutes appropriate follow-up?

Evaluation of current practice guidelines issued by various professional organizations has revealed significant differences in recommendations for long-term follow-up of patients with celiac disease (Silvester & Rashid, 2007). As information accumulates, broad guidelines for long-term management are beginning to emerge (Haines et al, 2008, AGA, 2006, Hill et al, 2005). While there is consensus on some aspects, others remain controversial.

Celiac disease has a wide clinical spectrum. In order to individualize the type of follow-up needed, it is important to stratify patients according to their risk of developing complications. Genetic factors strongly influence the development of celiac disease; specifically, the major histocompatibility complex class II antigens. About 90% of patients with celiac disease carry the HLA-DQ2 heterodimer encoded by alleles DQA1*05 and DQB1*02. The remainder have either HLA DQA1*05 or HLA DQB1*02, or express HLA-DQ8 encoded by alleles DQA1*03 and DQB1*0302. The HLA-DQ2 and DQ8 are within haplotypes also associated with other autoimmune disorders such as type-1diabetes and autoimmune thyroid disease. Patients with celiac disease who are homozygous for HLA-DQ2 tend to have more severe complications, including refractory celiac disease and enteropathy-associated T cell lymphoma (Al-Toma et al. 2006). The phenotype of patients who are homozygous for DQB1*02 tends to be associated with more severe symptoms, marked villous atrophy at diagnosis and slower recovery after instituting a gluten-free diet (Karinen et al. 2006, Jores et al. 2007). As our understanding of the genetics of celiac disease improves and HLA testing becomes more routinely available, it may be possible to identify patients who require more intensive follow-up.

Follow-up of patients with celiac disease should focus on three key areas; nutritional deficiencies, adherence to gluten-free diet and monitoring of complications. A proposed follow-up plan is listed in Table 1.

The physician's assessment at each visit should include a complete history, especially noting symptoms of abdominal pain, diarrhoea, weight loss, anorexia and fatigue. Physical examination should include measurement of weight, height and body mass index (BMI). Children should be serially evaluated with a growth chart to detect alterations in growth velocity. A complete, systemic examination should be performed in all patients.

The utility of serological testing and the usefulness of a repeat intestinal biopsy will be discussed later.

Yearly monitoring of thyroid function is recommended as thyroid disease develops commonly in celiac disease (Elstrom et al. 2008, Meloni et al. 2009). Hypothyroidism can be easily identified by laboratory tests (thyroid stimulating hormone, free thyroxine) and treated with hormone replacement therapy. Thyroid antibody testing may not be cost effective as it does not necessarily predict the development of clinical thyroid dysfunction. Also, currently there are no means of preventing the development of thyroiditis or other auto-immune disorders such as type-1 diabetes. There is controversy whether a gluten-free diet prevents autoimmune thyroiditis that is established or is in evolution (Meloni et al. 2009, Cassio et al, 2010).

The follow-up plan listed in Table 1 is the minimum recommended for an average, uncomplicated patient with celiac disease. If the patient remains ill, additional investigations

At Diagnosis (Physician and Dietitian)
- Education on celiac disease
- Gluten-free dietary counseling by a skilled dietitian
- Recommend family screening
- Recommend membership in a celiac support group
- Bone densitometry*
- Celiac serology (if not previously obtained)
- Other Routine Tests (complete blood count, iron studies, folate, thyroid function tests, liver enzymes, calcium, phosphate, vitamin D)
At 2 months (Physician and Dietitian)
- Assess symptoms and coping skills
- Dietary review
At 6 months (Physician and Dietitian)
- Assess symptoms
- Complete physical examination
- Dietary review
- Celiac serology
- Repeat Other Routine Tests (if previously abnormal)
At 12 months (Physician and Dietitian)
- Assess symptoms
- Complete physical examination
- Dietary review
- Celiac serology (if still positive)
- Repeat Other Routine Tests (if previously abnormal)
- Bone densitometry (if previously abnormal)
- Small intestinal biopsy*
Yearly (Physician and Dietitian)
- Assess symptoms
- Complete physical examination
- Dietary review
- Celiac serology
- Thyroid function tests
- Other Tests (as clinically indicated)

* Not recommended routinely for children. *See text*

Table 1. Proposed Routine Follow-up Plan for Patients with Celiac Disease

may be needed, as guided by the clinical findings. For example, micronutrients such as zinc should be measured in severe malnutrition. In patients with macrocytic anemia and normal folate, vitamin B12 status should be assessed by measuring serum cobalamin, homocystine and methylmalonic acid. Any abnormalities detected should be followed up with appropriate retesting after supplementation.

Celiac disease can be associated with other autoimmune disorders, such as type I diabetes mellitus or thyroiditis. If a patient suffers from one or more of these, follow-up should include relevant assessment and investigations.

Patients who remain symptomatic despite following a gluten-free diet may need to be seen more frequently, whereas those who were asymptomatic at diagnosis and remain so, may require less frequent visits.

5. Follow-up of paediatric patients

The general principles of management described above also apply to the paediatric population with a few notable differences. Growth sets children apart from adults. Celiac disease can adversely affect physical and neurodevelopmental growth, primarily due to nutritional deficiencies. Also, since very young children are unable to communicate their symptoms, a high index of suspicion should be maintained when inquiring about their health from the parents.

In children, all anthropometric measurements should be plotted as percentiles on growth charts. The BMI in children is not a fixed value but is age dependent and is expressed in percentiles. For children under three years of age, head circumference should also be measured. Poor growth implies a nutritional deficit. Normal growth is reassuring but does not rule out micronutrient deficiencies.

According to the revised guidelines of the European Society for Paediatric Gastroenterology and Nutrition, in children older than 2 years of age with symptoms suggestive of celiac disease, the characteristic histologic findings on small intestinal biopsy and unequivocal clinical resolution after institution of a gluten-free diet, the diagnosis can be considered definitive for lifelong celiac disease without need for further biopsies (Walker-Smith et al. 1990). A follow-up biopsy may be required only in selected patients in whom the diagnosis is in doubt, or if the child remains symptomatic despite being on a strict gluten-free diet.

In children with celiac disease, secondary nutritional problems such as iron deficiency, anemia and osteoporosis resolve completely after starting a gluten-free diet. Once corrected, routine follow-up laboratory testing for these conditions is not required.

6. Utility of serological testing in follow-up

Serological tests usually become negative within a year on a strict gluten-free diet and may be used to monitor compliance with the gluten-free diet. However, these tests are insufficiently sensitive to reflect occasional dietary transgressions (Kaukinen et al. 2002, 2007, Tursi et al. 2006). The degree and duration of gluten exposure will affect the results. Thus, these tests may be more useful in predicting non-adherence rather than strict adherence. Furthermore, normalization of the antibodies does not necessarily imply complete villous healing (Tursi et al. 2003). Some patients with normalized antibodies may have ongoing villous atrophy.

A persistently positive serological test after a patient has been on a gluten-free diet is highly indicative of ongoing gluten exposure and may indicate mucosal injury or development of refractory celiac disease. A negative test is reassuring only to a certain degree.

7. Role of routine repeat small intestinal biopsy

Small intestinal biopsy is the definitive way to document mucosal healing after starting a gluten-free diet. However, there is controversy as to whether all patients with celiac disease should undergo a follow-up biopsy to document intestinal healing. Some adult gastroenterologists routinely perform a follow-up biopsy in all patients after 12 months of starting a gluten-free diet. Others perform a biopsy only in selected cases.

Rates of mucosal healing are highly variable. In some studies, up to 40% of patients had persisting villous atrophy after two years (Tursi et al, 2006) and about 10% after five years on a gluten-free diet (Wahab et al. 2002). This raises the question of whether symptoms alone constitute a reliable guide to mucosal healing (Kaukinen et al. 2007). Ongoing villous atrophy can lead to nutritional problems such as osteoporosis and may increase the risk of developing complications such as lymphoma. Clinical symptoms, celiac serology and laboratory markers of inflammation are not robust enough measures to confirm mucosal healing. Until better non-invasive tests of mucosal healing can be developed, a repeat intestinal biopsy after a year of gluten-free diet is recommended.

Mucosal healing tends to be more rapid and more complete in children. Also, since endoscopy requires a general anesthetic in most cases, a repeat follow-up biopsy is not recommended in children with celiac disease who recover clinically and normalize their celiac antibody tests.

8. Non-responsive celiac disease

Most patients with celiac disease will improve and their symptoms will resolve after starting a gluten-free diet. However, some do not ... a phenomenon referred to as non-responsive celiac disease. Non-responsive celiac disease is defined as failure to respond to at least six months of treatment with a gluten-free diet (*primary*) or re-emergence of symptoms or laboratory abnormalities typical of celiac disease while continuing on treatment with a gluten-free diet (*secondary*). The six months of treatment duration with gluten-free diet is used an arbitrary cut off point since patients should have significant improvement by this time.

Non-responsive celiac disease is common. Among 603 patients followed at one health care facility over five years, 113 (19%) had non-responsive celiac disease (Leffler et al. 2007).

The causes of non-responsive celiac disease are listed in Table 2. Before embarking on any investigations, one must ensure that the diagnosis of celiac disease was correct in the first place. Of 55 patients referred to a tertiary care medical institution with a presumed diagnosis of non-responsive celiac disease, 6 (9.2%) did not have celiac disease (Abdulkarim et al. 2002). Some patients may self-diagnose and never undergo an intestinal biopsy. In others who do undergo intestinal biopsy, the specimen may get interpreted incorrectly. Furthermore, villous atrophy is not unique to celiac disease. Similar lesions can be seen in infectious, allergic or autoimmune enteropathy and in other disorders such as Crohn's disease and collagenous sprue.

-	Gluten exposure
-	Irritable bowel syndrome
-	Refractory celiac disease
-	Lactose intolerance
-	Pancreatic insufficiency
-	Microscopic colitis
-	Small intestinal bacterial overgrowth
-	Ulcerative jejunitis
-	Other co-existing conditions (gastroesophageal reflux disease, peptic ulcer, food allergy, eating disorder, inflammatory bowel disease, immunodeficiency)

Table 2. Causes of Non-Responsive Celiac Disease

Ongoing exposure to gluten in the diet is the most common cause of non-responsive celiac disease, occurring in 36% to 51% of patients (Leffler et al. 2007, Abdulkarim et al. 2002). The gluten exposure may be accidental or intentional. The recently proposed international definition of the gluten-free diet states that the gluten content should be less than 20 parts per million (ppm) i.e. less than 20 mg gluten in 1 kg of dry weight food product (Codex Alimentarius Commission, Standard 118-1979, July 2008). Although individuals may have varying degrees of gluten tolerance, ingestion of 50 mg of gluten daily over three months can be sufficient to cause injury to the small intestinal mucosa (Catassi et al. 2007). For example, an average slice of bread contains approximately 3.0-3.5 gm of gluten. Hence, an amount as little as 1/70th of a slice of bread consumed on a regular basis may lead to villous damage. Avoiding gluten contamination in diet is very difficult for many patients because there are many hidden sources of gluten in the diet. In some cases, the patient may be knowingly consuming gluten-containing foods and, for whatever reason, does not tell the physician. (Some patients feel guilty or embarrassed in admitting dietary transgressions!). Furthermore, patients may believe that occasional consumption of small quantities of gluten-containing foods is safe. A dietitian with expertise in gluten-free diet can help evaluate gluten ingestion in such cases.

After gluten ingestion, irritable bowel syndrome (IBS) is the second most common cause of non-responsive celiac disease. This is sometimes referred to as post-inflammatory IBS. A variety of symptoms including abdominal pain, diarrhoea and constipation can occur. The diagnosis is clinical and requires exclusion of other causes. The management is symptomatic and may include cognitive behavior therapy.

The villous atrophy present at the time of diagnosis of celiac disease may lead to secondary lactose intolerance, causing symptoms such as abdominal pain, gas, bloating and diarrhoea. A breath hydrogen test may provide objective evidence of lactase deficiency. A trial of a lactose-free diet or lactase enzyme supplements may help alleviate the symptoms. Patients require calcium and vitamin D supplements while on a lactose-free diet.

Microscopic colitis is an autoimmune inflammatory condition. There are two types, namely lymphocytic colitis and collagenous colitis. The main symptom is watery diarrhoea. A colonoscopy and biopsies are needed to make this diagnosis. Treatment includes a strict gluten-free diet and, in some cases drugs including 5-aminoslicylates, budesonide and azathioprine.

Pancreatic insufficiency may occur in some patients with celiac disease. The exact cause is unknown. Villous atrophy causing impaired secretion and action of enteric hormones such as enterokinase, cholecystokinin and secretin may play a role. Steatorrhoea and weight loss can occur. Tests for exocrine pancreatic insufficiency will be abnormal. Pancreatic enzyme replacement therapy and fat-soluble vitamin supplements should be prescribed. The problem is usually transient and pancreatic function recovers.

A damaged small intestinal mucosa provides a nidus for bacterial growth. Bacterial overgrowth in the small bowel can lead to diarrhoea and weight loss from steatorrhoea. Iron and vitamin B12 deficiency can occur. While the diagnosis is confirmed by a small bowel aspirate for bacterial colony counts, a course of empiric antibiotic therapy may be recommended. Bacterial overgrowth can be successfully treated with oral antibiotics.

Patients with celiac disease are at risk for developing other autoimmune disorders, most commonly autoimmune thyroid disease. Hypothyroidism can lead to a variety of symptoms that may mimic those of celiac disease, such as chronic fatigue and constipation. If celiac serology and intestinal biopsy are normal in a symptomatic patient who has good adherence to gluten-free diet, development of another autoimmune disorder should be considered.

An approach to the assessment of patients with non-responsive celiac disease is described in Table 3. If lymphoma is suspected, upper and lower gastrointestinal endoscopy, abdominal CT scan, capsule endoscopy, and possibly double-balloon enteroscopy should be considered.

-	Review of original diagnosis of celiac diagnosis
-	Careful review of gluten-free adherence by a skilled dietitian
-	Obtain IgA-tissue transglutaminase antibody (TTG)
-	If TTG abnormal, reinforce dietary adherence and reassess
-	If TTG normal (or remains abnormal on reassessment despite a strict gluten-free diet), obtain small intestinal biopsy to rule our refractory celiac disease
-	If biopsy normal, investigate for alternative diagnoses (Table 2)

Table 3. An Approach to Assessment of Non-Responsive Celiac Disease

9. Refractory celiac disease

Refractory celiac disease (RCD) or refractory sprue refers to initial or subsequent failure of a strict gluten-free diet to restore normal intestinal architecture and function in patients who have celiac-like enteropathy and have no evidence of other pathology including intestinal lymphoma.

Weight loss and diarrhoea are the most consistent symptoms of RCD. The diagnosis requires a small intestinal biopsy. Based on the histological appearance of the small intestinal mucosa, RCD is divided into two types. In RCD type-1 there is apparently a normal intraepithelial lymphocyte phenotype whereas in RCD type-2 there is monoclonal or polyclonal expansion of an aberrant intraepithelial lymphocyte population as shown by histochemical staining (Freeman, 2008). This latter type carries a high risk of overt enteropathy associated T cell lymphoma (EATL) and is associated with a greater mortality at two years (41%) compared to RCD type-I (14%).

Corticosteroid therapy may improve clinical symptoms in some patients with RCD but the response is not consistent. Patients with RCD type-1 often require immunosuppressive therapy. The treatment of RCD type-2 is unsatisfactory and the disease carries a high mortality with most patients dying within two years of diagnosis (Rubio-Tapia et al. 2009, Malamut et al. 2009). A variety of therapies have been tried including azathioprine, anti-tumor necrosis factor-alpha, cladribine, anti-CD-52, IL-15 antagonists and stem cell transplantation to replace the abnormal lymphocyte population. Because of the complex nature of therapy, RCD type-2 is best managed by centers with expertise in this condition.

10. Monitoring of complications

The two major complications of celiac disease that require careful monitoring include development of other autoimmune disorders and malignancy.

There is controversy whether a gluten-free diet prevents the development of other autoimmnune diseases (Ventura et al. 1999, Viljamaa et al. 2005, Sategna Guidetti et al. 2001). Molecular mimicry, one of the proposed mechanisms for autoimmunity, does implicate ongoing gluten exposure. Continued gluten ingestion may also contribute to systemic symptoms and development of other disorders like osteoporosis from production and circulation of pro-inflammatory cytokines (Fornari et al. 1998, Romaldini et al. 2002).

While a gluten-free diet may not completely eliminate risk of developing other autoimmune disorders, continued ingestion of gluten definitely increases the risk. This information may also help motivate patients to stay strictly gluten-free.

Patients with untreated celiac disease have a higher risk of developing malignancy compared to the general population. Such malignancies include lymphoma and oropharyngeal, esophageal and small intestinal cancer. A careful history, physical examination and appropriate investigations should be conducted in patients who are either non-adherent to the diet or who remain symptomatic despite following a strict gluten-free diet.

There is good evidence that a gluten-free diet is protective against the development of malignancy. Patients on a strict gluten-free diet for >5 years have the same overall risk for cancer as the general population (Cooper et al, 1982, Holmes et al. 1989). This information should be shared with patients to provide them with reassurance and encouragement for strict adherence to the diet.

11. Ongoing emotional and psychological support

The diagnosis of celiac disease can be overwhelming and coping with it challenging. Patients may feel depressed to learn that they can never eat wheat products again. Feelings of anxiety, anger, deprivation and frustration may develop. Eating in social situations can be especially problematic (Rashid et al. 2005, Zarkadas et al. 2006). Pressures from the extra time and cost involved in buying/preparing foods, along with competing priorities like family, job, etc. may further impair coping abilities and act as barriers to compliance. Dietary transgressions often occur in adolescents and young adults because of the need to conform to peers in social situations.

Long-term follow-up of patients with celiac disease will help monitor both their physical and psychological well being and maintain trust in the physician and dietitian. Normal physical examination and test results will provide patients on a strict gluten-free diet reassurance and encouragement. Abnormal test results can be a powerful motivator especially for those who do not get symptoms when they eat gluten-containing foods. Ongoing psychological support counseling improves compliance with gluten-free diet especially in patients with anxiety and depression (Addolorato et al. 2004).

A referral to a professional psychologist may be required in select cases to help improve the patient's coping skills.

12. Role of patient advocacy groups

Patient and family support and advocacy groups can help support patients with celiac disease who are starting a gluten-free diet. Models such as the Expert Patients Program in the United Kingdom in which individuals learn from each other how to cope with the challenges of a chronic condition can be used (Donaldson et al. 2003). Volunteer celiac support organizations in several countries provide excellent resources to their members and keep them updated on new developments. Physicians and patients have identified such organization as important sources of information (Zarkadas et al. 2006). Physicians should recommend their patients with celiac disease to become members of such support groups.

13. Conclusions

Celiac disease is not a trivial disorder. While most patients do well on a gluten-free diet, some do not. Complications including nutritional deficiencies, risk of developing other autoimmune disorders, refractory celiac disease and malignancy are important considerations. Symptoms alone do not provide a reliable guide to the presence of complications. In future, better stratification of risk factors for developing complications may allow for individualized follow-up plans for specific patients. All patients with celiac disease should have regular, systematic follow-up by a health care team that includes a physician and a dietitian.

14. References

Abdulkarim AS, Burgart LJ, See J et al. 2002. Etiology of Nonresponsive Celiac Disease: Results of a Systematic Approach. *Am J Gastroenterol*,97(8):2016-21.

Addolorato G, De Lorenzi G, Abenavoli L et al. 2004, Psychological support councelling improves gluten-free diet compliance in celiac disease. *Aliment Pharmacol Ther*, 20(7):777-782.

AGA-American Gastroenterological Association Institute medical position statement on the diagnosis and management of celiac disease. 2006. *Gastroenterology*, 131(6):1977-80.

Al-Toma A, Goerres MS, Meijer JW et al. 2006. Human leukocyte antigen-DQ2 homozygosity and the development of refractory celiac disease and enteropathy-associated T-cell lymphoma. *Clin Gastroenterol Hepatol*, 4:315-9.

Bardella MT, Molteni N, Prampolini L, et al. 1994. Need for follow up in coeliac disease. *Arch Dis Child*, 70:211-3.

Bebb JR, Lawson A, Knight T et al. 2006. Long-term follow-up of coeliac disease–what do coeliac patients want? *Aliment Pharmacol Ther*, 23:827-31.

Case S. 2005. The gluten-free diet: how to provide effective education and resources. *Gastroenterology*, 128(suppl 1):S128-S134.

Cassio A, Ricci G, Baronio F et al. 2010. Long-term clinical significance of thyroid autoimmunity in children with celiac disease. *J Pediatr*,156(2):292-5

Catassi C, Fabiani E, Iacono G, et al. 2007. A prospective, double-blind, placebo-controlled trial to establish a safe gluten threshold for patients with celiac disease. *Am J Clin Nutr*, 85:160-166.

Cooper BT, Holmes GK, Cooke WT. 1982. Lymphoma risk in coeliac disease of later life. *Digestion*, 23:89-92.

Donaldson L. 2003. Expert patients usher in a new era of opportunity for the NHS. *BMJ*, 14;326(7402):1279-80.

Elfstrom P, Montgomery SM, Kampe A et al. 2008. Risk of thyroid disease in individuals with celiac disease. *J Clinic Endocrinol Metab*, 93(10):3915-21.

Fornari MC, Pedreira S, Niveloni S, et al. 1998. Pre- and post-treatment serum levels of cytokines IL-1beta, IL-6, and IL-1 receptor antagonist in celiac disease. Are they related to the associated osteopenia? *Am J Gastroenterol*, 93:413-8.

Freeman HJ, Chopra A, Clandinin MT et al 2011. Recent advances in celiac disease. *World J Gastroenterol*, 17(18):2259-2272.

Freeman HJ. Refractory celiac disease and sprue-like intestinal disease. 2008. *World J Gastroenterol*, 14(6):828-830.

Haines ML, Anderson RP, Gibson RP. 2008. Systematic review:the evidence base for long-term management of celiac disease. *Aliment Pharmacol Ther*, 28:1042-1066.

Hill ID, Dirks MH, Liptak GS, et al. 2005. Guideline for the diagnosis and treatment of celiac disease in children: Recommendations of the North American Society for Pediatric Gastroenterology, Hepatology and Nutrition. *J Pediatr Gastroenterol Nutr*, 40(1):1-19.

Hogberg L, Grodzinsky E, Stenhammar L 2003. Better dietary compliance in patients with coeliac disease diagnosed in early childhood. *Scand J Gastroenterol*, 38:751-4.

Holmes GK, Prior P, Lane MR et al. 1989. Malignancy in coeliac disease– effect of a gluten free diet. *Gut*, 30:333-8.

Jores RD, Frau F, Cucca F et al. 2007. HLADQB1*0201 homozygosis predisposes to severe intestinal damage in celiac disease. *Scand J Gastroenterol*, 42:48–53.

Karinen H, Karkkainen P, Pihlajamaki J et al. 2006. Gene dose effect of the DQB1*0201 allele contributes to severity of celiac disease. *Scand J Gastroenterol*, 41:191-9.

Kaukinen K, Sulkanen S, Maki M, et al. 2002. IgA-class transglutaminase antibodies in evaluating the efficacy of gluten-free diet in coeliac disease. *Eur J Gastroenterol Hepatol*, 14:311-5.

Kaukinen K, Peraaho M, Lindfors K, et al. 2007. Persistent small bowel mucosal villous atrophy without symptoms in celiac disease. *Aliment Pharmacol Ther*, 25:1237-45.

Kupper C. 2005. Dietary guidelines and implementation for celiac disease. *Gastroenterology*, 128(suppl 1):S121-S127.

Lamontagne P, West GE, Galibois I. 2001. Quebecers with celiac disease: analysis of dietary problems. *Can J Diet Pract Res*, 62:175-81.

Leffler D, Dennis M, Hyett B et al. 2007. Etiologies and predictors of diagnosis in nonresponsive celiac disease. *Clin Gastroenterol Hepatol*,5(4):445-50.

Ljungman G, Myrdal U. 1993. Compliance in teenagers with coeliac disease–a Swedish follow-up study. *Acta Paediatr*, 82:235-8.

Malamut G, Afchain P, Verkarre V et al. 2009. Presentation and long-term followup of refractory celiac disease: comparison of type I with type II. *Gastroenterology*, 136(1):81-90.

Meloni A, Mandas C, Jores RD et al. 2009. Prevalence of autoimmune thyroiditis in children with celiac disease and effect of gluten withdrawal. *J Pediatr*, 155(1):51-5

NIH-National Institute of Health Consensus Development Conference Statement on Celiac Disease. June 28-30, 2004, 2005. *Gastroenterology*, 128:S1-S9.

Pietzak MM. 2005. Follow-up of patients with celiac disease: achieving compliance with treatment. *Gastroenterology*, 128:S135-41.

Rashid M, Cranney A, Zarkadas M et al. 2005. Celiac disease: Evaluation of the diagnosis and dietary compliance in Canadian children. *Pediatrics*, 116:e754-e759.

Romaldini CC, Barbieri D, Okay TS, et al. 2002. Serum soluble interleukin-2 receptor, interleukin-6, and tumor necrosis factor-alpha levels in children with celiac disease: response to treatment. *J Pediatr Gastroenterol Nutr*, 35:513-7.

Rubio-Tapia A, Kelly DG, Lahr BD et al. 2009. Clinical staging and survival in refractory celiac disease: a single center experience. *Gastroenterology*, 136(1):99-107.

Sategna Guidetti C, Solerio E, Scaglione N, et al. 2001. Duration of gluten exposure in adult coeliac disease does not correlate with the risk for autoimmune disorders. *Gut*, 49:502-5.

Silvester J, Rashid M 2010. Long-term management of patients with celiac disease: Current practices of gastroenterologists in Canada. *Can J Gastroenterol*, 24;(8):499-509.

Silvester J, Rashid M. 2007. Long-term follow-up of individuals with celiac disease: An evaluation of current practice guidelines. *Can J Gastroenterol*, 21(9):557-64.

Tursi A, Brandimarte G, Giorgetti GM. 2003. Lack of usefulness of anti-transglutaminase antibodies in assessing histologic recovery after gluten-free diet in celiac disease. *J Clin Gastroenterol*, 37:387-91.

Tursi A, Brandimarte G, Giorgetti GM et al. 2006. Endoscopic and histological findings in the duodenum of adults with celiac disease before and after changing to a gluten-free diet: a 2-year prospective study. *Endoscopy*, 38:702-7.

Ventura A, Magazzu G, Greco L. 1999. Duration of exposure to gluten and risk for autoimmune disorders in patients with celiac disease. SIGEP Study Group for Autoimmune Disorders in Celiac Disease. *Gastroenterology*,117:297-303.

Viljamaa M, Kaukinen K, Huhtala H, et al. 2005. Coeliac disease, autoimmune diseases and gluten exposure. *Scand J Gastroenterol*, 40:437-43.

Wahab PJ, Meijer JW, Mulder CJ. 2002. Histologic follow-up of people with celiac disease on a gluten-free diet: slow and incomplete recovery. *Am J Clin Pathol*, 118:459-63.

Walker-Smith JA, Guandalini S, Schmitz J et al. 1990. Revised criteria for diagnosis of coeliac disease. Report of Working Group of European Society of Paediatric Gastroenterology and Nutrition. *Arch Dis Child*, 65:909-11.

Zarkadas M, Cranney A, Case S et al. 2006. The impact of a gluten-free diet on adults with coeliac disease: Results of a national survey. *J Hum Nutr Diet*, 19:41-49.

10

On Treatment Outcomes in Coeliac Disease Diagnosed in Adulthood

Claes Hallert[1] and Susanne Roos[2]
[1]*Coeliac Centre at Norrkoping Hospital, Norrköping,*
[2] *Linköping University, ISV, Campus Norrkoping*
Sweden

1. Introduction

Coeliac disease (CD) is generally regarded as an intestinal disorder that can be fully treated by a gluten free diet (GFD). Indeed, this remains perfectly true in most medical aspects as regards the recovery of the small intestinal mucosa appearance, the blood count as well and the mineral bone density. In fact, life expectancy is similar to that of general population.

From a wider perspective, however, taking the subjective outcome of treatment into account the health-related quality of life (Hallert & Lohiniemi, 1999) and well-being i.e. patient-based perspectives refer to the perceived health state such as social, emotional, physical well-being or functioning, incorporating both positive and negative aspects of life. In Gastrointestinal (GI) disease the most relevant aspect of well-being pertains to relief of abdominal pain.

For adults struggling with a GFD for years to remain in clinical remission CD is not just associated with troublesome bowel complaints such as Indigestion, Diarrhoea, Constipation and Abdominal pain (Midhagen & Hallert, 2003). CD is also connected with a wide range of persistent symptoms outside the GI tract typically experienced by women diagnosed in adulthood that include various bodily pain syndromes and frank mood disorders (Ludvigsson et al., 2007), all making them apt to seek more health care services than women of same age in general population (Roos et al., 2011). Of interest considering the concept of CD in remission, a study compared health care costs per patient over 2 consecutive yrs of 137 women with CD treated median 7 yrs with 411 age-matched female population in Southeast Sweden using data derived from a local administrative database covering all health care services including prescribed drugs, imaging and lab. The results showed that the 93 per cent of the women CD used health-care services the 2-yr period amounting to mean Eur 5675 as compared with Eur 5414 for controls ($p<0.05$), the difference mainly accounted for by excessive use of hospital care (Eur 5864 *vs* Eur 5215) and prescription of drugs (Eur 993 *vs* Eur 702) (Hallert et al , 2011).

All of this is consistent with the idea that reduction in well-being is a feature of longstanding CD at least in women living in Sweden but not in men for largely unclear reasons (Roos et al., 2006).

2. Bowel symptoms *vs* well-being

A study addressing whether the high rate of GI symptoms would explain the poor well-being of women living on a GFD confirmed close negative correlations between the GI symptoms and psychological well-being as assessed by the Gastrointestinal Symptom rating Scale (GSRS) total score and the Psychological General Well-being (PGWB) index, respectively. However, looking at directions of relationships the study showed that women with a high rate of GI symptoms showed no lower well-being than men with high rate GI symptoms. Furthermore, women with reduced well-being had not higher rates of GI symptoms than men with reduced well-being. Awaiting further studies it was concluded that any causal interrelations of bowel symptoms and subjective poor health remain unproven (Roos et al., 2009).

3. Well-being and coping

The poorer treatment outcome of women with CD may to some extent reflect the way they cope with the disorder and what factors they believe adversely impact on the subjective well-being.

To this connection studies indicate that women living with CD understand well-being and quality of life quite differently than men with CD. Men living with CD for years tend to focus on bodily sensations like physical endurance and bowel symptoms and they are prone to use a problem-oriented coping strategy approach.

Women treated for CD, on the other hand, are seeking an emotionally oriented strategy and emphasise the social consequences of being a coeliac and refer to the value of food, role identification, social functioning and feeling restricted by constant fatigue. Women are generally more frustrated men by the various bothering bowel symptoms that continue to despite adhering closely to the GFD.

4. Everyday life with CD

It may rather be that the numerous dilemmas and restrictions in everyday life facing especially women living with CD account for much of their perceived disease burden, comprising concerns about having to abstain from important things in life and the possibility that the children may develop CD in addition to the unmet expectations of the treatment. (Hallert et al, 2003), amounting to a sense of frustration and disappointment beyond the early happy phase of remission. As rightly pointed out (Ciacci, 2010) being diagnosed with CD implies accepting to have got a chronic illness and in addition to this a tricky dietary treatment that must last for life. Most people are capable to handle the ensuing psychic reactions pretty uneventful, whereas some develop signs of depression suggestive of a coeliac profile comprising two principal characteristics, namely, reactiveness with anger and/or frustration and Pessimism including a cluster of symptoms signalling, powerlessness and constant fatigue.

In addition, women are inclined to express worries about having CD that affects all areas of life past, present and future when they do something that is outside the daily routines to such extent that the well-being of adults with CD in remission is in the same range as in adults with quiescent Crohn's disease.

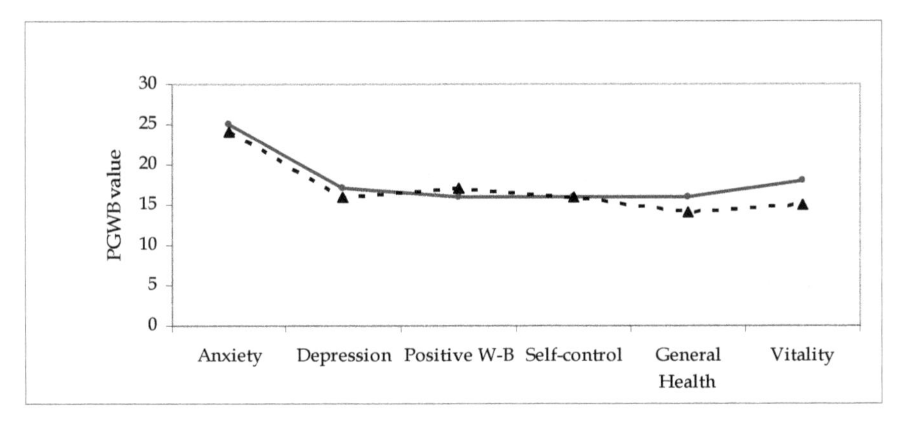

Fig. 1. Graph comparing dimensions of well-being in CD (solid line) and Crohns' disease (dotted line) (Stjernman, 2011).

For being a basically benign disorder these characteristics are an intriguing and unexpected feature of CD (Fera et al.(2003) that may be easily overlooked by gastroenterologists in charge. A tentative explanation for the poor treatment outcome of especially women living with CD diagnosed in adulthood may reside in the problematic transition into a life as a coeliac in association with poor insights into the nature of CD, sometimes, referred to as an allergy necessitating constant control of every dish that is often dated from the time of the diagnosis and rarely entertained since by the health care system, Yet current wisdom considers the once assumed fears of ingesting traces of gluten to be no longer valid (Collin et al., 2004). Gaining proper disease knowledge would thus be reassuring to most women and particularly when put into a structured education programme like a Coeliac School as outlined (Ring Jacobsson L et al., 2011).

5. The Coeliac School™

The Coeliac School an educational concept is based on the problem based learning pedagogy and includes weekly meetings in groups of 7-9 conducted by a tutor acting as a moderator. Each educational session is set to cover a predetermined topic presented as a scenario. The topics are decided by the group members according to specific needs and desires, thought promote active rather than passive learning. The group members were encouraged to perform self-studies between the meetings to find answers on raised issues. At the next meeting the group members were expected to evaluate and reflect upon the gathered information and to what extent it impacts on their daily life. Developing issues were treated by a new brainstorming allowing the group to invite an outside expert as needed. The benefits from taking part in the Coeliac School include improvement in mood and reduction in GI complaints as well opportunities to update diet knowledge.

A GFD is no single diet, nor simply foods devoid of gluten. Indeed, studies across Europe show that the composition of a GFD vary considerably between people and differ in several aspects from intakes as reported by general populations using food diaries. A study of adults in Sweden who had been on a GFD for 10 years revealed they had the same energy intake as general population controls of same age but lower daily intakes of fibres, niacin, folic acid, vitamin B-12, calcium, phosphorus and zinc. Moreover, clear discrepancies were observed between the groups in selecting foods among 28 food groups under study, particularly true for women (Grehn et al., 2001). A similar study conducted in UK showed generally adequate macronutrient intakes, while women tended have low daily intakes of fibre, magnesium, iron, zinc, manganese, selenium and folic acid but no differing energy intakes, suggesting they are prone to have sugary snack foods. (Wild et al, 2010).

There are good reasons to believe that a GFD is nutritionally unbalanced more often than routinely recognised in clinical practice, at risk to cause nutritional deficiencies that may be clinically important. Indeed, the low intakes of B vitamins in CD populations account for raised levels of plasma homocysteine, a marker of functional B vitamin deficiency. Lack of B vitamins may very well explain part of the depressive features of CD, gaining support by the results of a randomised controlled clinical trial adding 0.5 mg of vitamin B-12, 3 mg of vitamin B-6 and 0.8 mg of folic acid to the daily diet for six months that showed general improvement in well-being of adults on a GFD for many years, notably within Anxiety and Depression unlike for controls receiving placebo (Hallert et al., 2009). Accordingly, advising people to avoid of gluten should not be the sole focus of a GFD knowing eating oats, represents a major advance in CD therapy not only in adults (Högberg et al., 2004).

Indeed, oats is rich in dietary fibres and taking oats is generally found to raise the palatability of a GFD also largely appreciated for being cheap. Unfortunately. Oats is widely looked upon as cattle food that is at best just prejudice.

Over the past decade gluten intolerant sufferers have witnessed a vast increase in the availability of suitable foods in most Western countries only hampered by unfounded ideas that wheat starch or trace amounts of gluten can be harmful to the coeliac mucosa and thereby entertaining social phobia and restrictions in daily life. With an expanding food market on the internet novel gluten free products will be steadily entering the global arena. Rendering cereals like barley non toxic is however less likely to be seen in the near future.

6. Managing CD beyond remission

The ever growing prevalence of CD approaching 3 per cent (Myleus at al., 2009) represents an increasing challenge to any health provider to ensure that CD is successfully coped with by supporting CD sufferers to master every day life dilemmas through proper self-management i.e learning to take control rather being controlled by food absorbing the entire life (Sverker et al., 2005)

To date, nursing appears to be a neglected component of the follow-up of adults with CD. In fact it may add values to the care of adults with CD, knowing that in some countries only 60 per cent of patients have a high level of confidence in the information provided from a dietician or gastroenterologist. Even more so, 1,000 adult members of the German Celiac Society identified dissatisfaction with the doctor–patient communication as one of the strongest predictors of poor well-being (Häuser et al., 2007)

In our experience CD sufferers diagnosed in adulthood only rarely need monitoring of the diet adherence. Follow-up routines should rather focus on life adjustments, medical procedures to symptom control and measures to uncover depression signs preferably managed by a dedicated multi-disciplinary team as employed in the care of adults with other chronic disorders.

This is in good keeping with an observation (Dorn et al., 2010) that psychosocial factors more strongly affect well-being and bowel symptoms in CD than the appearance of the gut mucosa, underscoring the limitations of a biomedical model to help understanding adults living with CD in proven remission. This would allow for applying biopsychosocial approach in assessing health in CD since there is no underlying mucosal damage to treat. Instead CD sufferers may require attention to their psychosocial distress and worries that may include psychological support and treatment for the IBS-like symptoms.

7. Conclusions

CD is a benign yet sometimes a troublesome disorder of the GI tract often surrounded by obsolete patient's beliefs dated from the time of the diagnosis, making the condition especially hard to successfully cope with. This is apparently true for many women who are frustrated find the outcome of the long-term treatment and self-management worse than expected at start. The complexity of living with CD and remain well extends far beyond keeping the mucosa free from signs of inflammation. Given the increasing prevalence of CD across the globe improving the long-term health of these people represents a major challenge for any health care provider.

8. References

Ciacci, C. (2010). Depression and anxiety in celiac disease, pp. 227- 231, In: *Real life with Celiac disease Troubleshooting and Thriving Gluten Free;* The American Gastroenterological Association Publisher 2010 ISBN 978-1-60356-008-5

Collin, P. Thorell, L. & Kaukinen, K. (2004). The safe threshold for gluten contamination in gluten-free products. *Aliment Pharmcol Ther* Vol 19, pp.1277-1283.

Fera, T. Cascio, B. & Angelini, G. (2003). Affective disorders and quality of life in adult coeliac disease patients on a gluten-free diet. *Eur J Gastroenterol Hepatol* vol 15, pp.1287–92.

Grehn, S. Fridell, K. & Lilliecreutz, M. (2001). Dietary habits of Swedish adult coeliac patients treated by a gluten-free diet for 10 years. *Scand J Nutrition* Vol 45, pp.178-82.

Hallert C, Roos S, & Ring Jacobsson L. (2010). Coping and adapting to celiac disease, pp. 223-26. In: *Real life with Celiac disease Troubleshooting and Thriving Gluten Free;* The American Gastroenterological Association Publisher 2010 ISBN 978-1-60356-008-5.

Hallert, C. & Lohiniemi, S. (1999). Quality of life of celiac patients living on a gluten-free diet. (Ed.) *Nutrition* Vol 15, pp.795-97.

Hallert, C. & Roos, S. Grip, B. (2011). Swedish coeliac women in remission show raised health-care costs: Controlled study. *Proceedings of the UEGW, Stockholm, Sweden.*

Hallert, C. Grännö, C. & Hultén S. (2001). Living with coeliac disease - controlled study of the burden of illness. *Scand J Gastroenterol* Vol 37, pp. 39-42.

Hallert, C. Sandlund, O. & Broqvist, M. (2003). Perceptions of health-related quality of life of men and women living with c oeliac disease for 10 years. *Scand J Car Sci* Vol 17, pp.301-7.

Hallert, C. Svensson, M. & Tholstrup, J. (2009) B vitamins improve health in patients with coeliac disease living on a gluten- free diet. *Aliment Pharmacol Ther* Vol 29, pp. 811-16.

Högberg, L. Fälth-Magnussion, K. & Laurin, P. (2004). Oats to children with newly diagnosed coeliac disease: a randomized double blind study. *Gut,* Vol 53, pp.649-54.

Ludvigsson, JF. Reutfors, J. & Ösby, U. (2007). Coeliac disease and risk of mood disorders *J Affect Disord,* Vol 99, pp.117- 26.

Midhagen, G. & Hallert, C. (2003). High rate of gastrointestinal symptoms in celiac patients living on a gluten-free diet: controlled study. *Am J Gastroenterol,* Vol 98, 2023-26.

Ring Jacobsson, L. Friedrichsen, M. & Göransson, A. (2011). Does a Coeliac school increase psychological well-being in coeliac women living on a gluten-free diet? *J Clin Nursing* (in press)

Roos S. Wilhelmsson, S. & Hallert C. (2011). Well-being, self-image and bowel symptoms in women with long-standing coeliac disease J of Nursing and Health care of Chronic illness. (in press)

Roos, S. Kärner, A. & Hallert, C. (2006) Psychological well-being of adult coeliac patients treated for 10 years. *Dig Liv Dis* Vol 38, pp.77-82.

Roos, S. Wilhelmsson, S. & Hallert C. (2011). Swedish women with coeliac disease in remission use more health care services than other women: a controlled study Scand J of Gastroenterol, Vol 46,pp 13-19.

Roos, S. Wilhelmsson, S. & Hallert, C. (2011). Women with coeliac disease living on a gluten-free diet for years use more health-care than other Swedish women. *Scand J Gastroenterol* Vol 46, pp.13-19.

Stjernman, H. (2011). Crohn's disease in sickness and in health. MD *Thesis No.1228 Linkoping University, Linkoping,* Sweden.

Sverker, A. Hensing, G. & Hallert, C. (2005)'Controlled by food' - Lived experiences of coeliac disease. *J Hum Nutr Dietet* Vol 18, pp.171-80.

Permissions

The contributors of this book come from diverse backgrounds, making this book a truly international effort. This book will bring forth new frontiers with its revolutionizing research information and detailed analysis of the nascent developments around the world.

We would like to thank Peter Kruzliak, M.D., BSc., for lending his expertise to make the book truly unique. He has played a crucial role in the development of this book. Without his invaluable contribution this book wouldn't have been possible. He has made vital efforts to compile up to date information on the varied aspects of this subject to make this book a valuable addition to the collection of many professionals and students.

This book was conceptualized with the vision of imparting up-to-date information and advanced data in this field. To ensure the same, a matchless editorial board was set up. Every individual on the board went through rigorous rounds of assessment to prove their worth. After which they invested a large part of their time researching and compiling the most relevant data for our readers. Conferences and sessions were held from time to time between the editorial board and the contributing authors to present the data in the most comprehensible form. The editorial team has worked tirelessly to provide valuable and valid information to help people across the globe.

Every chapter published in this book has been scrutinized by our experts. Their significance has been extensively debated. The topics covered herein carry significant findings which will fuel the growth of the discipline. They may even be implemented as practical applications or may be referred to as a beginning point for another development.

The editorial board has been involved in producing this book since its inception. They have spent rigorous hours researching and exploring the diverse topics which have resulted in the successful publishing of this book. They have passed on their knowledge of decades through this book. To expedite this challenging task, the publisher supported the team at every step. A small team of assistant editors was also appointed to further simplify the editing procedure and attain best results for the readers.

Our editorial team has been hand-picked from every corner of the world. Their multi-ethnicity adds dynamic inputs to the discussions which result in innovative outcomes. These outcomes are then further discussed with the researchers and contributors who give their valuable feedback and opinion regarding the same. The feedback is then collaborated with the researches and they are edited in a comprehensive manner to aid the understanding of the subject.

Apart from the editorial board, the designing team has also invested a significant amount of their time in understanding the subject and creating the most relevant covers. They scrutinized every image to scout for the most suitable representation of the subject and create an appropriate cover for the book.

The publishing team has been involved in this book since its early stages. They were actively engaged in every process, be it collecting the data, connecting with the contributors or procuring relevant information. The team has been an ardent support to the editorial, designing and production team. Their endless efforts to recruit the best for this project, has resulted in the accomplishment of this book. They are a veteran in the field of academics and their pool of knowledge is as vast as their experience in printing. Their expertise and guidance has proved useful at every step. Their uncompromising quality standards have made this book an exceptional effort. Their encouragement from time to time has been an inspiration for everyone.

The publisher and the editorial board hope that this book will prove to be a valuable piece of knowledge for researchers, students, practitioners and scholars across the globe.

List of Contributors

Dorottya Nagy-Szakál, Katalin Eszter Müller, Kriszta Molnár, Ádám Vannay, Erna Sziksz, Beáta Szebeni, András Arató and Gábor Veres
First Department of Pediatrics, Semmelweis University, Budapest, Hungary

Hajnalka Győrffy
Second Department of Pathology, Semmelweis University, Budapest, Hungary

Ádám Vannay, Erna Sziksz and Beáta Szebeni
Research Group for Pediatrics and Nephrology, Semmelweis University and Hungarian Academy of Sciences, Budapest, Hungary

Mária Papp
Department of Medicine, University of Debrecen, Hungary

Erna Sziksz, Leonóra Himer, Beáta Szebeni, Tivadar Tulassay and Ádám Vannay
Research Group for Paediatrics and Nephrology, Semmelweis University and Hungarian Academy of Sciences, Budapest, Hungary

András Arató, Erna Sziksz, Leonóra Himer, Gábor Veres, Beáta Szebeni, Tivadar Tulassay and Ádám Vannay
First Department of Paediatrics, Semmelweis University, Budapest, Hungary

Vesna Stojiljković, Jelena Kasapović, Snežana Pejić, Ljubica Gavrilović and Snežana B. Pajović
Laboratory of Molecular Biology and Endocrinology, "Vinča", Institute of Nuclear Sciences, University of Belgrade, Belgrade, Serbia

Nedeljko Radlović
Department of Gastroenterology and Nutrition, University Children's Hospital, Belgrade, Serbia

Zorica S. Saičić
Department of Physiology, Institute of Biological Research "Siniša Stanković", University of Belgrade, Belgrade, Serbia

Peter Kruzliak
5th Department of Internal Medicine, University Hospital and Medical Faculty of Comenius University, Slovakia
Department of Physiology and Pathophysiology of the Slovak academy of Sciences, Bratislava, Slovakia

Mieczysław Szalecki
Clinic of Endocrinology and Diabetology, Children's Memorial Health Institute, Warsaw, Poland
Faculty of Health Sciences, Jan Kochanowski University, Kielce, Poland

Piotr Albrecht
Department of Pediatric Gastroenterology and Nutrition, Warsaw Medical University, Poland

Stefan Kluzek
Sport and Exercise Medicine, Oxford Deanery, Nuffield Orthopaedic Centre, Oxford, UK

Carlos Hernández-Lahoz
Neurology Services, Asturias Central University Hospital (HUCA), School of Medicine, University of Oviedo, Oviedo, Spain

Luis Rodrigo
Gastroenterology Services, Asturias Central University Hospital (HUCA), School of Medicine, University of Oviedo, Oviedo, Spain

Carolina Sousa, Ana Real, Mª de Lourdes Moreno and Isabel Comino
Department of Microbiology and Parasitology, Faculty of Pharmacy, University of Seville, Seville, Spain

Hugh J. Cornell
RMIT University, Melbourne, Australia

Teodor Stelmasiak
Glutagen Pty Ltd, Maribyrnong, Australia

Mohsin Rashid
Dalhousie University, Canada

Claes Hallert
Coeliac Centre at Norrkoping Hospital, Norrköping, Sweden

Susanne Roos
Linköping University, ISV, Campus Norrkoping, Sweden